Opportunities, Risks, and Future Directions of AI in Pulmonary Medicine

Rahul K. Patel
https://orcid.org/0000-0003-1175-0635
Illinois Institute of Technology, USA

Jayant B. Mehta
East Tennessee State University, USA

IGI Global
Scientific Publishing
Publishing Tomorrow's Research Today

Vice President of Editorial	Melissa Wagner
Director of Acquisitions	Mikaela Felty
Director of Book Development	Jocelynn Hessler
Production Manager	Mike Brehm
Cover Design	Jose Rosado

Published in the United States of America by
IGI Global Scientific Publishing
701 East Chocolate Avenue
Hershey, PA, 17033, USA
Tel: 717-533-8845 | Fax: 717-533-7115
Website: https://www.igi-global.com E-mail: cust@igi-global.com

Library of Congress Cataloging-in-Publication Data

LCCN: 2026016433 (CIP Data Pending)
ISBN13: 9798337377599
Isbn13Softcover: 9798337377605
EISBN13: 9798337377612
British Cataloguing in Publication Data
A Cataloguing in Publication record for this book is available from the British Library.

Table of Contents

Detailed Table of Contents

analysis of proprietary algorithms in consumer wearables shows promise for improved sleep staging and cardiorespiratory screening. AI offers greater reliability, reduced diagnostic delays, and enhanced accessibility via ambulatory studies. However, challenges include data security, algorithmic opacity, training bias, and risk of over-reliance. There remains a need for sustained clinician supervision, consistent with current American Academy of Sleep Medicine guidance. Ongoing model refinement and regulatory evolution will shape AI's responsible integration in sleep medicine.

This chapter explores the transformative role of artificial intelligence (AI) in the diagnosis, management, and prognosis of pulmonary infectious diseases, which continue to be a major global health burden. Diseases such as pneumonia, tuberculosis, COVID-19, and drug-resistant infections present persistent challenges, including delayed diagnosis, limited access to expert interpretation, and rising antimicrobial resistance. AI, particularly through machine learning and deep learning techniques, offers innovative solutions to address these challenges by enabling faster, more accurate, and data-driven clinical decision-making.

AI technology has changed the course of CC medicine both for mechanical ventilation and for respiratory failure in general, very quickly. This chapter will discuss four important aspects of AI in ICUs: 1) predicting early deterioration through predictive modelling; 2) automation to manage closed-loop ventilation systems (ventilators); 3) more accurate identification of patients with ARDS and identifying them by phenotype; and 4) integration of multimodal sources of data to support decision-

risk assessment. The combination of whole-slide imaging and AI technology in pathology assists in tumor grading and biomarker measurement and subtype identification. AI-powered predictive analytics assist in developing personalized treatment plans while they estimate treatment effectiveness and resistance patterns and patient survival rates.

Interstitial lung diseases represent a clinically challenging group of pulmonary disorders, for which early detection and accurate diagnosis are essential. High-resolution computed tomography provides detailed visualization of lung structures; however, manual interpretation is time-consuming and requires substantial specialized expertise. This chapter examines the integration of advanced artificial intelligence techniques with pulmonary imaging to automate the recognition of patterns in interstitial lung diseases. Three Vision Transformer architectures are systematically evaluated on high resolution chest imaging datasets to classify six primary pulmonary patterns. Attention maps, gradient-weighted class activation mapping visualizations, and performance metrics are employed to enhance interpretability and support clinical trust. The results demonstrate that the Swin Transformer provides superior accuracy and explainability. Furthermore, quantitative biomarkers facilitate objective monitoring of disease progression and support personalized treatment strategies.

Artificial intelligence (AI) is changing the way we look at pulmonary imaging by enhanced diagnosis and accurate findings for various lung disorders. The chapter deals with integration of AI in different modalities of medical imaging right from chest x-ray to computed tomography. In chest x-ray imaging, the AI algorithms can detect abnormalities, pneumonia, tuberculosis and nodules, often exceeding expectations of a radiologists. In computed tomography, AI integration facilitates lung cancer screening, achieving up to 99% accuracy in detecting the malignancies. It can also predict the malignancy accurately. Other than this it can quantify diseases like emphysema, fibrosis, airway modelling, COPD & ILD biomarkers. Combining the radionomics with clinical findings can estimate predictive models to provide personalised treatment plans. The chapter addresses AI tools utilized in existing workflow to assist effective aids in clinical judgements.

Naima Khan, Department of Computer Science and IT, Cholistan University of Veterinary and Animal Sciences, Bahawalpur, Pakistan
Hira Fatima, Department of Zoology, Division of Science and Technology, University of Education, Lahore, Pakistan
Iqra Rafique, Government College University, Faisalabad, Pakistan
Imrana Amir, Department of Zoology, University of Mianwali, Mianwali, Pakistan
Saima Nousheen, Department of Zoology, University of Mianwali, Mianwali, Pakistan
Zainab Abid, University of Managaement and Technology, Lahore, Pakistan
Adnan Afzal, Government College University, Faisalabad, Pakistan

Machine learning is increasingly transforming the management of asthma and chronic obstructive pulmonary disease (COPD) by enabling data-driven prediction, continuous monitoring, and outcome optimization. This chapter examines how machine learning models leverage clinical records, digital inhalers, wearable devices, and environmental data to predict exacerbations, assess disease control, and support personalized interventions. It highlights the impact of these approaches on clinical outcomes, healthcare utilization, and value-based care, while addressing challenges related to validation, interpretability, ethics, and equity. By exploring emerging research directions and implementation considerations, the chapter underscores the potential of machine learning to advance proactive and patient-centered respiratory care.

Shaik Aminabee, V.V. Institute of Pharmaceutical Sciences, Gudlavalleru, India

Pulmonary medicine is changing at an alarming rate due to the use of Artificial intelligence (AI) to improve the diagnosis of a disease, prediction, monitoring, and even the implementation of a personalized treatment plan. Innovative machine learning and deep learning models are being used in imaging analyses, pulmonary function test interpretation and clinical decision support systems and predict respiratory diseases, including chronic obstructive pulmonary disease, asthma, interstitial lung diseases, and lung cancer, earlier. Remote patient monitoring, tele-pulmonology, and precision medicine approaches are also aided with the help of AI innovations and enhance healthcare accessibility and outcomes. In spite of such promising innovations, there are still a number of challenges, such as the privacy of data, bias in algorithms, insufficient standardized regulatory frameworks, and inadequate clinical validation in practice. Clinician training, development of infrastructure and ethical governance are also important to integrate AI in regular pulmonary practice.

Preface

INTRODUCTION

Artificial intelligence (AI) has entered a defining stage in modern medicine. Rapid advances in machine learning, deep learning, computer vision, natural language processing, and predictive analytics now influence nearly every area of healthcare. Pulmonary medicine stands among the most rapidly evolving specialties within this transformation. Respiratory diseases remain major causes of morbidity and mortality worldwide, while healthcare systems continue facing increasing diagnostic complexity, workforce limitations, rising costs, and unequal access to specialized care. AI offers practical opportunities to improve diagnostic precision, optimize workflows, support clinical decision making, and advance personalized respiratory care.

Pulmonary medicine depends heavily on multidimensional data. Clinicians routinely integrate radiologic imaging, pulmonary function tests, laboratory findings, physiologic monitoring, pathology, genomics, and longitudinal clinical records. The increasing volume and complexity of these data create significant challenges for traditional clinical workflows. Diagnostic delays, interobserver variability, fragmented care coordination, and inconsistent access to specialists continue affecting patient outcomes globally. AI technologies now provide tools capable of addressing many of these limitations through automated pattern recognition, predictive modeling, and real time clinical analytics.

The role of AI in pulmonary medicine extends far beyond image interpretation. Current applications include automated radiologic analysis, disease phenotyping, risk stratification, early deterioration prediction, ventilator optimization, sleep study automation, pulmonary function interpretation, remote monitoring, precision oncology, and personalized therapeutic planning. AI systems increasingly integrate multimodal data from imaging, pathology, genomics, electronic health records, and wearable technologies. These developments are reshaping how respiratory diseases are diagnosed, monitored, and treated.

At the same time, important concerns remain unresolved. Questions involving algorithmic transparency, data quality, model generalizability, privacy protection, ethical governance, clinical validation, and regulatory oversight continue influencing adoption across healthcare systems. Responsible implementation requires collaboration among clinicians, researchers, engineers, policymakers, and healthcare organizations. AI should support clinical expertise rather than replace physician judgment. Sustainable integration depends on evidence-based deployment, rigorous validation, and continuous human oversight.

This book was developed to provide a comprehensive examination of the evolving relationship between AI and pulmonary medicine. The chapters collectively explore foundational concepts, disease specific applications, imaging innovations, predictive systems, and future directions. The contributors examine both opportunities and limitations while emphasizing clinically meaningful implementation. The goal is not only to describe technological advances, but also to evaluate how these tools may improve patient outcomes, healthcare delivery, and respiratory research.

This text is intended for a broad audience. Pulmonologists, intensivists, sleep medicine specialists, oncologists, radiologists, pathologists, pediatricians, respiratory therapists, biomedical researchers, medical students, residents, fellows, and healthcare administrators may all benefit from the discussions presented throughout this volume. Data scientists, engineers, and informatics professionals interested in healthcare applications of AI may also find value in understanding the clinical context of pulmonary diseases. The chapters were written to remain accessible to readers with varying levels of technical expertise while maintaining scientific rigor and clinical relevance.

CHAPTER OVERVIEW

Chapter 1 introduces the foundations of AI in pulmonary medicine. The chapter discusses how AI addresses challenges involving diagnosis, monitoring, and treatment planning across pulmonary diseases. Key applications include imaging phenotyping, radiomics, predictive modeling, wearable monitoring systems, and clinical decision support. The chapter also addresses ethical concerns, data quality, and regulatory considerations that influence implementation within healthcare systems. This chapter establishes the conceptual framework for the remainder of the book.

Chapter 2 examines the growing role of AI in sleep medicine. Sleep disorders remain highly prevalent and resource intensive to diagnose and manage. This chapter explains how deep learning and foundational models improve automated sleep staging and accelerate polysomnography interpretation. The discussion also evaluates AI integration within wearable technologies and ambulatory sleep studies. Important concerns regarding algorithmic opacity, clinician oversight, and current professional guidance are also reviewed.

Chapter 3 focuses on pulmonary infectious diseases. Pneumonia, tuberculosis, COVID 19, and drug-resistant infections continue presenting major global healthcare challenges. The chapter demonstrates how machine learning and deep learning techniques support faster diagnosis, improved imaging interpretation, and enhanced clinical decision making. AI driven approaches to infectious disease surveillance and antimicrobial resistance management are also explored.

Chapter 4 discusses the application of AI in critical care medicine and respiratory failure management. The chapter highlights predictive modeling for early clinical deterioration, automated ventilator systems, ARDS phenotyping, and multimodal data integration within intensive care units. The discussion emphasizes how AI may reduce physician cognitive burden while improving individualized treatment planning. Challenges involving interpretability, bias, and ethical implementation are also carefully examined.

Chapter 5 explores AI applications in pulmonary oncology, particularly lung cancer diagnosis and management. The chapter reviews AI-assisted radiomics, pathology analysis, imaging biomarkers, and personalized treatment approaches. Special attention is given to biomarker prediction, targeted therapies, prognostic modeling, and surgical decision support. The chapter demonstrates how AI may improve early detection and optimize precision oncology strategies.

Chapter 6 continues the discussion of pulmonary oncology through precision medicine applications. The chapter focuses on immunotherapy planning, radiation therapy optimization, survival prediction, and treatment monitoring. Emerging technologies such as explainable AI, federated learning, and digital twins are discussed as future innovations capable of further transforming lung cancer management.

Chapter 7 further evaluates AI driven lung cancer detection and diagnostic precision. The chapter discusses multimodal fusion models integrating imaging, pathology, and genomic data. AI applications involving low dose CT screening, nodule detection, tumor grading, biomarker analysis, and predictive analytics are reviewed. The chapter highlights the growing importance of integrated precision oncology systems.

Chapter 8 provides a broad examination of AI applications across pulmonary medicine. Topics include imaging analysis, pulmonary function interpretation, remote monitoring, tele pulmonology, and precision medicine approaches. The chapter also addresses major implementation barriers involving data privacy, algorithmic bias, infrastructure limitations, and clinician education. The discussion reinforces the need for ethical governance and clinical validation.

Chapter 9 focuses specifically on pulmonary imaging. The chapter reviews AI integration within chest radiography and computed tomography workflows. Applications include automated detection of pneumonia, tuberculosis, lung nodules, emphysema, fibrosis, and interstitial lung disease biomarkers. Radiomics and predictive analytics are discussed as tools supporting personalized treatment planning and improved diagnostic efficiency.

Chapter 10 examines machine learning applications in asthma and chronic obstructive pulmonary disease management. The chapter discusses predictive models using electronic records, wearable devices, environmental monitoring, and digital inhalers. AI supported approaches for exacerbation prediction, disease control assessment, and personalized interventions are evaluated. Ethical considerations, healthcare equity, and implementation challenges are also addressed.

Chapter 11 explores advanced AI techniques for interstitial lung disease imaging analysis. Vision Transformer architectures are evaluated for classification of pulmonary imaging patterns. Explainability tools, attention mapping, and quantitative biomarkers are discussed as methods supporting clinical trust and objective disease monitoring. The chapter demonstrates the growing importance of explainable AI within pulmonary diagnostics.

CONCLUSION

Collectively, the chapters in this volume demonstrate that AI is no longer a theoretical concept within pulmonary medicine. Many technologies now influence clinical workflows, research methodologies, and healthcare delivery systems. The field continues evolving rapidly as computational capabilities improve and multimodal datasets become increasingly accessible. However, technological advancement alone will not determine success. Clinical integration requires careful validation, ethical oversight, interdisciplinary collaboration, and ongoing physician engagement.

This book contributes to the field by providing a clinically grounded and multidisciplinary examination of AI in pulmonary medicine. The chapters combine technical innovation with practical clinical perspectives while acknowledging the challenges associated with implementation. By presenting both current applications and future directions, this text aims to support responsible adoption, stimulate further research, and encourage collaborative progress across respiratory medicine. The future of pulmonary care will increasingly depend on intelligent systems capable of supporting earlier diagnosis, personalized treatment, efficient workflows, and improved patient outcomes. This volume seeks to contribute meaningfully to that evolving future.

Jayant Mehta
East Tennessee State University, USA

Rahul K Patel
Illinois Institute of Technology, USA

Chapter 1

Introduction to the Opportunities, Risks, and Future Directions of AI in Pulmonary Medicine

Rahul K. Patel
http://orcid.org/0000-0003-1175-0635
Illinois Institute of Technology, USA

Jayant Mehta
East Tennessee State University, USA

Kunj R. Patel
http://orcid.org/0000-0002-5940-6844
Lake Erie School of Medicine, USA

Nikunj R. Patel
http://orcid.org/0009-0007-8056-6969
University of Wisconsin-Madison, USA

ABSTRACT

Artificial intelligence (AI) is transforming pulmonary medicine through improved diagnosis, monitoring, and treatment planning. Pulmonary diseases require interpretation of complex data from imaging, pulmonary function tests, and electronic health records. Traditional workflows often cause diagnostic delays, inconsistent interpretation, and fragmented care. AI addresses these gaps through automation, predictive modeling, and real time analytics. Current applications include imaging phenotyping, radiomics, diagnostic support systems, and wearable sensor monitoring. Predictive models support early detection and risk stratification, while decision tools

DOI: 10.4018/979-8-3373-7759-9.ch001

improve longitudinal management and personalized care. Key challenges include data quality, model generalizability, ethics, and regulatory oversight. This chapter reviews the rationale, evidence, and clinical role of AI in pulmonary medicine, with emphasis on responsible integration into healthcare systems and future research directions.

OVERVIEW OF PULMONARY MEDICINE

Pulmonary medicine covers the prevention, diagnosis, and treatment of diseases affecting the lungs and airways. Respiratory disorders are still a leading cause of illness and death worldwide. COPD, interstitial lung disease (ILD), pulmonary hypertension, lung cancer, and respiratory infections continue to strain healthcare systems. Imaging, pulmonary function testing, and molecular diagnostics have improved patient care, but important clinical challenges remain.

Many pulmonary diseases develop slowly and go undetected early on. COPD and ILD often present only after irreversible lung damage has already occurred, and those delays in diagnosis push patients toward worse outcomes. The field also generates a wide mix of data: radiographic imaging, spirometry, laboratory tests, pathology, genomics, and physiologic monitoring. Clinicians have to integrate all of this in real time at the bedside, often under pressure.

Rising rates of chronic respiratory disease have put more pressure on healthcare infrastructure and staff. Aging populations, air pollution, tobacco use, and occupational exposures keep pushing incidence upward worldwide. Scalable, data-driven approaches that improve efficiency and diagnostic precision are increasingly necessary in this setting (Antão et al., 2024).

Imaging sits at the center of modern respiratory care. High-resolution computed tomography (CT) and chest radiography give detailed structural views of the lung, but interpretation still varies considerably between readers. AI systems are increasingly used to address this, helping make image interpretation more consistent and reducing diagnostic delays (Saha et al., 2023).

FUNDAMENTALS OF ARTIFICIAL INTELLIGENCE

Artificial intelligence (AI) refers to computational systems that can perform tasks usually requiring human cognition, including pattern recognition, prediction, classification, natural language processing, and decision support. Machine learning is a branch of AI in which algorithms learn from data rather than from explicit programming, using past examples to predict future outcomes. Deep learning is a further subset that uses multilayer neural networks to find complex patterns in large datasets.

Healthcare uses of AI have grown rapidly over the past decade. Medical imaging, predictive analytics, EHR analysis, and clinical decision support are among the most active areas. Pulmonary medicine maps onto AI's strengths unusually well, since respiratory care depends heavily on image analysis, physiologic signals, and tracking patients over time.

Machine learning models can process large datasets much faster than traditional statistical methods. Supervised learning classifies outcomes using labeled data, unsupervised learning finds patterns in unlabeled data, and reinforcement learning improves through iterative feedback. Deep learning, especially convolutional neural networks, has performed well in radiologic interpretation and pulmonary image analysis (Saha et al., 2023).

AI is increasingly used for both diagnosis and risk prediction in respiratory disease. Algorithms can now help identify pulmonary embolisms, airflow obstruction, and fibrotic lung disease faster than traditional workflows allow. Automated systems also improve severity stratification and prediction of exacerbation risk (Allena & Khanal, 2023).

Generative AI and large language models have pushed clinical interest further. These systems can summarize medical literature, draft clinical documentation, and retrieve biomedical knowledge that used to fall entirely on physicians. The capabilities are genuine, but they come with real questions about reliability, transparency, bias, and clinical accountability. Current evidence supports cautious integration with continued physician oversight (Bubeck et al., 2023).

AI systems depend heavily on good data, which is hard to come by in medicine. Incomplete or inaccurate datasets, demographic imbalance, and inconsistent labeling can all reduce model reliability and may disproportionately affect minority groups. Validation has to be careful, reporting has to be transparent, and clinicians, engineers, and data scientists have to actually work together.

CONVERGENCE OF PULMONARY MEDICINE AND ARTIFICIAL INTELLIGENCE

Pulmonary medicine and AI are converging as part of the wider move toward precision medicine and digital healthcare. Respiratory medicine produces a lot of data that machine learning can work with, both structured and unstructured: pulmonary function tests, imaging datasets, wearable sensor outputs, environmental exposure measurements, and electronic health records.

AI is finding a foothold across pulmonary subspecialties. In obstructive airway disease, machine learning models help with early detection of COPD and asthma from spirometry and symptom patterns. Automated detection improves diagnostic efficiency and may reduce the downstream costs of late diagnosis (Xu et al., 2023).

In pulmonary imaging, AI increasingly helps radiologists identify nodules, infiltrates, fibrosis, and vascular abnormalities. Algorithms sometimes pick up subtle features that get missed on routine reads. These systems improve reproducibility and support earlier intervention (Saha et al., 2023).

Interstitial lung disease is another active area. Image analysis tools can quantify fibrotic progression and help classify idiopathic pulmonary fibrosis patterns, and newer systems combine imaging, histopathology, and genomic data to tighten diagnostic confidence and speed up the workup (Handa, 2023).

Pulmonary hypertension has seen similar growth. Bibliometric work shows rising global research activity around AI-driven prediction and risk stratification models for the condition (Foguem & Keleko, 2023).

The limitations are not minor. Many AI models lack external validation across diverse populations, which creates real gaps in care quality. Black-box algorithms can be hard to interpret at the bedside. Patient privacy, algorithmic bias, and accountability continue to drive regulatory debate. Clinicians need a working sense of both what these tools can do and where they fail and have to let that shape how they actually use them in practice.

Pulmonary medicine is much more likely to end up with human-AI collaboration than with fully autonomous systems. AI can improve efficiency, reduce diagnostic variability, and support more personalized care, but physician judgment, clinical context, and direct conversation with patients are not going to be replaced.

DATA ECOSYSTEMS AND DIGITAL INFRASTRUCTURE IN PULMONARY MEDICINE

Clinical and Biomedical Data Sources

Modern pulmonary medicine produces large amounts of heterogeneous clinical data. It comes from electronic health records (EHRs), pulmonary function testing, imaging platforms, laboratory systems, and physiologic monitoring devices. AI systems rely on these datasets to identify disease patterns and predict clinical outcomes, and pulling these sources together forms the foundation of digital pulmonary medicine.

EHRs hold longitudinal patient information, including demographics, medications, laboratory results, clinical notes, and hospitalization records. These records support predictive modeling in chronic obstructive pulmonary disease (COPD), asthma, pulmonary fibrosis, and critical care medicine (Khemasuwan et al., 2020). AI systems can analyze both structured and unstructured EHR data to identify early disease progression and exacerbation risk (Mlodzinski et al., 2020). EHR systems often use inconsistent formats and coding standards, however, which limits interoperability across institutions and undercuts how well models trained at one site transfer to another.

Pulmonary function testing provides essential physiologic information. Spirometry, lung volumes, and diffusion capacity measurements all contribute to diagnosis and longitudinal disease monitoring. The American Thoracic Society has emphasized the importance of integrating standardized pulmonary function data into interoperable digital infrastructures (McCormack et al., 2021). AI-assisted interpretation of pulmonary function tests has shown potential for automated disease classification and improved diagnostic consistency (Mekov et al., 2020). Imaging further expands these datasets through chest radiography and computed tomography (CT), and deep learning models increasingly analyze imaging biomarkers tied to emphysema, interstitial lung disease, lung nodules, and pulmonary infections (Khemasuwan et al., 2020).

Some biomedical datasets now reach beyond conventional hospital systems. Genomic sequencing, proteomics, and biomarker profiling all feed into precision pulmonology, and combining these multimodal datasets lets AI systems identify phenotypic and molecular disease signatures. Fusing imaging and EHR data through deep learning has improved predictive accuracy compared with using either data type alone (Huang et al., 2020). The shift toward multimodal clinical ecosystems is reshaping how pulmonary data is used.

Patient Generated and Environmental Data

The rapid expansion of wearable technologies and mobile health systems has opened up new dimensions of respiratory monitoring. Patient generated health data now include physiologic signals, symptom reports, medication adherence records, and environmental exposure measurements, all of which support continuous monitoring outside the clinic.

Wearable devices can collect respiratory rate, oxygen saturation, heart rate variability, activity levels, and sleep patterns. These technologies provide long term physiologic information that episodic clinic visits simply cannot capture. Continuous respiratory monitoring has shown promise for asthma management, COPD exacerbation prediction, and remote patient surveillance (Alam et al., 2020). Consumer wearables and smartphones increasingly support passive data collection with minimal patient burden, such as newer versions of the Apple Watch (Low, 2020). AI algorithms can sift through these streams and flag physiologic deterioration before the patient feels anything different.

Smart inhalers and mobile respiratory applications also contribute valuable adherence and behavioral data. These tools track medication usage patterns, inhaler technique, and symptom frequency, and remote symptom monitoring integrated into EHR systems has shown benefits for chronic disease management and longitudinal care coordination (Gandrup et al., 2020). AI driven monitoring platforms may reduce hospitalization rates through earlier intervention and more personalized treatment adjustments.

Environmental data further strengthen pulmonary AI ecosystems. Air pollution, occupational exposures, pollen levels, and climate variables strongly affect respiratory health outcomes, and combining environmental exposure datasets with clinical information makes predictive modeling possible for asthma exacerbations and respiratory emergencies. Real time environmental surveillance can sharpen individualized risk assessment and improve public health planning.

Plenty of practical problems are still unresolved. Many wearable devices lack standardized data exchange capabilities and clear regulatory approval pathways (Muzny et al., 2020). Sensor accuracy varies between manufacturers, and proprietary software ecosystems make it hard to combine data at scale or trust that what gets combined is comparable. None of that has stopped patient generated and environmental data from becoming an increasingly important part of pulmonary medicine infrastructure.

Challenges in Data Integration

Digital ecosystems offer real opportunities, but major barriers still limit effective implementation. Data integration is one of the biggest challenges in AI-enabled pulmonary medicine, since healthcare systems often store information in fragmented and incompatible formats across multiple vendors and institutions.

Interoperability is a central obstacle because health information systems often lack standardized communication protocols and semantic consistency across datasets. Standards like HL7, DICOM, SNOMED CT, and LOINC improve structured data exchange, but adoption is uneven across healthcare environments (Peng et al., 2020). Pulmonary function laboratories, imaging archives, wearable platforms, and EHR systems often operate independently, with no smooth integration pathways between them.

Data quality also affects AI performance. Missing values, inconsistent annotations, incomplete documentation, and measurement variability can all introduce bias into machine learning models, and pulmonary datasets may contain demographic imbalances that reduce how well a model generalizes across populations. AI systems trained on narrow datasets risk producing inaccurate predictions when used in more diverse clinical settings (Khemasuwan et al., 2020). Without external validation and standardized reporting, these models cannot really be trusted in practice.

Privacy and cybersecurity are part of the same picture. Respiratory datasets often contain sensitive personal health information (PHI), and large-scale data sharing raises real concerns about unauthorized access, data breaches, and patient consent. Federated learning and privacy-preserving AI frameworks may reduce some of these risks by enabling distributed model training without centralized data transfer, but the regulatory and ethical landscape is still catching up.

Healthcare organizations also face operational hurdles during AI integration. Clinical workflow disruption, infrastructure costs, and limited technical expertise can all slow adoption, and getting implementation right depends on clinicians, engineers, informaticians, and policymakers actually working together rather than past each other. Pulmonary medicine therefore depends not just on better algorithms, but on reliable, interoperable, and ethically governed digital infrastructure that holds up in everyday clinical use.

OPPORTUNITIES OF AI ACROSS PULMONARY CARE

AI in Diagnosis and Disease Classification

AI has broadened diagnostic capability in pulmonary medicine. Machine learning and deep learning systems now support image interpretation, disease classification, and early detection of respiratory disorders. They work with large datasets from computed tomography (CT), chest radiography, bronchoscopy, and pulmonary function testing, and can pick out subtle radiographic patterns that clinicians may miss on routine reads (Khemasuwan et al., 2020).

In lung cancer screening, AI-assisted imaging is already pulling its weight. Deep convolutional neural networks (CNNs) can improve nodule detection and malignancy prediction on chest CT, and AI can also help identify interstitial lung disease phenotypes and emphysematous changes with high reproducibility. Functional lung imaging combined with AI provides quantitative measurement of ventilation and perfusion abnormalities, which may support earlier diagnosis of chronic obstructive pulmonary disease (COPD) and pulmonary fibrosis (San José Estépar, 2022).

Machine learning also improves pulmonary function assessment. Algorithms can predict spirometric abnormalities, classify airflow limitation, and estimate disease progression trajectories from multidimensional physiologic data, which supports more precise diagnosis and individualized disease characterization (Giri et al., 2021).

During the COVID-19 pandemic, AI systems quickly gained attention for rapid triage and severity prediction. Models analyzed chest imaging and clinical variables to distinguish COVID-19 pneumonia from other respiratory conditions, and these tools helped sustain diagnostic workflows during periods of overwhelming healthcare demand (Khemasuwan et al., 2020).

None of this removes the need for external validation and integration into real clinical environments. Generalizability is the recurring problem: algorithms trained on narrow datasets often perform poorly across diverse populations, and a model that works at one hospital may not work at the next. Clinician oversight is essential.

AI for Monitoring and Personalized Treatment

AI is increasingly used for longitudinal monitoring and individualized respiratory care. Pulmonary medicine now generates continuous streams of physiologic and behavioral data through wearable devices, smart inhalers, telemonitoring systems, and remote sensors, and AI algorithms can process these streams in real time to flag patterns linked to clinical deterioration.

Predictive analytics has become a major focus. Machine learning models can identify patients at increased risk for COPD exacerbations, respiratory failure, or hospital readmission. These systems track trends in oxygen saturation, respiratory rate, medication adherence, environmental exposure, and symptom progression, so deterioration can sometimes be caught early enough to act on before patients decompensate (Levenson et al., 2020).

AI also feeds into personalized treatment strategies. In acute respiratory distress syndrome (ARDS), investigators increasingly use machine learning to pull out biological and clinical sub-phenotypes, with the aim of matching therapy to the patient rather than treating a heterogeneous population as if it were one group (Wick et al., 2021).

Precision pulmonology may also improve medication selection and ventilator management. AI systems can integrate genomic, radiographic, physiologic, and clinical variables to guide individualized therapy. In mechanically ventilated patients, machine learning models help predict ventilator-associated complications and optimize ventilator settings, which may reduce complications and improve outcomes in critical care (Sharma et al., 2021).

Remote patient monitoring has expanded quickly. Smart inhalers and wearable biosensors let clinicians track adherence and respiratory status outside the clinic.

AI-based monitoring systems can also generate automated alerts when predefined risk thresholds are crossed, which may cut emergency department visits and tighten chronic disease management.

There are real concerns to sit with: algorithm transparency, data privacy, and uneven access to digital technologies. Without careful governance and validation, the technology widens the gap between patients who already have good care and patients who don't.

AI in Critical Care and Pulmonary Research

AI applications in pulmonary critical care continue to grow. Intensive care units produce huge volumes of physiologic data from monitors, ventilators, laboratory systems, and electronic health records, and AI systems can pull these high-dimensional datasets together to support clinical decision making and early recognition of physiologic instability.

Machine learning algorithms have shown promise for predicting sepsis, respiratory decompensation, and prolonged mechanical ventilation. AI-supported telemetry systems analyze physiologic trends continuously and may detect deterioration earlier than conventional monitoring approaches (Maslove et al., 2021).

Clinical decision support systems increasingly fold AI-driven predictions into intensive care workflows. These tools help clinicians with triage decisions, ventilator management, sedation strategies, and mortality prediction, and AI models may also flag high-risk patients who could benefit from earlier escalation of care (Yoon et al., 2022).

Pulmonary research also benefits from AI-enabled analytics. Large language models, natural language processing, and predictive modeling support rapid analysis of scientific literature and EHR data. AI helps with identifying disease phenotypes, finding biomarkers, and recruiting patients for clinical trials, which can speed up translational research and compress the timeline from bench to bedside.

AI also supports drug discovery and therapeutic development. Machine learning algorithms can identify candidate molecules, predict treatment responses, and analyze molecular interactions more efficiently than traditional methods, which may help advance therapies for pulmonary fibrosis, lung cancer, and ARDS.

Critical care AI still needs cautious, methodical implementation. Studies have raised concerns about overfitting, lack of external validation, and poor reproducibility across institutions, and when models with those problems get deployed, patients can be harmed in real ways (van de Sande et al., 2021). What pushes the field forward is transparent methodology, multicenter validation, and clinicians, engineers, and regulators working through the rough edges together rather than each in their own silo.

RISKS, LIMITATIONS, AND ETHICAL CONSIDERATIONS

Technical and Clinical Limitations

AI systems have performed well in pulmonary imaging, respiratory monitoring, and clinical prediction. The technical limitations are also real. Many AI models rely heavily on retrospective datasets from limited populations, and those datasets often fail to represent diverse patient groups, healthcare systems, or disease patterns. Models trained that way tend to fall apart once they're deployed somewhere different from where they were built (Gallifant et al., 2022).

Algorithmic bias is a major concern in pulmonary medicine. Chest radiograph algorithms can systematically underdiagnose disease in underserved populations. Seyyed-Kalantari et al. (2021) showed that several chest imaging algorithms had reduced sensitivity among disadvantaged patient groups, which can deepen existing inequities in respiratory care, especially for patients who already struggle to access healthcare.

Model interpretability is another limitation. Many deep learning systems function as "black box" models, and clinicians often receive predictions without understanding the reasoning behind them. That lack of transparency erodes physician trust and makes clinical decision making harder. Explainability matters particularly in pulmonary medicine because respiratory disorders usually require complex longitudinal assessment involving imaging, pulmonary function testing, and symptom progression (Kerasidou, 2021).

Validation and reproducibility are also significant challenges. AI systems may perform well during internal testing and fail during external validation. In respiratory critical care, systematic reviews have flagged inconsistent reporting standards, poor methodological transparency, and elevated bias risk in AI-assisted mechanical ventilation studies (Gallifant et al., 2022). Clinicians want solid evidence before they start trusting an algorithm with high-stakes pulmonary care, and that's a fair ask.

Workflow disruption is worth taking seriously too. Excessive alerts and recommendations can contribute to clinician fatigue, and in pulmonary critical care settings physicians already wade through large volumes of physiologic data. A poorly designed AI system can add cognitive burden rather than reduce it. Integration that actually works has to be built around how clinicians think and move through their day, not bolted on top of it.

Ethical and Legal Challenges

The ethical implications of AI in pulmonary medicine go beyond technical performance. Patient autonomy, privacy, accountability, and transparency all come into play. AI systems often need large quantities of sensitive health data, including imaging studies, spirometry results, genomic data, and wearable device information, and mishandling any of it can damage patient confidentiality and trust.

Transparency and explainability matter ethically because patients and clinicians increasingly want to understand the reasoning behind AI-generated recommendations. Kerasidou (2021) emphasized that explainability directly shapes trust in medical AI systems. Without enough transparency, clinicians may hesitate to lean on algorithmic outputs in critical pulmonary decisions like lung cancer diagnosis or ventilator management.

Legal accountability is another unresolved issue. Working out who is responsible gets hard when AI-assisted decisions contribute to patient harm, and liability may involve clinicians, hospitals, software developers, or device manufacturers. Autonomous medical AI systems add further regulatory uncertainty because current legal frameworks were not designed with continuously learning algorithms in mind (Saenz et al., 2023).

Ethical concerns also come up around informed consent. Many patients may not fully understand how AI systems analyze data or generate recommendations. Meaningful consent requires transparency about algorithm use, data collection, and potential risks, and multi-stakeholder research has highlighted the importance of keeping human oversight within clinical pathways to preserve accountability and ethical decision making (Redrup Hill et al., 2023).

Bias mitigation matters too. Algorithms trained on imbalanced datasets can reinforce disparities related to race, socioeconomic status, geography, or healthcare access, so ethical governance has to include continuous monitoring, fairness assessment, and inclusive data collection. Zhang and Zhang (2023) point to data quality, opacity, bias, and responsibility attribution as the things that ultimately decide whether a medical AI system can be trusted.

Equity and Access Concerns

AI technologies can improve access to pulmonary care through remote monitoring, predictive analytics, and automated diagnostics. The same technologies can also widen existing healthcare disparities when access to digital infrastructure is uneven. Patients in rural or resource-limited regions often lack advanced imaging systems, wearable devices, and the reliable broadband internet that AI-enabled care depends on.

The digital divide falls hardest on the people who can least absorb it: older adults, low-income communities, and underserved racial groups. If AI systems are mainly developed from data collected at large academic centers, they will not address the needs of marginalized populations well. Health equity depends on building representative datasets and developing models inclusively from the start.

Bias monitoring matters more now than it used to in healthcare AI governance. Proactive algorithm surveillance can help spot disparities before widespread clinical harm occurs (Sendak et al., 2023), and continuous auditing can check whether pulmonary AI systems maintain equitable performance across demographic groups.

Strategies for improving equity include federated learning, diverse data partnerships, and fairness-focused validation methods. Federated learning lets institutions collaborate without sharing raw patient data directly, which broadens dataset diversity while protecting privacy. Health equity frameworks also recommend involving clinicians, ethicists, patients, and underserved communities during AI development and deployment (Berdahl et al., 2023).

Responsible implementation means balancing innovation against patient safety and fairness. Pulmonary medicine increasingly depends on complex digital systems for diagnosis, monitoring, and treatment planning, and AI clearly opens up new possibilities. Whether those possibilities translate into actual benefit for patients depends on how the technology is governed, validated, deployed, and overseen by humans who can still say no.

CLINICAL INTEGRATION AND HEALTHCARE TRANSFORMATION

AI Assisted Clinical Decision Making

AI is increasingly part of pulmonary medicine workflows. AI systems help clinicians with imaging interpretation, risk prediction, and diagnostic prioritization, and they improve efficiency during heavy clinical workloads. Use in pulmonary and critical care settings now goes well beyond experimental.

AI-driven clinical decision support systems improve diagnostic appropriateness and workflow coordination. Studies have shown improved imaging utilization after AI-supported decision support was added to clinical practice (Chepelev et al., 2021). These systems cut unnecessary imaging while supporting guideline adherence, and they may reduce resource overuse in pulmonary diagnostics, particularly during workup of pulmonary embolism and thoracic abnormalities.

Pulmonary imaging is a major area of AI integration. Deep learning systems now help identify pulmonary infections, pneumothorax, interstitial lung disease, and chronic obstructive pulmonary disease. One clinical implementation study described successful integration of an AI pneumothorax detection algorithm directly into thoracic radiology workflows; the system prioritized urgent chest radiographs and sped up clinical review (Pierce et al., 2021).

AI also feeds into pulmonary and critical care decision making through predictive analytics. Machine learning models analyze physiologic data, laboratory findings, and imaging patterns at the same time, which supports earlier detection of respiratory deterioration and intensive care complications. Recent reviews argue that AI systems may improve triage, mechanical ventilation management, and longitudinal disease monitoring in pulmonary medicine (Friedman et al., 2024).

None of this removes the need for human oversight. A poorly validated AI system can introduce bias, false predictions, and workflow disruption, and clinicians have to interpret algorithmic output within broader clinical context. Human factors research showed that usability strongly influences adoption of AI-assisted decision support tools in pulmonary embolism diagnosis (Salwei et al., 2021a). When the interface was poor, clinicians trusted the tool less and used it less effectively.

AI integration also changes the physician-patient interaction. Automated documentation and predictive systems may reduce administrative burden, but clinicians are still the ones responsible for shared decision making and the conversation in the room. Trustworthy implementation requires transparent algorithms and explainable outputs, because once patients lose confidence in how their care is being decided, getting it back is hard.

AI and Value Based Pulmonary Care

Healthcare systems increasingly prioritize value-based care models. These frameworks focus on clinical outcomes, cost reduction, and efficient use of resources. Pulmonary medicine carries a substantial economic burden, since chronic respiratory diseases often need repeated hospitalization and long-term management.

AI technologies can support value-based pulmonary care through earlier intervention and predictive monitoring. Machine learning models identify patients at high risk for exacerbation, hospital readmission, or respiratory decline, and earlier recognition lets clinicians start preventive treatment before things get worse.

COPD is one of the most expensive pulmonary conditions globally. Hospitalizations from acute exacerbations drive a large share of those costs. Quality improvement initiatives have shown that standardized, technology-supported care pathways improve outcomes and reduce avoidable utilization (Tsao et al., 2022), and AI-assisted systems may strengthen those approaches through automated risk stratification and personalized monitoring.

Remote monitoring technologies also contribute to value-based respiratory care. Smart inhalers, wearable sensors, and home spirometry systems generate continuous physiologic data, and AI algorithms can analyze these streams to flag worsening symptoms and slipping adherence. Catching problems earlier can reduce emergency visits and ICU admissions.

Value-based pulmonary care also depends on better use of imaging and diagnostic testing. AI-enabled decision support systems cut unnecessary testing while improving diagnostic precision. After AI was added to imaging workflows, appropriateness improved measurably and waste went down within healthcare systems (Chepelev et al., 2021).

Professional societies are leaning into high-value pulmonary care strategies. Reviews in CHEST emphasized that physicians need to participate actively in value-based healthcare transformation through evidence-based interventions and efficient resource stewardship (Wahidi et al., 2023). AI may support those goals by improving standardization and reducing unwarranted variation in pulmonary practice.

Cost-effectiveness is the part nobody has nailed down yet. Many AI systems require substantial infrastructure investment, integration costs, and ongoing validation, so institutions have to decide whether the outcome improvements justify the spending. Until longer-term studies catch up, the economic case for AI in pulmonary medicine is going to keep being argued one institution at a time.

Education and Workforce Development

The expansion of AI in pulmonary medicine demands real workforce adaptation. Clinicians now run into AI-assisted imaging systems, predictive analytics platforms, and automated documentation tools during routine practice, and medical education has to evolve alongside that change.

AI literacy matters now. Clinicians need to understand what algorithms do well, where they fail, how bias creeps in, and what the ethical stakes are. Respiratory medicine reviews have emphasized that inadequate understanding of AI can erode clinician trust and undercut effective adoption in obstructive lung disease management (Antão et al., 2024).

Future pulmonary physicians will likely need interdisciplinary training. Their education should cover data interpretation, digital health systems, and the basics of machine learning. Those competencies help clinicians critically evaluate AI-generated recommendations rather than accept output uncritically.

Healthcare organizations also have to prepare existing professionals for workflow transformation. Resistance to adoption often comes from limited training and unclear implementation strategies. Human-centered integration improves clinician acceptance and usability, and studies of AI-supported pulmonary embolism decision tools showed that successful implementation depended heavily on workflow alignment and clinician engagement (Salwei et al., 2021b).

Interdisciplinary collaboration matters more than it used to. Pulmonary specialists, data scientists, engineers, and informaticians have to work together during system design and validation, because tools built without clinical input tend to fail at the bedside no matter how well they perform in testing.

AI may also reshape workforce structure within pulmonary medicine. Automation may cut down on repetitive administrative tasks and free clinicians up for more direct patient care, but clinicians still hold the oversight responsibility and the ethical accountability. The point is to give physicians better tools to think with, not to take the thinking out of their hands.

EMERGING INNOVATIONS AND FUTURE DIRECTIONS

Precision and Predictive Pulmonology

AI is changing pulmonary medicine through precision and predictive approaches. Modern pulmonary care increasingly depends on large-scale integration of imaging, physiologic measurements, genomics, environmental exposures, and electronic health records. Machine learning systems can pick out subtle disease patterns that are hard to spot through conventional analysis, and that supports earlier diagnosis, personalized treatment selection, and prediction of how disease will progress (Khemasuwan et al., 2020).

Predictive analytics has become a major focus in chronic respiratory diseases like chronic obstructive pulmonary disease (COPD), asthma, pulmonary fibrosis, and pulmonary hypertension. AI models can estimate hospitalization risk, exacerbation probability, and mortality from multidimensional clinical datasets, which can improve preventive intervention and reduce avoidable admissions. Machine learning also enhances pulmonary imaging interpretation through automated identification of radiographic abnormalities and quantitative analysis of CT scans (Mlodzinski et al., 2020).

Adaptive learning systems are another major innovation. They keep updating predictive models as new patient data comes in. Real-time physiologic monitoring through wearable devices and smart inhalers lets AI systems pick up deterioration before clinical symptoms worsen, which shifts respiratory care from reactive to proactive. The longer-term promise of precision pulmonology is treatment planning that tracks each patient as they actually change over time, instead of relying on a snapshot from the last clinic visit.

Advanced Technologies in Respiratory AI

Generative AI is one of the more active fronts in healthcare innovation right now. Large language models and generative AI systems can summarize clinical notes, assist with documentation, support literature synthesis, and help clinicians communicate with patients. In pulmonary medicine, these tools may help physicians interpret complex datasets and generate evidence-based recommendations. Clinical implementation still needs careful oversight, though, because hallucinations, bias, and inaccurate outputs are real concerns.

Federated learning has also become increasingly important in respiratory medicine. Traditional AI development usually requires centralized patient data collection, which creates privacy and regulatory headaches. Federated learning lets institutions train AI models collaboratively without directly sharing patient-level data: instead of moving the data, model parameters are exchanged while the data stay where they are. This improves privacy protection while allowing larger and more diverse training datasets (Rieke et al., 2020; Xu et al., 2021).

Federated learning may be especially valuable in pulmonary medicine because respiratory diseases often vary by geography, environment, and demographics. Multi-institutional collaboration can therefore improve model generalizability and reduce algorithmic bias. Privacy-preserving AI frameworks also help with regulatory compliance and enable international research collaborations. The catch is the technical overhead: communication efficiency, model synchronization, and uneven data quality across institutions globally are all real problems that don't go away on their own.

Digital twins are another promising innovation in pulmonary medicine. A digital twin is a dynamic virtual representation of an individual patient that integrates physiologic data, imaging, biomarkers, and computational models. Pulmonary digital twins may simulate respiratory mechanics, gas exchange, airflow dynamics, and treatment responses in real time, which could let clinicians try out therapeutic strategies virtually before applying them to the actual patient (Gonsard et al., 2024).

Potential applications include optimizing ventilator settings in critical care, predicting fibrosis progression, and individualizing bronchodilator selection. Digital twins may also help untangle the complex gene-environment interactions involved in chronic lung disease. The barriers are practical: computation demands are heavy, data integration is messy, and high-quality longitudinal datasets are still scarce.

Edge computing and Internet of Things (IoT) technologies also support future respiratory AI systems. Smart respiratory devices can collect continuous physiologic information while processing selected data locally rather than sending everything to centralized cloud infrastructure, which reduces latency and may improve real-time monitoring in home-based pulmonary care. Combining wearable sensors with AI-driven analytics may expand remote respiratory management and tele-pulmonology services.

Research Priorities and Global Collaboration

Future progress in pulmonary AI depends on rigorous clinical validation and multidisciplinary collaboration. Many existing AI studies are still retrospective and rely on limited datasets. Prospective multicenter validation studies are needed before widespread clinical implementation, and external validation across diverse patient populations matters especially because algorithmic performance can drop when models encounter demographic or environmental differences they didn't see during training (Mekov et al., 2020).

International collaboration is going to matter more for respiratory AI development. Large global datasets can improve model robustness and help identify rare disease patterns that smaller local datasets simply can't capture. Shared research frameworks may also accelerate innovation in pulmonary imaging, intensive care monitoring, and respiratory epidemiology. Harmonizing regulatory standards and data governance policies across healthcare systems is still tough, though, and that part isn't getting solved quickly.

Ethical considerations will shape how future AI integration plays out. Transparency, interpretability, accountability, and fairness keep showing up as the core issues, and black-box algorithms can erode clinician trust and complicate decision making in high-risk pulmonary settings. Researchers therefore need to prioritize explainable AI systems that let clinicians see how predictions are generated. Human oversight will remain essential even as automation expands.

Educational reform belongs on the same list. Pulmonary clinicians increasingly need familiarity with AI principles, data interpretation, and algorithm limitations, so interdisciplinary training across medicine, data science, engineering, and bioinformatics may become necessary within pulmonary education programs. That kind of training could support responsible AI adoption and strengthen collaboration between clinicians and computational scientists.

Emerging AI technologies could significantly transform pulmonary medicine over the coming decades. Precision medicine, federated learning, generative AI, and digital twin systems may together improve diagnosis, monitoring, and therapeutic personalization. But thc transformation is conditional, not automatic. It depends on validation that actually holds up, governance that takes ethical questions seriously, and clinical and technical disciplines sticking with the collaboration past the point where it gets hard.

CONCLUSION

Summary of Opportunities and Risks

AI is now a major presence in pulmonary medicine. Recent advances have improved disease detection, pulmonary imaging analysis, pulmonary function interpretation, and predictive monitoring. AI systems can help clinicians identify interstitial lung disease, pulmonary hypertension, and respiratory failure patterns more efficiently (Saha et al., 2023). Collaborative models that pair explainable AI with pulmonologist expertise have also improved interpretation accuracy in pulmonary function testing (Das et al., 2023). Taken together, these developments suggest AI can sharpen diagnostic precision and support more personalized respiratory care.

The downsides matter too. AI systems depend heavily on data quality, dataset diversity, and external validation, and bias in training data can drag down performance for underrepresented populations. Limited interpretability creates barriers to clinician trust and regulatory adoption on top of that. Several studies have emphasized the need for explainable and transparent AI frameworks in pulmonary medicine and medical imaging (Champendal et al., 2023; Mamalakis et al., 2023). Ethical concerns around accountability, patient privacy, cybersecurity, and informed consent continue to shape implementation decisions in healthcare systems (Satapathy et al., 2023). The point of these tools is to extend what a physician can do, not to take the physician's place at the bedside.

Vision for Responsible AI Enabled Pulmonary Medicine

The future of pulmonary medicine will likely involve close collaboration between clinicians, data scientists, engineers, and policymakers. Responsible AI integration requires transparent algorithms, standardized validation procedures, and continuous post-deployment monitoring. International frameworks increasingly emphasize fairness, robustness, explainability, and usability as central principles for trustworthy medical AI systems (Lekadir et al., 2023). These matter especially in pulmonary medicine, where respiratory diseases often require longitudinal monitoring and high-stakes clinical decisions.

Future AI systems may support precision pulmonology through multimodal data integration. Combining imaging, pulmonary function testing, genomics, and environmental exposure data could improve individualized disease prediction and treatment planning, and advances in generative AI and computational physiological modeling may further enhance critical care decision support and mechanical ventilation optimization (Warnaar et al., 2023). At the same time, institutions have to weigh innovation against ethical oversight and equitable access. AI tools should stay accessible across diverse healthcare settings, including the low-resource environments where pulmonary disease burden is highest.

Clinician education will also shape successful implementation. Pulmonologists need to understand what AI-assisted systems can and can't do, and training programs should therefore include data literacy, algorithm interpretation, and ethical evaluation. Automated systems aren't going to replicate the way clinicians weigh context, factor in what matters to a particular patient, and reason through cases with colleagues, so human oversight is going to stay essential. In the end, responsible adoption depends on physicians and patients trusting each other through whatever the technology adds to the picture.

Roadmap for the Remaining Chapters of the Book

The remaining chapters of this book will examine the expanding role of AI across pulmonary medicine in greater detail. These subsequent chapters will explore machine learning fundamentals, imaging applications, pulmonary function interpretation, critical care monitoring, predictive analytics, and precision medicine strategies. Additional sections will also address wearable technologies, telemedicine integration, digital biomarkers, and AI assisted research methodologies.

The book will also examine ethical, legal, and regulatory considerations influencing clinical adoption, and topics such as explainability, bias mitigation, cybersecurity, and governance frameworks will receive focused attention. Emerging innovations including generative AI, federated learning, and digital twin technologies will also be discussed in relation to future respiratory care. Collectively, these chapters aim to provide clinicians, researchers, and trainees with a comprehensive understanding of how AI may transform pulmonary medicine while maintaining scientific rigor, patient safety, and ethical responsibility.

REFERENCES

Alam, R., Peden, D. B., & Lach, J. C. (2020). Wearable respiration monitoring: Interpretable inference with context and sensor biomarkers. arXiv. PMID: N/A. https://doi.org//arXiv.2007.01413DOI: 10.1101/2020.07.04.20146456

Allena, N., & Khanal, S. (2023). The algorithmic lung detective: Artificial intelligence in the diagnosis of pulmonary embolism. *Cureus*, *15*(12), e51006. DOI: 10.7759/cureus.51006 PMID: 38259362

Antão, J., de Mast, J., Marques, A., Franssen, F. M. E., Spruit, M. A., & Deng, Q. (2024). Demystification of artificial intelligence for respiratory clinicians managing patients with obstructive lung diseases. *Expert Review of Respiratory Medicine*, *17*(12), 1207–1219. DOI: 10.1080/17476348.2024.2302940 PMID: 38270524

Berdahl, C. T., Baker, L., Mann, S., Osoba, O., & Girosi, F. (2023). Strategies to improve the impact of artificial intelligence on health equity: Scoping review. JMIR AI, 2, e42936. PMID: N/A. https://doi.org/DOI: 10.2196/42936

Bubeck, S., Chandrasekaran, V., Eldan, R., Gehrke, J., Horvitz, E., Kamar, E., Lee, P., Lee, Y. T., Li, Y., Lundberg, S., Nori, H., Palangi, H., Ribeiro, M. T., & Zhang, Y. (2023). Sparks of artificial general intelligence: Early experiments with GPT 4. arXiv. PMID: N/A. https://doi.org//arXiv.2303.12712DOI: 10.48550

Champendal, M., Muller, H., Prior, J., & dos Reis, C. S. (2023). A scoping review of interpretability and explainability concerning artificial intelligence methods in medical imaging. *European Journal of Radiology*, *169*, 111159. DOI: 10.1016/j.ejrad.2023.111159 PMID: 37976760

Chepelev, L. L., Wang, X., Gold, B., Bonzel, C. L., Rybicki, F. J., Uyeda, J. W., & Sheikh, A. (2021). Improved appropriateness of advanced diagnostic imaging after implementation of clinical decision support mechanism. Journal of Digital Imaging, 34, 397–403. PMID: N/A. https://doi.org/DOI: 10.1007/s10278-021-00433-6

Das, N., Happaerts, S., Gyselinck, I., Staes, M., Derom, E., Brusselle, G., Burgos, F., Contoli, M., Dinh-Xuan, A. T., Franssen, F. M. E., Gonem, S., Greening, N., Haenebalcke, C., Man, W. D.-C., Moisés, J., Peché, R., Poberezhets, V., Quint, J. K., Steiner, M. C., & Janssens, W. (2023). Collaboration between explainable artificial intelligence and pulmonologists improves the accuracy of pulmonary function test interpretation. *The European Respiratory Journal*, *61*(5), 2201720. DOI: 10.1183/13993003.01720-2022 PMID: 37080566

Foguem, G. T., & Keleko, A. T. (2023). Artificial intelligence applied in pulmonary hypertension: A bibliometric analysis. *AI and Ethics*, *3*(4), 1063–1093. Advance online publication. DOI: 10.1007/s43681-023-00267-8 PMID: 37360147

Friedman, S. H., Long, K. J., Sexauer, S., Menon, A. A., & Kilb, E. F. (2024). Role of Artificial Intelligence in Assisting Pulmonary and Critical Care Clinical Decision-Making. *American Journal of Respiratory and Critical Care Medicine*, *210*(5), 662–664. DOI: 10.1164/rccm.202402-0331RR PMID: 38924771

Gallifant, J., Zhang, J., Arias Lopez, M. D. P., Zhu, T., Camporota, L., Celi, L. A., & Formenti, F. (2022). Artificial intelligence for mechanical ventilation: Systematic review of design, reporting standards, and bias. *British Journal of Anaesthesia*, *128*(2), 343–351. DOI: 10.1016/j.bja.2021.09.025 PMID: 34772497

Gandrup, J., Ali, S. M., McBeth, J., van der Veer, S. N., & Dixon, W. G. (2020). Remote symptom monitoring integrated into electronic health records: A systematic review. *Journal of the American Medical Informatics Association : JAMIA*, *27*(11), 1752–1763. DOI: 10.1093/jamia/ocaa177 PMID: 32968785

Giri, P. C., Chowdhury, A. M., Bedoya, A., Chen, H., Lee, H. S., Lee, P., Henriquez, C., MacIntyre, N. R., & Huang, Y. C. T. (2021). Application of machine learning in pulmonary function assessment: Where are we now and where are we going? *Frontiers in Physiology*, *12*, 678540. DOI: 10.3389/fphys.2021.678540 PMID: 34248665

Gonsard, A., Genet, M., & Drummond, D. (2024). Digital twins for chronic lung diseases. European Respiratory Review, 33(174), 240159. PMID: N/A. https://doi.org/DOI: 10.1183/16000617.0159-2024

Handa, T. (2023). The potential role of artificial intelligence in the clinical practice of interstitial lung disease. *Respiratory Investigation*, *61*(6), 702–710. DOI: 10.1016/j.resinv.2023.08.006 PMID: 37708636

Huang, S. C., Pareek, A., Seyyedi, S., Banerjee, I., & Lungren, M. P. (2020). Fusion of medical imaging and electronic health records using deep learning: A systematic review and implementation guidelines. *NPJ Digital Medicine*, *3*(1), 136. DOI: 10.1038/s41746-020-00341-z PMID: 33083571

Kerasidou, A. (2021). Ethics of artificial intelligence in global health: Explainability, algorithmic bias and trust. *Journal of Oral Biology and Craniofacial Research*, *11*(4), 612–614. DOI: 10.1016/j.jobcr.2021.09.004 PMID: 34567966

Khemasuwan, D., Sorensen, J. S., & Colt, H. G. (2020). Artificial intelligence in pulmonary medicine: Computer vision, predictive model and COVID-19. *European Respiratory Review : an Official Journal of the European Respiratory Society, 29*(157), 200181. DOI: 10.1183/16000617.0181-2020 PMID: 33004526

Lekadir, K., Feragen, A., Fofanah, A. J., Frangi, A. F., Buyx, A., ... (2023). FUTURE AI: International consensus guideline for trustworthy and deployable artificial intelligence in healthcare. arXiv. PMID: N/A. https://doi.org//arXiv.2309.12325DOI: 10.48550

Levenson, A. R., Morales Nebreda, L., Alexander, M. J., & Schroedl, C. J. (2020). Harnessing machine learning to improve patient outcomes in pulmonary and critical care medicine. *American Journal of Respiratory and Critical Care Medicine, 202*(1), 30–39. DOI: 10.1164/rccm.201912-2486RR PMID: 32752881

Low, C. A. (2020). Harnessing consumer smartphone and wearable sensors for clinical cancer research. npj. *Digital Medicine, 3*(1), 140. DOI: 10.1038/s41746-020-00351-x PMID: 33134557

Mamalakis, M., Dwivedi, K., Sharkey, M., Alabed, S., Kiely, D., & Swift, A. J. (2023). A transparent artificial intelligence framework to assess lung disease in pulmonary hypertension. Scientific Reports, 13, 3812. PMID: N/A. https://doi.org/ DOI: 10.1038/s41598-023-30503-4

Maslove, D. M., Elbers, P. W. G., & Clermont, G. (2021). Artificial intelligence in telemetry: What clinicians should know. *Intensive Care Medicine, 47*(2), 150–153. DOI: 10.1007/s00134-020-06295-w PMID: 33386857

McCormack, M. C., Bascom, R., Brandt, M., Burgos, F., Butler, S., Caggiano, C., Dimmock, A. E. F., Fineberg, A., Goldstein, J., Guzman, F. C., Halldin, C. N., Johnson, J. D., Kerby, G. S., Krishnan, J. A., Kurth, L., Morgan, G., Mularski, R. A., Pasquale, C. B., Ryu, J., & Drummond, M. B. (2021). Electronic health records and pulmonary function data: Developing an interoperability roadmap. An official American Thoracic Society workshop report. *Annals of the American Thoracic Society, 18*(1), 1–11. DOI: 10.1513/AnnalsATS.202010-1318ST PMID: 33385224

Mekov, E., Miravitlles, M., & Petkov, R. (2020). Artificial intelligence and machine learning in respiratory medicine. *Expert Review of Respiratory Medicine, 14*(6), 559–564. DOI: 10.1080/17476348.2020.1743181 PMID: 32166988

Mlodzinski, E., Stone, D. J., & Celi, L. A. (2020). Machine learning for pulmonary and critical care medicine: A narrative review. *Pulmonary Therapy, 6*(1), 67–77. DOI: 10.1007/s41030-020-00110-z PMID: 32048244

Muzny, M., Henriksen, A., Giordanengo, A., Muzik, J., Grøttland, A., Blixgård, H., Hartvigsen, G., & Årsand, E. (2020). Wearable sensors with possibilities for data exchange: Analyzing status and needs of different actors in mobile health monitoring systems. *International Journal of Medical Informatics*, *133*, 104017. DOI: 10.1016/j.ijmedinf.2019.104017 PMID: 31778885

Peng, C., Goswami, P., & Bai, G. (2020). A literature review of current technologies on health data integration for patient centered health management. *Health Informatics Journal*, *26*(3), 1926–1951. DOI: 10.1177/1460458219892387 PMID: 31884843

Pierce, J. D., Rosipko, B., Youngblood, L., Gilkeson, R. C., Gupta, A., & Bittencourt, L. K. (2021). Seamless integration of artificial intelligence into the clinical environment: Our experience with a novel pneumothorax detection artificial intelligence algorithm. *Journal of the American College of Radiology*, *18*(11), 1497–1505. DOI: 10.1016/j.jacr.2021.08.023 PMID: 34597622

Rieke, N., Hancox, J., Li, W., Milletarì, F., Roth, H. R., Albarqouni, S., Bakas, S., Galtier, M. N., Landman, B. A., Maier-Hein, K., Ourselin, S., Sheller, M., Summers, R. M., Trask, A., Xu, D., Baust, M., & Cardoso, M. J. (2020). The future of digital health with federated learning. *NPJ Digital Medicine*, *3*(1), 119. DOI: 10.1038/s41746-020-00323-1 PMID: 33015372

Saha, P. K., Nadeem, S. A., & Comellas, A. P. (2023). A survey on artificial intelligence in pulmonary imaging. *Wiley Interdisciplinary Reviews. Data Mining and Knowledge Discovery*, *13*(6), e1510. DOI: 10.1002/widm.1510 PMID: 38249785

Salwei, M. E., Carayon, P., & Hoonakker, P. L. T. (2021a). Workflow integration analysis of a human factors-based clinical decision support in the emergency department. Applied Ergonomics, 97, 103498. PMID: N/A. https://doi.org/DOI: 10.1016/j.apergo.2021.103498

Salwei, M. E., Carayon, P., & Hoonakker, P. L. T. (2021b). Usability barriers and facilitators of a human factors engineering-based clinical decision support technology for diagnosing pulmonary embolism. International Journal of Medical Informatics, 158, 104657. PMID: N/A. https://doi.org/DOI: 10.1016/j.ijmedinf.2021.104657

San José Estépar, R. (2022). Artificial intelligence in functional imaging of the lung. *The British Journal of Radiology*, *95*(1132), 20210527. DOI: 10.1259/bjr.20210527 PMID: 34890215

Satapathy, P., Padhi, B. K., & Al Khathlan, N. (2023). Artificial intelligence in respiratory therapy: Opportunities and ethical challenges. *Respiratory Medicine*, *217*, 107342. DOI: 10.1016/j.rmed.2023.107342 PMID: 37380092

Sendak, M., Balu, S., & Hernandez, A. F. (2023). Proactive algorithm monitoring to ensure health equity. JAMA Network Open, 6(12), e2345022. PMID: N/A. https://doi.org/DOI: 10.1001/jamanetworkopen.2023.45022

Seyyed-Kalantari, L., Zhang, H., McDermott, M. B. A., Chen, I. Y., & Ghassemi, M. (2021). Underdiagnosis bias of artificial intelligence algorithms applied to chest radiographs in under served patient populations. *Nature Medicine*, *27*(12), 2176–2182. DOI: 10.1038/s41591-021-01595-0 PMID: 34893776

Sharma, M., Taweesedt, P. T., & Surani, S. (2021). Utilizing artificial intelligence in critical care: Adding a handy tool to our armamentarium. *Cureus*, *13*(6), e15531. DOI: 10.7759/cureus.15531 PMID: 34268051

Tsao, M., Laikijrung, C., Tran, A., Pon, T., Roach, D., Liu, B., & Le, K. (2022). Optimizing quality of care in patients admitted with chronic obstructive pulmonary disease exacerbation. *Chronic Respiratory Disease*, *19*, 14799731211073348. DOI: 10.1177/14799731211073348 PMID: 35041553

van de Sande, D., van Genderen, M. E., Huiskens, J., Gommers, D., & van Bommel, J. (2021). Moving from bytes to bedside: A systematic review on the use of artificial intelligence in the intensive care unit. *Intensive Care Medicine*, *47*(7), 750–760. DOI: 10.1007/s00134-021-06446-7 PMID: 34089064

Wahidi, M. M., Haywood, H. B., Bass, G. D., Nathanson, I., Chowdhury, A., & Sangvai, D. (2023). Value-based care for chest physicians. *Chest*, *163*(5), 1193–1200. DOI: 10.1016/j.chest.2022.12.041 PMID: 36627080

Warnaar, R. S. P., Mulder, M. P., Fresiello, L., Cornet, A. D., & Heunks, L. M. A. (2023). Computational physiological models for individualised mechanical ventilation: A systematic literature review focussing on quality, availability, and clinical readiness. Critical Care, 27, 268. PMID: N/A. https://doi.org/DOI: 10.1186/s13054-023-04549-9

Wick, K. D., McAuley, D. F., Levitt, J. E., Beitler, J. R., Annane, D., Riviello, E. D., Calfee, C. S., & Matthay, M. A. (2021). Promises and challenges of personalized medicine to guide ARDS therapy. *Critical Care*, *25*(1), 404. DOI: 10.1186/s13054-021-03822-z PMID: 34814925

Xu, J., Glicksberg, B. S., Su, C., Walker, P., Bian, J., & Wang, F. (2021). Federated learning for healthcare informatics. *Journal of Healthcare Informatics Research*, *5*(1), 1–19. DOI: 10.1007/s41666-020-00082-4 PMID: 33204939

Xu, S., Deo, R. C., Soar, J., Barua, P. D., Faust, O., Homaira, N., Jaffe, A., Kabir, A. L., & Acharya, U. R. (2023). Automated detection of airflow obstructive diseases: A systematic review of the last decade (2013–2022). *Computer Methods and Programs in Biomedicine, 241*, 107746. DOI: 10.1016/j.cmpb.2023.107746 PMID: 37660550

Yoon, J. H., Pinsky, M. R., & Clermont, G. (2022). Artificial intelligence in critical care medicine. Critical Care, 26(1), 75. PMID: N/A. https://doi.org/DOI: 10.1186/s13054-022-03915-3

Zhang, J., & Zhang, Z. M. (2023). Ethics and governance of trustworthy medical artificial intelligence. BMC Medical Informatics and Decision Making, 23, 7. PMID: N/A. https://doi.org/DOI: 10.1186/s12911-023-02103-9

Chapter 2

Use of Artificial Intelligence in Treatment and Management of Sleep Disorders

Subhendu Rath
http://orcid.org/0000-0002-1625-8175
University of Kentucky, USA

Jillian Prier
University of Michigan, USA

Kunj R. Patel
http://orcid.org/0000-0002-5940-6844
Lake Erie School of Medicine, USA

Nikunj R. Patel
http://orcid.org/0009-0007-8056-6969
University of Wisconsin-Madison, USA

ABSTRACT

This chapter examines the role of artificial intelligence (AI) in sleep medicine. Sleep disorders are highly prevalent and carry substantial morbidity. Sleep studies, particularly in-lab polysomnography (PSG), require significant resources and laboratory access, followed by manual scoring prior to interpretation. Recent advances in deep learning and foundational models have enabled automated sleep staging, often matching human scorers and accelerating study analysis. AI-enhanced analysis of proprietary algorithms in consumer wearables shows promise for improved sleep staging and cardiorespiratory screening. AI offers greater reliability, reduced

DOI: 10.4018/979-8-3373-7759-9.ch002

diagnostic delays, and enhanced accessibility via ambulatory studies. However, challenges include data security, algorithmic opacity, training bias, and risk of over-reliance. There remains a need for sustained clinician supervision, consistent with current American Academy of Sleep Medicine guidance. Ongoing model refinement and regulatory evolution will shape AI's responsible integration in sleep medicine.

ARTIFICIAL INTELLIGENCE IN SLEEP DISORDERS

The use of artificial intelligence (AI) has influenced most of the fields of healthcare, including sleep medicine. The most common sleep disorders include sleep-disordered breathing and insomnia (Wickwire and Collop, 2010). Sleep disorders also include less common conditions such as parasomnias and sleep-related movement disorders, such as restless legs syndrome. Obstructive sleep apnea, the most prevalent form of sleep-disordered breathing, affects approximately 17% of females and 34% of males (Gottlieb and Punjabi, 2020). Definitive diagnosis of sleep disorders typically requires polysomnography, a resource-intensive overnight study that records neurophysiological and cardiorespiratory parameters. Polysomnography (PSG) is a multichannel overnight recording that simultaneously captures brain activity using electroencephalography (EEG), eye movements using electrooculography (EOG), muscle tone using electromyography (EMG), heart rhythm using electrocardiography (ECG), airflow, respiratory effort, and blood oxygen saturation. Because nearly every sleep disorder discussed in this paper manifests as abnormalities in one or more of these signals, polysomnography serves as both the diagnostic reference standard and the primary source of labeled training data for the AI models reviewed here. While polysomnography is an effective tool in detecting the presence of sleep disorders, there is limited availability and high cost for many patients. Since there is not a more affordable and accessible option in the detection of sleep disorders in real-time, there is a potential demand for AI-driven, wearable-based, and home-monitoring alternatives discussed later in this paper. Bhatt et al. (2025) observed that recent advances in AI with the foundational models trained on large datasets have improved automated signal analysis and interpretation. Foundation models are large-scale neural networks pre-trained on broad, often unlabeled datasets and subsequently fine-tuned for specific downstream tasks. In sleep medicine, foundation models trained on large-scale datasets of physiological recordings can learn general representations of EEG, ECG, and respiratory signals that transfer effectively to specialized tasks such as sleep stage classification, apnea detection, and arousal scoring. This transfer-learning approach reduces the need for large, hand-labeled datasets at every individual clinic or device manufacturer, allowing smaller institutions to deploy high-performing models without building their own. Similarly,

Demrozi et al. (2023) observed that home-based monitoring devices have improved accessibility and enabled earlier diagnosis and treatment initiation for many sleep disorders. Home-based monitoring devices allow patients to collect multiple nights of physiological data in their natural sleep environment. This is clinically significant for sleep disorders because a single in-laboratory study captures only one night, potentially missing the night-to-night variability in conditions such as obstructive sleep apnea and periodic limb movement disorder. Furthermore, doctors can monitor responses to changes in sleep patterns post-treatment. By generating longitudinal datasets at scale, these devices can supply the volume and diversity of input that AI models require to detect subtle temporal patterns to triage patient complaints more efficiently for confirmatory polysomnography.

AI-based computer applications continue to expand across approaches to care in sleep medicine. Sun et al. (2017) and Nikkonen et al. (2021) showed that AI deep learning models extend the capabilities of automated sleep staging and apnea detection with high correlations to expert scoring respectively. This algorithm allows physicians to detect sleep apnea in real time, and stratify the severity of sleep apnea, informing possible treatment. Deep learning models, particularly convolutional and recurrent architectures, can learn the distinctive waveform morphologies that define each sleep stage directly from raw EEG without hand-engineered features such as sleep spindle detection. Given these models can process entire overnight recordings consistently, they can reduce inter-rater variability that has historically limited manual scoring, flagging apneic and hypopneic events in real time and enabling severity stratification directly informing treatment selection (e.g. CPAP, oral-appliance, or surgical referral). Similarly, Baron et al. (2018) suggested that wearable devices using photoplethysmography and accelerometry provide an option for screening without the need for laboratory testing, allowing for rapid screening and observation of suspected sleep apnea. Photoplethysmography (PPG) uses light absorption changes in the skin to derive pulse rate, pulse waveform morphology, and indirectly oxygen saturation, while accelerometry detects body motion to distinguish wake from sleep periods. Together, these two low-cost sensors can approximate several signals normally obtained by polysomnography: the autonomic surges associated with apneic events appear as PPG-derived heart-rate variability changes, with limb movements and arousals appearing as accelerometry spikes. AI models trained on PPG and accelerometry data can therefore screen for sleep apnea, estimate sleep stages, and detect movement disorders without electrodes, dramatically lowering the barrier to widespread, longitudinal screening. Hanif et al. (2026) demonstrated AI-driven approaches to CPAP management. This includes unsupervised phenotyping of usage patterns and supervised adherence prediction, which can enhance individualized titration and treatment optimization, as well as allow physicians to precisely cater treatment according to the severity of the disease, addressing pressure intolerance, treatment-emergent central sleep apnea, or poor adherence. CPAP titration requires balancing pressure high enough to splint the upper airway without causing patient discomfort, mask leak, or central apneas from over-ventilation. AI-driven decision support systems analyze night-by-night residual apnea-hypopnea indices, leak data, and pressure response curves from auto-titrating CPAP machines to recommend pressure adjustments tailored to each patient's airway mechanics. This is particularly valuable in sleep medicine given the multifactorial nature of OSA as a disease, with multiple factors that predispose patients to OSA, such as upper airway collapsibility, loop gain, and arousal threshold. As a result, a single continuous pressure setting often results in either undertreatment or poor adherence. Espie et al. (2012) demonstrated that adaptive, automated algorithms can deliver personalized cognitive behavioral therapy for insomnia through fully automated digital platforms, with treatment regimens that progressively adjust to patient-reported sleep data. Adaptive algorithms in digital CBT-I platforms continuously adjust therapeutic regimens based on the patient's daily sleep diary entries and wearable-derived sleep metrics, if available. This addresses a core challenge in insomnia treatment: prescribed sleep windows must be progressively titrated as sleep efficiency improves, a process that traditionally requires weekly therapist contact. By automating this titration, these algorithms make the first-line treatment for chronic insomnia available at a larger scale despite the well-documented shortage of trained CBT-I therapists. There are advances due to AI-based systems in detecting or reducing effects of sleep disorders. However, challenges remain in deploying such systems to be used for diverse populations. Consistent validation of benefits compared to standard testing is still inconsistent. Requirements for patient security, such as data privacy, regulatory oversight, and clinical integration, need further development to ensure safe and effective deployment of AI-based systems.

SLEEP STAGING

Sleep is categorized in five stages including Wake, Stage 1, Stage 2, Stage 3, and Rapid Eye Movement (REM) sleep. Stages 1, 2, and 3 are collectively referred to as non-rapid eye movement (NREM) sleep. These stages are typically scored manually according to standardized criteria outlined in The Manual for the Scoring of Sleep and Associated Events, a modern scoring system that evolved from the Rechtschaffen and Kales framework (Sun et al., 2017). Despite this standardization of scoring, inter-rater variability persists when only one technologist performs the scoring test (Danker-Hopfe et al., 2009; Younes et al., 2018). EEG records cortical electrical activity used to perform polysomnographic sleep staging: theta activity marks NREM1, sleep spindles and K-complexes mark NREM2, delta waves mark

NREM3, and low-voltage mixed-frequency activity marks REM. Given manual EEG scoring represents the most time-intensive component of sleep study and the principal source of inter-rater variability, EEG is the signal modality where AI has produced the most direct clinical impact. Convolutional networks trained on millions of EEG epochs now match or exceed expert agreement, freeing technologists to focus on pathological events that still benefit from human review. Stage 1 (NREM1) represents light sleep, is characterized by theta activity on electroencephalogram (EEG), and accounts for approximately 5% of total sleep time. Stage 2 (NREM2), the longest stage, shows sleep spindles and K complexes, and accounts for about 45% of sleep time. Stage 3 (NREM3) represents deep sleep, characterized by delta waves, and accounts for roughly 25% of sleep time. Parasomnias, such as sleepwalking and night terrors, occur predominantly in NREM3. NREM3 durations are affected by substances including alcohol and sedatives, resulting in reduction of sleep time in this stage. About 25% of sleep time is in the REM sleep stage, which has also been associated with dreaming. Reduced REM latency is observed in narcolepsy, while REM-related behavior abnormalities are associated with neurodegenerative disorders such as Parkinson's Disease and Lewy Body Dementia. Artificial intelligence offers measurable improvements in sleep staging Danker-Hopfe et al. (2009) found that agreement across scorers is quantified using kappa statistics and the typical values range from 0.68 to 0.76. Younes and Hanly (2016) argued that AI models improve consistency by identifying attributes such as sleep spindles, K complexes, and delta wave activity. In addition, Patanaik et al. (2018) and Sun et al. (2017) concluded that large-scale datasets and deep learning approaches enhance classification accuracy and reduce scoring time of sleep staging. These systems with artificial intelligence models help sleep technologists and clinicians in standardizing sleep disorder classification by reducing subjective variability in the measurement due to human interpretation and errors, however testing and validation is required with diverse and broader populations with sleep disorders. Systems also need to be expanded to include the requirement for integration with clinical workflows.

RESPIRATORY EVENTS

Events within standardized scoring frameworks that incorporate airflow signals from nasal pressure transducers and thermistors are called respiratory events (Zou et al., 2025). Nasal pressure transducers measure the small pressure fluctuations at the nostrils caused by inspiration and expiration, while thermistors detect temperature changes from inhaled colder versus exhaled warmer air. Together they characterize airflow morphology with sufficient resolution to distinguish complete cessations, known as apneas, from partial reductions, known as hypopneas, and to differentiate obstructive from central events when interpreted alongside respiratory effort signals. These channels are the input substrate that AI respiratory-event detectors operate on, and recent neural networks have shown that even single-channel nasal pressure can be sufficient for accurate event scoring, opening the door to simplified home apnea testing (Zou et al., 2025). Understanding and analyzing such events are fundamental requirements for the diagnosis of sleep-disordered breathing. These events are manually scored by technologists and clinicians as a standard practice, though it is constrained by time demands and inter-scorer variability. Artificial intelligence systems have demonstrated usefulness in overcoming these limitations. Nikkonen et al. (2021) demonstrated that the neural network models using multimodal inputs, including oximetry and respiratory effort signals, have achieved substantial agreement with expert scorers, with kappa values approaching 0.73. Multimodal neural networks combine signals from different physiological modalities. For example, pulse oximetry tracks oxygen desaturations, while respiratory effort belts, around the chest and abdomen, detect paradoxical breathing, learning the patterns that distinguish obstructive from central apneas, true events from artifact, and clinically significant from incidental desaturations. This fusion is particularly important for sleep-disordered breathing because no single channel reliably captures every event type, with the kappa values approaching expert agreement reported in this paper reflecting the model's ability to cross-reference modalities at a level similar to an experienced human scorer. Additional studies by ElMoaqet et al. (2020) using deep recurrent neural networks have shown that even single-channel respiratory signals can support accurate event detection. Recurrent neural networks (RNNs), and their long short-term memory (LSTM) variants, are designed to model sequential data by maintaining an internal state that carries information forward across time steps. This makes them well suited to respiratory event detection because the diagnostic features of apneas and hypopneas are inherently temporal patterns rather than instantaneous waveform features. Achieving accurate detection from a single channel substantially simplifies home sleep apnea testing hardware and reduces patient burden, expanding screening reach to populations underserved by laboratory polysomnography. Biswal et al. (2018) showed that deep recurrent-convolutional neural networks trained on both in-laboratory and unattended home polysomnography (from the MGH and Sleep Heart Health Study datasets) can score sleep stages, apneic events, and limb movements at expert level. So far, there are limited improvements in terms of slight reductions in accuracy compared to in-laboratory polysomnography however the performance remains comparable to expert human scoring, indicating that additional research and development in AI based approaches will improve scalability and efficiency in diagnostic pathways for sleep-disordered breathing.

Central Disorders of Hypersomnolence

Lopez et al. (2017) reported that the central disorders of hypersomnolence present diagnostic challenges due to variability in testing conditions and limited reliability of repeated assessments. The diagnosis of narcolepsy heavily relies on the measurements such as REM latency and sleep-onset transitions, which are susceptible to external influences with traditional approaches. Stephansen et al. (2018) argued that AI-based approaches have shown promise in improving diagnostic precision. Liu et al. (2008) also demonstrated that the Neural network analyses incorporating sleep stage transitions and REM latency have enabled accurate classification of narcolepsy. This research consistently suggests that the additional AI models integrating electroencephalographic data and pupillometry have demonstrated insight into the diagnosis of narcolepsy compared with healthy controls, with such approaches providing objective and data-driven solutions to reduce diagnostic delay and variability.

Pupillometry measures pupil diameter and its fluctuations, which reflect autonomic arousal state and are abnormally unstable in narcolepsy due to dysregulation of wake-promoting hypocretin/orexin signaling. When AI models combine these autonomic signals with EEG features such as REM latency and sleep-onset transitions, they capture two complementary dimensions of the disorder, central nervous system instability and autonomic dysregulation, producing more reliable narcolepsy classifications than either modality alone. In this way, AI models reduce the diagnostic delays that patients routinely experience with central hypersomnolence.

SLEEP DISORDERS

REM-Sleep Behavior Disorder

REM Sleep Behavior Disorder is linked with an increased risk of neurodegenerative conditions such as Lewy Body Dementia, with the diagnosis requiring clinical history and electrophysiological evaluation to confirm the increased muscle tone during REM sleep. This confirmation process requires detailed inspection of electromyographic (EMG) signals, especially from submentalis and anterior tibialis leads, to identify tonic and phasic EMG activity (Goldstein et al., 2020). Submentalis EMG, placed under the chin, captures the postural muscle atonia that normally accompanies REM sleep, while anterior tibialis EMG, placed over the shin, captures leg movements relevant to PLMD. The diagnostic basis of REM Sleep Behavior Disorder rests on detecting the absence of expected REM atonia, which is a labor-intensive task across an entire night's worth of data. AI algorithms that quantify tonic and phasic EMG activity can screen lengthy recordings faster than manual review and, when combined with clinician oversight, can flag patients at elevated risk for synucleinopathies such as Parkinson's disease, Lewy body dementia. This is particularly important given these neurodegenerative diseases can have RBD as a possible prodromal symptom. Quantitative thresholds are not explicitly confirmed and are under refinement with additional data and research, however normative values have been proposed (Frauscher et al., 2012). Frauscher et al. (2014) confirmed that automated detection systems have demonstrated utility in identifying abnormal REM motor activity using algorithmic analysis of these signals. Additionally, integration of AI based system with manual review further improved results in terms of more specificity and reduced false positives. As a result, AI model-based tools could reduce manual burden and help with earlier identification of patients at risk for neurodegenerative disease with additional accuracy and efficiency.

Insomnia

Morin & Jarrin (2022) explained that insomnia is defined by persistent difficulty initiating or maintaining sleep, or early awakening, occurring at least three nights per week for at least three months, with associated functional impairment. Furthermore, statistics showed that chronic insomnia affects approximately 10 to 15% of adults, while transient symptoms occur in up to 30 to 35% of the adult population (Morin & Jarrin, 2022). First-line treatment for insomnia is cognitive behavioral therapy for insomnia (CBT-I), which targets maladaptive behaviors and cognitive distortions to reduce adverse effects of the disorder in patients. There are limited number of CBT-I trained therapists. As a result, AI-supported digital CBT-I platforms can be effective in improving efficiency and accuracy of both the diagnosis and management of chronic insomnia. These AI systems use machine learning models to modify interventions such as sleep restriction, stimulus control, and cognitive restructuring based on patient-reported data. Espie et al. (2019) have confirmed that randomized controlled trials have demonstrated significant improvements in insomnia severity and sleep latency, with outcomes comparable to therapist-delivered CBT-I.

AI has also been applied to understand and characterize the pathophysiology of insomnia. Perlis et al. (2022) reviewed evidence that insomnia involves hyperarousal phenotypes characterized by high-frequency EEG activity, autonomic dysregulation, and neuroendocrine markers such as elevated cortisol. These are features that machine learning approaches can use to detect disease severity through abnormalities in heart rate variability and sympathetic nervous system activation. These AI system-aided approaches complement symptom-based diagnosis and guide personalized treatment strategies. In addition, different sets of AI tools, such as large language models (LLM), are being researched to enhance patient engagement, symptom detection, and delivery of psychoeducation, however currently with limited clinical validation. LLMs are neural networks trained on vast text corpora that can generate fluent, context-aware natural language responses. In sleep medicine, they offer the potential to deliver psychoeducation about sleep hygiene, conduct conversational symptom screening, and provide between-session support for patients undergoing CBT-I, which are functions that traditionally require clinician time. Given insomnia and circadian disorders rely heavily on subjective symptom narratives, LLMs may be particularly suited to eliciting and structuring patient histories, though the paper notes appropriately that clinical validation remains preliminary and that hallucination and safety risks require careful oversight.

Obstructive Sleep Apnea: Endotyping, Phenotyping, and Treatment Optimization

Obstructive sleep apnea (OSA) is a disorder with many etiologies. Upper airway collapsibility, neuromuscular responsiveness and ventilatory control instability are some of the factors associated with OSA. The apnea-hypopnea index (AHI) is one of the conventional metrics for OSA. However, it can be ineffective in failing to foresee treatment response, symptom severity, or longstanding cardiovascular outcomes. Zinchuk, Gentry, Concato, and Yaggi (2017) argued that large-scale, multivariate datasets from polysomnography, physiological measurements, and clinical parameters can be integrated using AI. Such integration will result in more precise OSA endotyping. With the help of machine learning models, it is possible to identify separate OSA phenotypes with differing symptom profiles, comorbidities, and treatment responses. OSA endotyping refers to identifying the underlying physiological mechanism driving an individual's apnea, such as anatomical airway collapsibility, low arousal threshold, high loop gain, or poor neuromuscular compensation, with different potential therapies for each potential contribution. Machine learning models, such as clustering and supervised classifiers operating on multi-dimensional polysomnographic and clinical data, can uncover these subgroups in more detail compared to the traditional apnea-hypopnea index. This directly informs treatment selection. For example, anatomically driven OSA may favor surgical or mandibular advancement approaches, while high-loop-gain phenotypes may respond to oxygen therapy or specific pharmacologic agents, allowing the kind of precision medicine that this paper highlights. For example, patients with anatomical airway collapse may experience better outcomes with surgical interventions while the patients with high arousal thresholds may benefit from continuous positive airway pressure (CPAP) and pharmacotherapy. AI-driven phenotyping makes it possible to help patients with such individualized treatment strategies beyond conventional approaches.

It can be a major challenge to implement effective treatment plans with poor adherence to CPAP. Hanif et al. (2026) reported the application of AI tools for predicting and improving adherence by analyzing early patterns of usage, demographics, and symptoms. They reviewed AI-based predictive models showing strong performance during the first week of CPAP data, with several models achieving area under the curve (AUC) values exceeding 0.85 for long-term adherence prediction. Furthermore, deep analysis provides additional insights when CPAP devices with embedded sensors and telemonitoring with AI modeling are used for generating continuous data related to sleep data streams such as residual apnea-hypopnea index, mask leak, pressure settings, and usage duration. Modern CPAP machines record nightly residual apnea-hypopnea index, mask leak, pressure delivered, and usage hours, transmitting this data to cloud platforms via cellular or Wi-Fi connections. AI models can detect early markers of treatment failure such as rising residual events, escalating leaks, and shrinking nightly use in advance before patient report, allowing for more proactive intervention. Given CPAP adherence in the first month can be a meaningful predictor of long-term use, this early-warning capability is particularly impactful for patients with newly diagnosed OSA. AI-powered platforms can analyze this to detect clinically relevant irregularities and deviations such as positional OSA, mask leaks, or declining adherence. AI integration provides comprehensive views of treatment response with natural language processing allowing automated analysis of patient-reported symptoms. Jahrami et al. (2025) and De Zambotti et al. (2023) concluded that these approaches enhance precision medicine for OSA, improving clinical efficiency and data-driven intervention proactively.

Sleep-Related Movement Disorders

Two of the most prevalent sleep-related movement disorders are restless legs syndrome (RLS) and periodic limb movement disorder (PLMD). RLS is a neurological sensorimotor disorder characterized by an uncomfortable urge to move that typically worsens at rest, intensifies in the evening, and is relieved by movement. PLMD includes repetitive, stereotyped limb movements during sleep with a movement frequency threshold of five episodes per hour in children or fifteen per hour in adults. PLMD is scored manually via the anterior tibialis electromyogram (EMG) channel during polysomnography. Like challenges in sleep staging and respiratory event scoring, manual scoring of periodic limb movements is also a labor-intensive process prone to inter-rater variability.

Automated detection algorithms for PLMD have been developed using signal processing applied to EMG channels, with deep learning approaches recently demonstrating high accuracy. Carvelli et al. (2020) reported that a convolutional neural network trained on anterior tibialis EMG data achieved sensitivity and specificity exceeding 90% relative to expert manual scoring, effectively distinguishing true limb movements from artifacts. Convolutional neural networks (CNNs) detect local waveform shapes through learned filters that slide across the input signal, making them well suited to identifying the stereotyped, brief muscle bursts that characterize periodic limb movements. The reported >90% sensitivity and specificity by Carvelli et al. (2020) reflects the CNN's ability to distinguish true PLMs from common artifacts such as voluntary repositioning, blanket adjustments, or electrode noise which is a discrimination that previously required tedious manual review. Automated CNN-based PLM scoring across full nights also enables large-scale cohort studies linking PLMD to cardiovascular and neurodegenerative outcomes, which was previously prohibitive due to manual scoring time. In addition to improving accuracy, AI-enabled tools provide standardized scoring over entire study durations resulting in reduced variability from human scorers and enabling large-scale research with clinical associations across thousands of patients.

Natural language processing (NLP) functionality of AI systems have been applied to large electronic health record (EHR) datasets to analyze unstructured clinical notes and structured diagnostic codes for extracting possible RLS cases. Trenkwalder et al. (2016) argued that the RLS diagnosis are subjective, and it relies on the urge to move, worsening at rest, relief with movement, and circadian pattern. In addition, the NLP models can facilitate epidemiological studies, disease surveillance, and quality improvement initiatives in sleep medicine. NLP enables AI systems to parse unstructured text such as clinical notes, patient-reported symptom diaries, and survey responses, converting into structured data suitable for analysis. In sleep medicine this is especially valuable because conditions such as restless legs syndrome, insomnia, and circadian rhythm disorders are diagnosed largely by patient-reported phenomenology that can be difficult to capture in structured fields. Applying NLP to large EHR datasets can identify undiagnosed RLS and insomnia cases through descriptions in the documentation of outside providers, collecting symptom data across thousands of patients to support epidemiological research and quality improvement.

Future AI applications may include polysomnographic data as an input from the wearable devices and integrating these data with EHR. This workflow with effective analysis and interpretation can predict severity of RLS and effectiveness of treatment response, as well as identifying phenotypic subgroups that respond to specific approaches of interventions, such as pharmacologic or behavioral. Machine learning models could also detect subtle and temporal patterns in limb movement frequency or periodicity, correlating them with comorbidities beyond sleep disorders, such as cardiovascular disease, diabetes, and neurodegenerative conditions. Moreover, AI-driven tools can be embedded in home monitoring devices to provide continuous, real-time feedback for alerting patients or clinicians reporting any abnormal PLM activity, enhancing personalized therapy management and adherence. Overall, AI advancements promise major transformations in both clinical care and research in sleep-related movement disorders by improving efficiency, diagnostic accuracy, standardizing scoring, therapy personalization, and enabling large-scale longitudinal analyses.

Circadian Rhythm Sleep-Wake Disorders

Circadian rhythm sleep-wake disorders (CRSWDs) result from misalignment between the endogenous circadian clock and the desired sleep-wake schedule, due to extrinsic and intrinsic abnormalities within the circadian timing system. Delayed sleep-wake phase disorder, advanced sleep-wake phase disorder, non-24-hour sleep-wake rhythm disorder, shift work sleep disorder, and jet lag disorder are some of the common CRSWDs. Zhu and Zee (2012) reasoned that accurate diagnosis of these disorders remains challenging. This difficulty arises from the need for longitudinal assessment of sleep timing over days to weeks, reliance on subjective patient reports, and the absence of a single-night objective test comparable to polysomnography used in other sleep disorders.

Conventionally, actigraphy has served as the primary method for assessing circadian rhythms, offering continuous monitoring of rest and activity patterns over extended time periods, providing objective and threshold-based evaluation. Actigraphy uses a wrist-worn accelerometer to record movement continuously over days to weeks, with rest-activity patterns serving as a proxy for sleep-wake timing. This is a commonly used objective method for assessing circadian rhythm sleep-wake disorders given diagnosing conditions, such as delayed sleep-wake phase disorder or non-24-hour rhythm, requires longitudinal data that polysomnography cannot provide. When combined with machine learning, actigraphy outputs can identify circadian features such as inter-day stability, intra-day variability, and relative amplitude that correlate with melatonin onset and clock gene expression, supporting precise chronotherapy. Integration of machine learning algorithms with actigraphy provides significant advances over conventional threshold-based scoring, enabling extraction of nuanced circadian features such as inter-day stability and intra-day variability, as well as relative amplitude. In addition, AI models have further been correlated with peripheral clock gene expression to accurately validate circadian phase estimation. Depner et al. (2020) demonstrated that machine learning algorithms combining wrist actigraphy with photosensitive biomarkers has improved estimation of dim-light melatonin onset, which is considered the gold-standard circadian phase marker compared with traditional actigraphy methods.

The new generation of devices in consumer-grade wearables with photoplethysmography, accelerometers, and temperature sensors provides passive, long-term capture of sleep and physiological data at population scales that can be used by AI models to understand and interpret individual sleep cycles and traditional norms.

The combination of these three sensors captures complementary dimensions of sleep physiology. For example, PPG provides cardiac and autonomic information, accelerometry tracks movement and posture, and skin temperature reflecting core body temperature rhythms directly tied to circadian phase. Worn passively for months, these devices generate larger scale, longitudinal datasets needed to model normal sleep variation, identify circadian misalignment in shift workers and jet-lagged travelers, and link sleep patterns to comorbidities such as metabolic syndrome and mood disorders, normally more challenging with traditional testing. AI-driven analytics of these datasets provide actionable insights such as the identification of circadian misalignment patterns, with personalization of chronotherapy interventions, as well as epidemiological analysis of associated comorbidities including metabolic syndrome, mood disorders, and cancer. Trained machine learning models can optimize the timing of light therapy, melatonin administration, and behavioral interventions specific to personalized circadian profiles. Integration of natural language processing with various relevant data sources such as patient-reported outcomes and wearable data can further enhance prediction, detection, and monitoring of CRSWDs, enabling more precise circadian medicine. Jahrami et al. (2025) and De Zambotti et al. (2023) concluded that, due to the shift from population-based protocols, common treatments to individualized circadian management accuracy and compliance of treatment have improved.

Wearables

Laboratory polysomnography remains the most accurate test for majority of sleep disorders, particularly sleep-disordered breathing, parasomnias, and sleep-related movement disorders. This technique requires specialized equipment as well as the expertise of trained sleep technicians to administer the tests. Strassberger et al. (2023) demonstrated substantial night-to-night variability in polysomnography-derived physiologic traits in patients with moderate to severe OSA, supporting the need for multi-night recording to capture true disease severity. Actigraphy is often preferred for longitudinal assessment of sleep and wake pattern in more natural setting (Ancoli-Israel et al., 2003). These complex sets of prerequisites make laboratory-based methods less efficient and more cumbersome.

At the same time, modern technological innovations have expanded access to sleep-related data using sensors for measuring heart rate, photoplethysmography, heart rate variability, and skin temperature as a part of consumer wearables, with measurements able to be collected both in long-term and day-to-day settings. Most of these wearable devices rely on proprietary methods to estimate sleep stages which are obstacles to transparency and standardization efforts. Centralized artificial intelligence platforms can enable analysis of large-scale pattern and longitudinal phenotyping with more generalizable methods. De Zambotti et al. (2023) and Jahrami et al. (2025) proposed that the meeting clinical standards and method transparency are essential for credibility and clinical adoption. Oks et al. (2025) also recognized and emphasized the need for rigorous testing and quality assurance for integration into clinical workflows.

AI-DRIVEN INNOVATIONS IN SLEEP DISORDER MANAGEMENT

As we discussed so far, Artificial intelligence (AI) has rapidly expanded in providing effective and efficient approaches for addressing the needs of sleep medicine by offering new tactics in the engagement, diagnosis, treatment, and monitoring of patients. Sleep evaluation methods were mostly laboratory-based, with limitations being resource-intensive, prone to human error, and limited in scalability before wearables with AI integration. AI uses machine learning (ML) and deep learning (DL) techniques to analyze complex physiological data streams at scale resulting in better accuracy and efficiency, with continuous long-term monitoring and the support for personalized interventions. Recent studies conducted by Aziz et al. (2025) showed that AI applications can be superior compared to human performance in many areas of sleep medicine, however also noting challenges in generalizability, data quality, and clinical integration. A simple and clinically relevant common AI architecture for automated sleep diagnosis can be organized into sequential modules as shown in figure 1, where each module reflects how physiological signals are processed and translated into clinical outputs. The following sections discuss various AI-based model architectures for addressing specific sleep disorders discussed in earlier sections based on this common AI architecture.

Figure 1. Overview of architecture of AI based automated diagnosis for sleep disorders

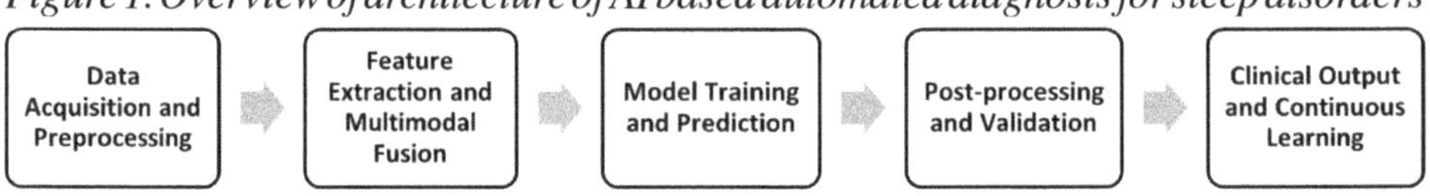

AI System Architecture for Automated Diagnosis

Similar to the architecture in Figure 1, a simplified AI framework for digital phenotyping in sleep medicine uses the same core layers. Goldstein et al. (2020) described the layered structure of AI systems used in sleep medicine, in which physiological data flow through acquisition, feature extraction, model training, and clinical output stages. However, each layer is adapted to process data specific to Automated Diagnosis.

Data Acquisition and Preprocessing

In this first layer, data related to physiological signals are collected from polysomnography or wearable devices. Type of data includes EEG, ECG, airflow, respiratory effort, and oximetry. These data are synchronized and segmented into standard epochs and processed for removal of artifact. To be prepared for analysis, data are normalized and transformed into time-series or time–frequency representations for AI model input.

Feature Extraction and Multimodal Fusion

Deep learning models extract meaningful trends and features from each data stream. Complex sets of data layers are identified for understanding local waveform and frequency patterns. While processing the data, temporal dependencies are conserved through a sequence-aware processing mechanism. Topographies from various sensory system data are further integrated into unified data streams for analysis across physiological systems.

Model Training and Prediction

Within AI System, labeled datasets with known sleep stages and respiratory events are used for training the supervised learning models. During the training phase, the model generates predictions for sleep stages, apnea–hypopnea events, and related abnormalities according to the acceptable confidence level. After initial training, optimization methods to improve accuracy and generalization across diverse datasets are used to fine tune the decision making for more scenarios and conditions.

Post-processing and Validation

Output from the previous phase is refined in the post processing layer of the AI system based on clinical practice rules, smoothing techniques, and pre-validated thresholds. This step ensures the physiological accuracy of the recommendations. During the internal validation phase results are evaluated against current diagnostic standards including manual scoring and metrics. Manual scoring for sleep diagnostics includes sensitivity, specificity, and agreement indices for external validation across independent data streams to ensure generalizability and clinical reliability.

Clinical Output and Continuous Learning

Final outputs from the AI-enabled sleep study systems include reports on sleep staging, apnea indices, and annotation of events of specific interest to integrate AI system into wider clinical workflows. Such reports are human interpretable to draw attention to relevant signal features to be used for clinician review. Any improvement opportunities are fed back to AI model for continuous learning updates. In addition, AI models are also trained continuously by feeding them new data regarding evolving patient populations.

AI System Architecture for Wearable-Based Screening and Digital Phenotyping

Similar to the architecture in Figure 1, a simplified AI framework for wearable-based screening uses the same core layers. Zhai et al. (2024) outlined how deep learning architectures are layered onto wearable sensor pipelines to translate raw signals into clinically interpretable sleep metrics. However, each layer is adapted to process data specific to wearable-based screening. Given wearables are mainly consumer products, the outputs from wearable-based systems are presented as clinically relevant with user-friendly metrics. For example, conditions such as obstructive sleep apnea scores related to estimated sleep duration, sleep efficiency, fragmentation indices to derive overall risk scores that can be shared with a physician to support clinical decision-making and guide further diagnostic evaluation. Wearables can be connected to the Internet through mobile applications. Connectivity enables possibility of conducting deep analysis using centralized AI tools, integrated dashboards, longitudinal monitoring, and remote clinical review. Data streams from ongoing wearable devices in use are continuously included into corrective or tuning feedback loops. These feedback loop mechanisms allow periodic model recalibration and performance improvement. AI-based individualized recalibration specifically uses individual variability to target improvement opportunities, while generalized improvement is based on device differences and evolving usage patterns as identified by Zhai et al. (2024).

Data Acquisition and Preprocessing

Wearable devices collect accelerometry, photoplethysmography, light exposure, heart rate, and respiratory pattern signals. This raw data is susceptible to real-world artifacts such as signal noise due to motion. Data are cleaned through filtering, normalization, and external noise removal. These data quality checks at the source ensure that only reliable data segments are used for downstream data analysis.

Feature Extraction and Multimodal Fusion

Physiological signals related to the heart rate, activity levels, and sleep fragmentation indices are derived from the cleaned signals. Wearables usually have many sensors and data streams captured from these multiple sensors, which can be combined to capture complementary aspects of sleep physiology. These combined data streams represent a more accurate and complete picture compared to individual sensor inputs.

Model Training and Prediction

Specialized versions of AI models, such as machine learning models including convolutional neural networks, random forests, or support vector machines, are trained on labeled datasets validated against polysomnography. Random forests build ensembles of decision trees and aggregate their predictions to produce robust classifications that resist overfitting, while support vector machines find optimal boundaries between classes in high-dimensional feature spaces. These traditional machine learning methods remain valuable in sleep applications where datasets are smaller, features are well understood (e.g., heart-rate variability metrics, actigraphy summary statistics), and interpretability matters more than raw accuracy. They are often the first models deployed in wearable-based screening, where computational constraints and the need to explain outputs to clinicians and patients favor simpler architectures over deep networks. These AI models are trained to recognize the patterns within sleep stages and sleep disorders data streams. They are also training to distinguish sleep disturbance patterns that can identify significant events related to circadian misalignment and signs of relapse. Once trained, AI systems can alert clinician teams with predictions and recommendations based on sleep duration, fragmentation, and apnea events.

Post-processing and Validation

Post processing and validation are performed for data streams related to photoplethysmography, accelerometry, and peripheral oxygen saturation that originate from wearables. This sub-system of AI uses temporal smoothing and rule-based corrections to ensure physiological consistency. It also corrects wearable device-specific anomalies to account for variability in sensor quality, skin contact, and signal dropout. Finally, the wearable device-based AI model output is validated for sensitivity, specificity, and confidence using polysomnography and similar clinically annotated metrics. Measurements are recalibrated for wider population usage irrespective of the hardware and software platforms. Threshold specific adjustments are also made using established standards and regulatory requirements for confirming accuracy.

Clinical Output and Continuous Learning

Clinical outputs from this layer of the system include sleep efficiency, disturbance indices, and risk scores, presented as metrics for ease of use. Clinical outputs are also integrated into clinical systems and mobile platforms for periodic monitoring. Feedback loops are used for redirecting the AI system for continuous AI model improvement as new data becomes available or inaccuracies are found.

This simplified AI architecture for wearable based screening and digital phenotyping provides new functionalities in terms of continuous long-term monitoring and actionable insights while minimizing operational complexity.

Clinical Decision Support

AI-enabled clinical decision support systems are integrated with electronic health records (EHRs) systems to identify hidden trends. Oks et al. (2025) emphasized that AI-based clinical decision support tools should integrate with EHR data and PAP device output to assist sleep specialists rather than replace clinical judgment. Such systems aid sleep specialists to assist in making more effective clinical decisions. These EHR systems use ML-derived recommendations in treatment planning, including optimization of positive airway pressure (PAP) therapy titration. For example, AI models examine usage patterns and deviations from PAP devices to recommend exact interventions to care teams. AI-driven decision support systems improve narcolepsy management by identifying sleep-onset REM episodes that are hard to recognize with human efforts. In addition, ML models can modify treatment approaches by considering sleep metrics, comorbid conditions, and patient-reported outcomes. However, the implementation of these systems requires careful architecture of AI systems including user interfaces, internal decision-making algorithms, and integration with existing clinical workflows. SHAP (Shapley Additive Explanations) is one of the explainable AI (xAI) methods typically used in AI implementation to make overall systems clinician-friendly, transparent and trustworthy which helps drive the adoption of typical AI-enabled clinical decision support architecture (Lundberg & Lee, 2017). SHAP assigns each input feature a numerical contribution to a model's prediction, drawing on game-theoretic principles to attribute importance fairly across correlated features. In sleep medicine this matters because clinicians cannot act on a black-box recommendation that an AI flags a patient as high risk for CPAP non-adherence or as having an unusual sleep-stage distribution. They need to know which signals (e.g., early-week usage hours, mask leak, baseline AHI) drove the prediction. xAI methods such as SHAP, attention visualization, and saliency mapping make AI outputs auditable, support clinician trust, and are increasingly required by regulatory frameworks such as the FDA's Software as a Medical Device guidance.

Data Acquisition and Preprocessing

Initial data for clinical decision support systems are acquired from electronic health records, polysomnography, PAP devices, and patient-reported outcomes. These datasets include demographics, medical comorbidities, medication use, sleep metrics, and PAP adherence patterns in many different formats. Datasets may be subjective in nature that require additional preprocessing. Preprocessing involves data synchronization, handling missing values, normalization, and alignment of records received from multiple sources.

Feature Extraction and Multimodal Fusion

In this layer of AI systems, clinical and physiological data related to apnea/hypopnea indices, PAP usage, sleep metrics, and comorbidity profiles are identified and categorized. Sub-systems also extract the patterns of behavior and long-term changes in symptoms. These data related to various behavioral interests are combined to represent the interactions between clinical variables (cause) and sleep data (effect).

Model Training and Prediction

Machine learning models are trained on pre-labeled data for decision making. Pre-labeled data include PAP non-adherence, treatment response, and diagnostic patterns. AI models use supervised learning for performing data analysis and produce targeted recommendations as well as sequential recommendations.

Post-processing and Validation

Predicted recommendations are further refined using regulatory and clinical regulations to ensure compliance, as well as accuracy, calibration, and clinical utility. External validation is performed using publicly available datasets from regulatory and research bodies to ensure generalizability.

Clinical Output and Continuous Learning

Outputs are presented as recommended treatments, risk scores, and alerts for high-risk patients. AI-based systems provide information as clinical output with reasoning and support using xAI. Sub-systems provision continuous learning by providing access to external data sources for new patient data, treatment options, and clinical practices to improve accuracy and personalization.

Behavioral Interventions

One of the most refined AI applications in behavioral sleep medicine are digital cognitive behavioral therapy for insomnia (dCBT-I) platforms. These platforms use adaptive AI algorithms to customize therapy related to techniques and pace based on inputs from patient provided sleep diary and behavioral patterns. Bai et al. (2024) performed a meta-analysis of digital CBT interventions and concluded that the dCBT-I produces clinically meaningful improvements in sleep onset latency, sleep quality, and insomnia severity, with comparable effect sizes to clinician-delivered CBT in selected populations. These findings highlight the promise of AI-based tools to reduce barriers including the constraints of therapist availability and geographic access. AI-based behavioral intervention systems use real-time sensor data to personalize recommendations related to the optimal sleep timing, stimulus control approaches, and relaxation exercises. Hybrid AI behavioral intervention models provide recommendations for therapy size and focus areas based on individual self-reported symptoms, data from wearable systems, behavioral responses, and patient engagement patterns. More research is needed to explore the effectiveness and efficiency of these AI-enhanced behavioral tools compared to traditional therapy in various conditions and population types. Our proposed AI-based behavioral intervention system architecture includes subsystems that look like following:

Data Acquisition and Preprocessing

One of the main sources of data acquisition for behavioral intervention AI systems are collected from patients such as their observational notes, symptom questionnaires, session data, and change patterns. Additional inputs may include automated and wearable machine collected sleep times, durations, activity levels, and heart rate variation data. Collected data are standardized to create consistent profiles of sleep behavior and treatment plans.

Feature Extraction and Multimodal Fusion

This layer of AI systems extracts key features from patterns in the data related to sleep onset latency, wake after sleep onset, sleep efficiency, and deviations from prescribed behavioral strategies. This layer also quantifies the observations related to the frequency of platform use and intervention response. These features and observations are combined with physiological data from wearables to provide comprehensive insight of patient behavior and treatment response.

Model Training and Prediction

In this layer of AI system, machine learning models are trained to identify patterns associated with optimal intervention strategies as input and treatment response as output. ML algorithms use therapy approach, pace, and intensity to determine personalized individual progress and engagement. Predictive models identify potential for suboptimal response or risk of dropout to recommend the early strategy adjustments.

Post-processing and Validation

In this sublayer of AI systems, AI model outputs are refined using clinically recognized behavioral therapy principles. Validation is performed against clinical results related to insomnia severity and sleep quality. Accuracy of the AI system is measured using provisional and sustained positive patient impact.

Clinical Output and Continuous Learning

Personalized therapy recommendations, measurable progress, and feedback on sleep patterns are examples of clinical outputs delivered at this layer of the AI platforms. Patients receive recommendations on sleep scheduling, stimulus control, and relaxation techniques. Finally, continuous learning sub-layers update recommendations based on ongoing patient data, allowing dynamic adjustment of therapy to improve adherence, effectiveness, and long-term outcomes.

Remote Monitoring

Typically, AI systems have back-end processing units that can be hosted in the cloud. Cloud portions of AI systems leverage the access to advanced AI capabilities, massive data processing power and storage needed for larger scale data analysis. Cloud platforms provide large-scale storage for large amounts of data continuously from thousands of distributed CPAP machines, wearables, and homc monitors. This architecture can make population-level remote monitoring more accessible, given a centralized AI back end can simultaneously analyze nightly streams from multiple patients, flag anomalies in real time, integrate updates to model weights as new training data accumulates, and deliver alerts to clinicians through dashboards or EHR integrations. Without cloud infrastructure, the longitudinal, scalable monitoring this paper describes for OSA, insomnia, and circadian disorders would not be operationally practical. As a result, back-end AI portions of the system can be used as AI-enabled remote monitoring platforms. Back-end AI systems aggregate continuous data streams from many sources to detect the smallest level of treatment deviations, sleep disturbances, and physiological anomalies. Remote monitoring AI models can flag even the smallest elevation of residual apnea indices, mask leak, or decreases in usage. As a result, immediate alerts to clinical teams can facilitate more timely interventions. In this way, remote monitoring AI tools extend care beyond regular clinic visits, potentially adding to the telemedicine model (Sparrow et al., 2010; Zou et al., 2025).

Remote monitoring AI tools track long term sleep metrics that could predict medical conditions beyond sleep disorders such as cardiovascular or metabolic dysfunction. Predictive analytics from remote monitoring AI can allow clinicians to identify at-risk patients proactively and adjust treatment plans. Additionally, AI functionalities such as advanced natural language processing (NLP) can capture patient-reported symptom data in many different languages to improve the overall quality of clinical care.

Methods for Underpinning AI Models

AI-enabled applications in sleep medicine leverage a range of computational methods as previously discussed in various AI architecture, based on supervised learning approaches to ensure human oversight continues during development.

Deep learning architecture, such as CNNs and recurrent neural networks (RNNs), are another type of AI implementation that can be widely used in medical AI applications. Medical data can be high volume and complex in nature, with deep learning techniques effective in examining patterns in complex time-series data. Deep learning of multidimensional approaches combines physiological and behavioral datasets to provide more accurate predictions.

One of the newer additions in medical AI applications is explainable AI methods (xAI). Doshi-Velez and Kim (2017) argued that interpretable machine learning is essential for clinical adoption, requiring transparency at each layer of the decision-making process. Medical diagnosis requires a high degree of transparency and clinician interpretability of the AI decision making processes at each layer. xAI can be used with supervised and deep learning models to provide oversight from clinicians, external observers, and regulators.

LIMITATIONS AND CHALLENGES

AI systems for sleep disorders promise efficiency and effectiveness, however there are still limitations for use in routine clinical practice.

Given that collecting data from vast data sources requires a great deal of technological infrastructure, AI systems tend to be more prevalent in developed countries. This can result in dataset bias and limited generalizability. Available input datasets may not reflect broader patient demographics.

Technological advancements have advanced at a rapid rate, which can result in sensor variability and data quality variations from wearables. As a result, this can limit the quality of analysis, with impacts on AI model performance.

Given AI development has occurred at a rapid pace, regulatory bodies around the world have varying levels of oversight and formal regulatory frameworks.

Medical records and data have strict security requirements, with continuous physiologic monitoring from wearables representing challenges in adhering to established security standards.

Birrer et al. (2024) considered many of these limitations and proposed that additional validation efforts, data management practices, and transparent regulatory standards are essential to ensure safe and unbiased deployment of AI technologies in sleep medicine.

ETHICAL CONSIDERATIONS, LIMITATIONS, AND IMPLEMENTATION CHALLENGES

Several ethical, technical, and practical limitations require careful consideration before widespread deployment of AI systems in sleep medicine.

Unintentional algorithmic bias represents an important ethical concern. Many AI models are trained on datasets derived from academic sleep laboratories or developed economies that could overrepresent specific demographic groups, with less reliable performance in underrepresented geographic and demographic groups. Sjoding et al. (2020) and Obermeyer et al. (2019) reasoned that proactive mitigation is needed by implementing diversified training datasets, continuous bias monitoring, and fairness tuning.

AI model operation may not be readily interpretable, which can be challenging for clinicians. Deep learning systems provide high predictive accuracy however their complexity can limit clinician understanding of their decision-making process. Doshi-Velez and Kim (2017) studied and concluded that explainable AI (XAI) methods can provide post-hoc interpretations with attention mechanisms, saliency mapping, and SHAP value analysis, improving transparency and trust in clinical settings.

AI is trained in sensitive physiologic values, wearable device data, and patient information. This can be stored, transmitted, and processed at many different locations, which represents significant data privacy and security concerns. Rieke et al. (2020) concluded that federated learning approaches without sharing raw patient information could represent a method for protecting patient privacy during AI model development while still providing training data diversity. Federated learning trains a single AI model across multiple institutions by sending model updates instead of raw patient data to a central coordinator, allowing each site's data to remain behind its institutional firewall. This is particularly relevant to sleep medicine because polysomnographic recordings, wearable streams, and EHR data are subject to HIPAA, GDPR, and similar protections, and because no single sleep center has a sufficiently diverse dataset to train models that generalize across age, sex, race, body habitus, and comorbidity profiles. Federated learning therefore directly addresses two challenges this paper raises: privacy and dataset bias.

There are efforts to address many of these ethical considerations and limitations. Oks et al. (2025) explained that the American Academy of Sleep Medicine stressed that AI should supplement, rather than replace, clinician decisions using continuous performance monitoring under clinician supervision. Regulatory oversight, such as the U.S. Food and Drug Administration's (FDA) Software as a Medical Device (SaMD) framework is working on addressing these challenges to ensure AI tools meet safety and efficacy standards before clinical use.

SUMMARY

Artificial intelligence (AI) has initiated measurable changes in sleep medicine for diagnosis, monitoring, and treatment strategies, expanding the field with advancements in automated analysis, wearable-based screening, digital phenotyping, and decision-support systems. These developments have improved efficiency and analysis of complex physiological sleep data. At the same time, AI also enabled the possibility of scalable individualized care strategies, on a level that has been previously difficult to implement.

Traditional sleep diagnostics rely heavily on polysomnography, which requires manual scoring of multiple physiologic channels. This process is time intensive with the potential for inter-rater variability, which AI-based systems can improve. Jahrami et al. (2025) concluded that convolutional and recurrent neural networks have been trained on large polysomnographic datasets to classify sleep stages and identify respiratory events with human level expertise, reducing inconsistencies and shortening analysis time. Zhang et al. (2022) further reported that deep learning models demonstrate high sensitivity and specificity for sleep staging and apnea detection when supplied with electroencephalographic, electrocardiographic, and respiratory data for analysis and interpretation.

Wearable technologies extend patient access to medical data outside of traditional clinical settings. They collect continuous data streams related to photoplethysmography, accelerometry, and heart rate. AI systems can use these data streams to assess sleep duration, fragmentation, and respiratory disturbances. Birrer et al. (2024) summarized that wearable device-based screening models showed acceptable level of detection capabilities when compared with polysomnographic standards. De Zambotti et al. (2023) emphasized that long term data collected using wearable devices capture periodic rhythm disruption and behavioral changes associated with insomnia and neurobehavioral impairment. Despite these benefits, inconsistencies in sensors and data quality are still challenges that need to be further addressed. In addition, widespread clinical adoption requires endorsement across diverse populations.

AI-enabled clinical decision support systems utilize electronic health records with sleep metrics to develop more effective therapy plans. As per Hanif et al. (2026) and Aziz et al. (2025), AI system predictive models can identify patients at risk of nonadherence to treatment plans, allowing for early and targeted interventions. AI-based remote monitoring systems further allow for care beyond the boundaries of traditional clinic settings to enhance telemedicine capabilities. Natural language processing methods can incorporate multilingual patient-reported symptoms resulting in more effective assessments.

Behavioral sleep medicine has also benefited from AI integration, used to deliver digital cognitive behavioral therapy for insomnia based on patient input and engagement patterns. Bai et al. (2024) found that randomized trials improved insomnia severity and sleep onset latency. AI platforms for behavioral interventions provide evidence-based care in settings with limited specialist availability. Integration with wearables for data collections further personalizes behavioral recommendations.

Several challenges include algorithmic bias from a lack of diverse populations in AI-model training and variability of wearable data. Sjoding et al. (2020) showed that photoplethysmography-based oximetry may be less accurate in individuals with darker skin tones, leading to data inaccuracies. There needs to be more work to obtain diverse datasets to address systematic bias of established datasets.

Interpretability also limits clinical adoption since many AI systems with deep learning models can provide challenges in trusting recommendations from a process that not all clinicians fully understand. However, Doshi-Vclcz and Kim (2017) suggested that explainable AI methods can improve transparency of deep learning systems. Regulations are also addressing these concerns with additional requirements for AI-based medical software related to validation, transparency, and oversight.

Data privacy remains a critical consideration, as AI systems depend on large volumes of sensitive health information that must comply with established regulatory standards such as HIPAA and GDPR. Federated learning offers one approach to preserve privacy while enabling model development across distributed datasets. This approach avoids central data storage and supports broader collaboration.

Oks et al. (2025) argued that clinical judgment requires physician oversight, with the American Academy of Sleep Medicine recommending that AI tools assist rather than replace clinicians.

Overall, AI-based systems in sleep medicine have enhanced diagnostic precision, expanded healthcare reach, and augmented sleep disorder management. However, integration of AI system into routine sleep medicine practice depends on vigilant quality assurance, ethical safeguards, and applicability within clinical workflows to continue shaping the future of medical applications.

FUTURE DIRECTIONS

Progress with AI usage in sleep medicine will depend on the conjunction of physiological data stream analysis, digital phenotyping outputs, and emerging genetic markers to offer more precise characterization of sleep disorders (Jahrami et al., 2025).

Another possible future direction is development of models that are both interpretable and unbiased to strengthen assurance and safety in real-world settings. As these AI systems move closer to routine care, their design must reflect not only technical superiority but also impartiality across populations.

Sustained progress requires coordinated efforts across multiple domains, with clinicians, data scientists, ethicists, and regulatory bodies collaborating to shape standards and guidelines for quality assurance, deployment, and oversight. These partnerships are necessary to ensure that advances in artificial intelligence translate into measurable benefits while maintaining ethical and clinical integrity.

REFERENCES

Ancoli-Israel, S., Cole, R., Alessi, C., Chambers, M., Moorcroft, W., & Pollak, C. P. (2003). The role of actigraphy in the study of sleep and circadian rhythms. *Sleep, 26*(3), 342–392. DOI: 10.1093/sleep/26.3.342 PMID: 12749557

Aziz, S., Ali, A. A. M., & Aslam, H.. (2025). Wearable artificial intelligence for sleep disorders: Scoping review. *Journal of Medical Internet Research, 27*, e65272. DOI: 10.2196/65272 PMID: 40327852

Bai, N., Cao, J., Zhang, H., Liu, X., & Yin, M. (2024). Digital cognitive behavioural therapy for patients with insomnia and depression: A systematic review and meta-analysis. *Journal of Psychiatric and Mental Health Nursing, 31*(4), 654–667. DOI: 10.1111/jpm.13024 PMID: 38226714

Baron, K. G., Duffecy, J., Berendsen, M. A., Cheung Mason, I., Lattie, E. G., & Manalo, N. C. (2018). Feeling validated yet? A scoping review of the use of consumer-targeted wearable and mobile technology to measure and improve sleep. *Sleep Medicine Reviews, 40*, 151–159. DOI: 10.1016/j.smrv.2017.12.002 PMID: 29395985

Bhatt, A., Sengupta, S., Abolhassani, A., Brower, D., Forehand, C., Keats, K., Kwon, Y., & Healy, W. J. (2025). Awakening sleep medicine: The transformative role of artificial intelligence in sleep health. *Current Sleep Medicine Reports, 11*(1), 13. Advance online publication. DOI: 10.1007/s40675-025-00328-w

Birrer, V., Elgendi, M., Lambercy, O., Giggins, O. M., & Penders, J. (2024). Evaluating reliability in wearable devices for sleep staging. npj. *Digital Medicine, 7*(1), 74. DOI: 10.1038/s41746-024-01016-9 PMID: 38499793

Biswal, S., Sun, H., Goparaju, B., Westover, M. B., Sun, J., & Bianchi, M. T. (2018). Expert-level sleep scoring with deep neural networks. *Journal of the American Medical Informatics Association : JAMIA, 25*(12), 1643–1650. DOI: 10.1093/jamia/ocy131 PMID: 30445569

Carvelli, L., Olesen, A. N., Brink-Kjær, A., Leary, E. B., Peppard, P. E., Mignot, E., Sørensen, H. B. D., & Jennum, P. (2020). Design of a deep learning model for automatic scoring of periodic and non-periodic leg movements during sleep validated against multiple human experts. *Sleep Medicine, 69*, 109–119. DOI: 10.1016/j.sleep.2019.12.032 PMID: 32062037

Danker-Hopfe, H., Anderer, P., Zeitlhofer, J., Boeck, M., Dorn, H., Gruber, G., Heller, E., Loretz, E., Moser, D., Parapatics, S., Saletu, B., Schmidt, A., & Dorffner, G. (2009). Interrater reliability for sleep scoring according to the Rechtschaffen & Kales and the new AASM standard. *Journal of Sleep Research, 18*(1), 74–84. DOI: 10.1111/j.1365-2869.2008.00700.x PMID: 19250176

De Zambotti, M., Goldstein, C., Cook, J. D., Menghini, L., Altini, M., Cheng, P., & Robillard, R. (2023). State of the science and recommendations for using wearable technology in sleep and circadian research. *Sleep (Basel), 47*(4), zsad325. Advance online publication. DOI: 10.1093/sleep/zsad325 PMID: 38149978

Demrozi, F., Borzì, L., & Olmo, G. (2023). Wearable sensors for supporting diagnosis, prognosis, and monitoring of neurodegenerative diseases. *Electronics (Basel), 12*(6), 1269. DOI: 10.3390/electronics12061269

Depner, C. M., Cheng, P. C., Devine, J. K., Khosla, S., De Zambotti, M., Robillard, R., Vakulin, A., & Drummond, S. P. A. (2020). Wearable technologies for developing sleep and circadian biomarkers: A summary of workshop discussions. *Sleep (Basel), 43*(2), zsz254. Advance online publication. DOI: 10.1093/sleep/zsz254 PMID: 31641776

Doshi-Velez, F., & Kim, B. (2017). Towards a rigorous science of interpretable machine learning. arXiv preprint arXiv:1702.08608. https://arxiv.org/abs/1702.08608

ElMoaqet, H., Eid, M., Glos, M., Ryalat, M., & Penzel, T. (2020, September 4). *Deep recurrent neural networks for automatic detection of sleep apnea from single channel respiration signals*. MDPI. https://www.mdpi.com/1424-8220/20/18/5037

Espie, C. A., Emsley, R., Kyle, S. D., Gordon, C., Drake, C. L., Siriwardena, A. N., Cape, J., Ong, J. C., Sheaves, B., Foster, R., Freeman, D., Costa-Font, J., Marsden, A., & Luik, A. I. (2019). Effect of digital cognitive behavioral therapy for insomnia on health, psychological well-being, and sleep-related quality of life: A randomized clinical trial. *JAMA Psychiatry, 76*(1), 21–30. DOI: 10.1001/jamapsychiatry.2018.2745 PMID: 30264137

Espie, C. A., Kyle, S. D., Williams, C., Ong, J. C., Douglas, N. J., Hames, P., & Brown, J. S. (2012). A randomized, placebo-controlled trial of online cognitive behavioral therapy for chronic insomnia disorder delivered via an automated media-rich web application. *Sleep (Basel), 35*(6), 769–781. DOI: 10.5665/sleep.1872 PMID: 22654196

Frauscher, B., Gabelia, D., Biermayr, M., Stefani, A., Hackner, H., Mitterling, T., Poewe, W., & Högl, B. (2014). Validation of an integrated software for the detection of rapid eye movement sleep behavior disorder. *Sleep (Basel)*, *37*(10), 1663–1671. DOI: 10.5665/sleep.4076 PMID: 25197814

Frauscher, B., Iranzo, A., Gaig, C., Gschliesser, V., Guaita, M., Raffelseder, V., Ehrmann, L., Sola, N., Salamero, M., Tolosa, E., Poewe, W., Santamaria, J., & Högl, B. (2012). Normative EMG values during REM sleep for the diagnosis of REM sleep behavior disorder. *Sleep (Basel)*, *35*(6), 835–847. DOI: 10.5665/sleep.1886 PMID: 22654203

Goldstein, C., Berry, R. B., Kent, D. T., Kristo, D. A., Seixas, A., Redline, S., & Westover, M. B. (2020). Artificial intelligence in sleep medicine: Background and implications for clinicians. *Journal of Clinical Sleep Medicine : JCSM : Official Publication of the American Academy of Sleep Medicine*, *16*(4), 609–618. DOI: 10.5664/jcsm.8388 PMID: 32065113

Gottlieb, D. J., & Punjabi, N. M. (2020). Diagnosis and management of obstructive sleep apnea. *Journal of the American Medical Association*, *323*(14), 1389–1400. DOI: 10.1001/jama.2020.3514 PMID: 32286648

Hanif, U., Vitrac, J., Marinho, P., Jennum, P., Gozal, D., Mignot, E., & Elbaz, M. (2026). Rethinking CPAP adherence with artificial intelligence. *Sleep (Basel)*, •••, zsag097. Advance online publication. DOI: 10.1093/sleep/zsag097 PMID: 41947377

Jahrami, H., Husain, W., Trabelsi, K., Penzel, T., Hirshkowitz, M., Razjouyan, J., BaHammam, A. S., & Sharafkhaneh, A. (2025). Artificial intelligence and sleep medicine II: A scoping review of applications, advancements, and future directions. *Sleep Medicine Reviews*, *85*, 102212. DOI: 10.1016/j.smrv.2025.102212 PMID: 41330180

Liu, D., Pang, Z., & Lloyd, S. (2008). A neural network method for detection of obstructive sleep apnea and narcolepsy based on pupil size and EEG. *IEEE Transactions on Neural Networks*, *19*(2), 308–318. DOI: 10.1109/TNN.2007.908634 PMID: 18269961

Lopez, R., Doukkali, A., Barateau, L., Evangelista, E., Chenini, S., Jaussent, I., & Dauvilliers, Y. (2017). Test-retest reliability of the multiple sleep latency test in central disorders of hypersomnolence. *Sleep (Basel)*, *40*(12), zsx164. Advance online publication. DOI: 10.1093/sleep/zsx164 PMID: 29099966

Lundberg, S. M., & Lee, S.-I. (2017). A unified approach to interpreting model predictions. *Advances in Neural Information Processing Systems*, *30*, 4765–4774.

Morin, C. M., & Jarrin, D. C. (2022). Epidemiology of insomnia: Prevalence, course, risk factors, and public health burden. *Sleep Medicine Clinics*, *17*(2), 173–191. DOI: 10.1016/j.jsmc.2022.03.003 PMID: 35659072

Nikkonen, S., Korkalainen, H., Leino, A., Myllymaa, S., Duce, B., Leppänen, T., & Toyras, J. (2021). Automatic respiratory event scoring in obstructive sleep apnea using a long short-term memory neural network. *IEEE Journal of Biomedical and Health Informatics*, *25*(8), 2917–2927. DOI: 10.1109/JBHI.2021.3064694 PMID: 33687851

Obermeyer, Z., Powers, B., Vogeli, C., & Mullainathan, S. (2019). Dissecting racial bias in an algorithm used to manage the health of populations. *Science*, *366*(6464), 447–453. DOI: 10.1126/science.aax2342 PMID: 31649194

Oks, M., Sachdeva, R., Davenport, M., Husain, A. M., Kalra, M., Krishnan, V., Le, T., Parekh, A. A., Park, H., Prasad, B., Ryals, S. M., Zia, S., Anastasi, M., Shelgikar, A. V., Abbasi-Feinberg, F., Abreu, A. R., Bandyopadhyay, A., Gurubhagavatula, I., Kapur, V. K., & Wickwire, E. M. (2025). Artificial intelligence in sleep medicine: An updated American Academy of Sleep Medicine position statement. *Journal of Clinical Sleep Medicine : JCSM : Official Publication of the American Academy of Sleep Medicine*, *21*(11), 1953–1962. DOI: 10.5664/jcsm.11832 PMID: 40742116

Patanaik, A., Ong, J. L., Gooley, J. J., Ancoli-Israel, S., & Chee, M. W. L. (2018). An end-to-end framework for real-time automatic sleep stage classification. *Sleep (Basel)*, *41*(5). Advance online publication. DOI: 10.1093/sleep/zsy041 PMID: 29590492

Perlis, M. L., Posner, D., Riemann, D., Bastien, C. H., Teel, J., & Thase, M. (2022). Insomnia. *Lancet*, *400*(10357), 1047–1060. DOI: 10.1016/S0140-6736(22)00879-0 PMID: 36115372

Rieke, N., Hancox, J., Li, W., Milletarì, F., Roth, H. R., Albarqouni, S., Bakas, S., Galtier, M. N., Landman, B. A., Maier-Hein, K., Ourselin, S., Sheller, M., Summers, R. M., Trask, A., Xu, D., Baust, M., & Cardoso, M. J. (2020). The future of digital health with federated learning. *NPJ Digital Medicine*, *3*(1), 119. DOI: 10.1038/s41746-020-00323-1 PMID: 33015372

Sjoding, M. W., Dickson, R. P., Iwashyna, T. J., Gay, S. E., & Valley, T. S. (2020). Racial bias in pulse oximetry measurement. *The New England Journal of Medicine*, *383*(25), 2477–2478. DOI: 10.1056/NEJMc2029240 PMID: 33326721

Sparrow, D., Aloia, M., Demolles, D. A., & Gottlieb, D. J. (2010). A telemedicine intervention to improve adherence to continuous positive airway pressure: A randomised controlled trial. *Thorax*, *65*(12), 1061–1066. DOI: 10.1136/thx.2009.133215 PMID: 20880872

Stephansen, J. B., Olesen, A. N., Olsen, M., Ambati, A., Leary, E. B., Moore, H. E., Carrillo, O., Lin, L., Han, F., Yan, H., Sun, Y. L., Dauvilliers, Y., Scholz, S., Barateau, L., Hogl, B., Stefani, A., Hong, S. C., Kim, T. W., Pizza, F., & Mignot, E. (2018). Neural network analysis of sleep stages enables efficient diagnosis of narcolepsy. *Nature Communications*, *9*(1), 5229. DOI: 10.1038/s41467-018-07229-3 PMID: 30523329

Strassberger, C., Hedner, J., Sands, S. A., Tolbert, T. M., Taranto-Montemurro, L., Marciniak, A., Zou, D., & Grote, L. (2023). Night-to-night variability of PSG-derived physiological endotypic traits in patients with moderate to severe Obstructive Sleep Apnea. *Chest*. Advance online publication. DOI: 10.1016/j.chest.2022.12.029 PMID: 36610664

Sun, H., Jia, J., Goparaju, B., Huang, G. B., Sourina, O., Bianchi, M. T., & Westover, M. B. (2017). Large-scale automated sleep staging. *Sleep (Basel)*, *40*(10), zsx139. Advance online publication. DOI: 10.1093/sleep/zsx139 PMID: 29029305

Trenkwalder, C., Allen, R., Béné Harbé, E., Bhatt, D., Bhattacharyya, A., & Bhattacharyya, B.. (2016). Restless legs syndrome associated with major diseases. *Neurology*, *86*(14), 1336–1343. DOI: 10.1212/WNL.0000000000002542 PMID: 26944272

Wickwire, E. M., & Collop, N. A. (2010). Insomnia and sleep-related breathing disorders. *Chest*, *137*(6), 1449–1463. DOI: 10.1378/chest.09-1485 PMID: 20525657

Younes, M., & Hanly, P. J. (2016). Minimizing interrater variability in staging sleep by use of computer-derived features. *Journal of Clinical Sleep Medicine : JCSM : Official Publication of the American Academy of Sleep Medicine*, *12*(10), 1347–1356. DOI: 10.5664/jcsm.6186 PMID: 27448418

Younes, M., Kuna, S. T., Pack, A. I., Walsh, J. K., Kushida, C. A., Staley, B., & Pien, G. W. (2018). Reliability of the American Academy of Sleep Medicine rules for assessing sleep depth in clinical practice. *Journal of Clinical Sleep Medicine : JCSM : Official Publication of the American Academy of Sleep Medicine*, *14*(2), 205–213. DOI: 10.5664/jcsm.6934 PMID: 29351821

Zhai, B., Elder, G. J., & Godfrey, A. (2024). Challenges and opportunities of deep learning for wearable-based objective sleep assessment. npj. *Digital Medicine*, *7*(1), 85. DOI: 10.1038/s41746-024-01086-9 PMID: 38575794

Zhang, C., Yu, W., Li, Y., Sun, H., Zhang, Y., & De Vos, M. (2022). CMS2-Net: Semi-supervised sleep staging for diverse obstructive sleep apnea severity. *IEEE Journal of Biomedical and Health Informatics*, *26*(7), 3447–3457. DOI: 10.1109/JBHI.2022.3156585 PMID: 35255000

Zhu, L., & Zee, P. C. (2012). Circadian rhythm sleep disorders. *Neurologic Clinics*, *30*(4), 1167–1191. DOI: 10.1016/j.ncl.2012.08.011 PMID: 23099133

Zinchuk, A. V., Gentry, M. J., Concato, J., & Yaggi, H. K. (2017). Phenotypes in obstructive sleep apnea: A definition, examples and evolution of approaches. *Sleep Medicine Reviews*, *35*, 113–123. DOI: 10.1016/j.smrv.2016.10.002 PMID: 27815038

Zou, D., Lisik, D., Bailly, S., & Verbraecken, J. (2025). Redefining telemedicine in obstructive sleep apnea management through artificial intelligence. *Frontiers in Sleep*, *4*, 1678077. DOI: 10.3389/frsle.2025.1678077 PMID: 41425184

Chapter 3
Artificial Intelligence in Pulmonary Infectious Diseases:
Pneumonia Diagnosis, Tuberculosis Diagnosis, and Antimicrobial Resistance Prediction

Milind Chunkhare
http://orcid.org/0000-0001-9299-2075
Symbiosis International (Deemed to be) University, India

Bhageswar Madire
Symbiosis International (Deemed to be) University, India

Vaishnavi Deshmukh
Symbiosis International (Deemed to be) University, India

ABSTRACT

This chapter explores the transformative role of artificial intelligence (AI) in the diagnosis, management, and prognosis of pulmonary infectious diseases, which continue to be a major global health burden. Diseases such as pneumonia, tuberculosis, COVID-19, and drug-resistant infections present persistent challenges, including delayed diagnosis, limited access to expert interpretation, and rising antimicrobial resistance. AI, particularly through machine learning and deep learning techniques, offers innovative solutions to address these challenges by enabling faster, more accurate, and data-driven clinical decision-making.

DOI: 10.4018/979-8-3373-7759-9.ch003

1. INTRODUCTION

Infectious diseases are one of the primary causes of illness and death worldwide(Michaud, 2009). Consider it as pneumonia, which people are contracting in their communities, to tuberculosis, which is difficult to cure with medicine, to the flu, which recurs annually, and viral infection outbreaks that affect the lungs. Our bodies combat all types of germs in the lung. Although we have come a long way in making medicines that are capable of combating infection, understanding what kind of germs are causing people to be sick, and taking care of people who are very sick, there are still many things that doctors need to combat. These issues include the failure to diagnose diseases due to uncertainty about the nature of the disease, leading to prescribing medicine without absolute certainty about the problem, and the increasing prevalence of germs resistant to available medicines. These are not mere problems. They imply that people must remain in the hospital longer than they need to, somebody loses that they should not need to, and that we are being deprived slowly of the medicines we have been depending on all along to make people well(Rosenfeld et al., 1957).It is due to these issues that artificial intelligence is increasingly being employed in clinics(*Revolutionizing Healthcare: The Role of Artificial Intelligence in Clinical Practice | BMC Medical Education | Springer Nature Link*, n.d.).

Artificial intelligence is not potentially a thing that could be in the future it is the present and it is assisting us. We have become much more skillful in the last two decades at using computers to screen large volumes of data, and we have achieved significant progress in what is known as machine learning. This implies that we can develop computer models that can identify patterns in diseases that people cannot perceive and will be able to predict how the patient will go before it happens and recommend a treatment that is individualized to that particular patient. Education where artificial intelligence meets lung infection is an advancing field in medicine.

In this chapter, we examine the manner in which artificial intelligence is being utilized in a bid to assist us with all kinds of lung infections. We will start with pneumonia, which has been studied the most using artificial intelligence. We then discuss tuberculosis, which is a major problem worldwide and requires new tools that can help diagnose tuberculosis, particularly in localities that lack many resources. This time, we will look at the utilization of artificial intelligence during the COVID-19 pandemic, which not only proved that artificial intelligence could be just as effective in the real world but also accelerated its further advancement(Vaishya et al., 2020). Finally, we will consider how machine learning can assist us in combating germs that are resistant to medicines, which will be a huge challenge in the future. In this chapter, we will consider both what can and cannot be done with the help of artificial intelligence in medicine and highlight what doctors, researchers, and health systems should know when they begin using these new technologies.

2. PNEUMONIA DETECTION AND SEVERITY PREDICTION

Figure 1. Schematic representation of AI-based pneumonia detection and severity prediction using clinical and imaging data

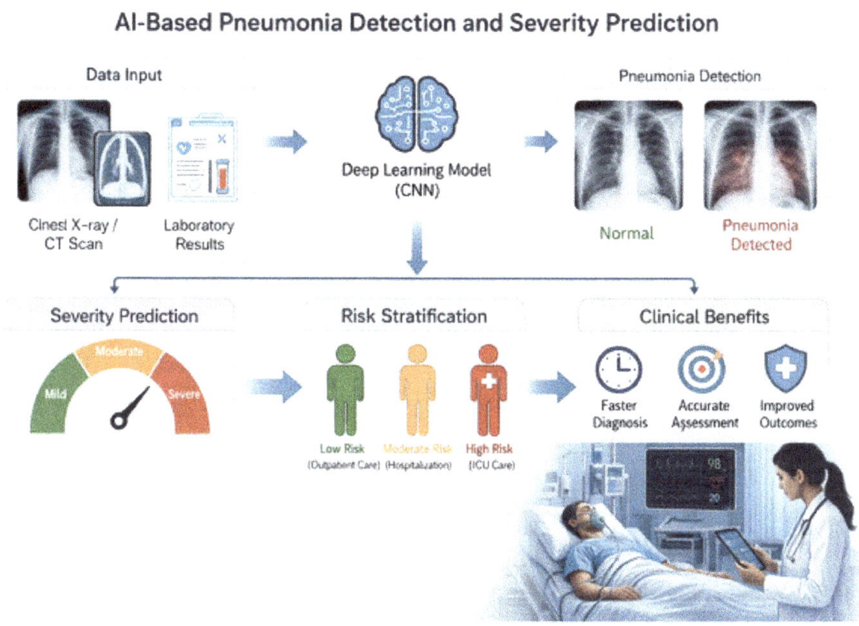

2.1. The Diagnostic Challenge of Pneumonia

Pneumonia is an infection in the lungs. It is extremely poor with children below the age of five years. Many adults and immunodeficient individuals are forced to visit the hospital due to pneumonia(Vaishya et al., 2020). Doctors have a time diagnosing pneumonia. Such symptoms may also manifest themselves in such conditions as heart issues or blood clots. That makes it tough for doctors to figure out what's wrong, with the patient(*Integrative Physiology of Pneumonia | Physiological Reviews | American Physiological Society*, n.d.).

Doctors usually start by taking a chest X-ray. Chest X-rays are easy to do and not too expensive. They are helpful. Not all the time the picture is clear. The doctor may not have a lot of experience. This may result in errors. Diagnosing pneumonia early. Correctly is very important for reducing the number of people who get sick around the world especially among children under five years old. Pneumonia is a reason why many people in this group die. It is hard to tell if someone has pneumonia or something else like fluid in the lungs or lung cancer just by looking at pictures of their lungs(*Integrative Physiology of Pneumonia | Physiological Reviews | American Physiological Society*, n.d.).

To make diagnosis easier researchers are using computer programs called deep learning architectures like modified convolutional neural networks to help doctors tell the difference between pneumonia and other diseases. Some of these programs like CheXNet are very good at looking at pictures of lungs. Can even do better than human doctors at diagnosing problems(Rajpurkar et al., 2017a).

Pictures of the lungs in CT scans are taken. They are able to detect issues that are missed with X-rays. The ct scans are costly and harmful in the use of radiation. They are not readily available(Sluimer et al., 2006).

The other issue is to determine what has caused the pneumonia. Physicians tend to commence treatment without having the certainty since lab results take time. This may make people use antibiotics even without need due to the same.

These problems can have consequences. Patients may not get the treatment. The excessive use of antibiotics may cause them to be weakened. Worse of treatment, in case of delayed or incorrect treatment of the pneumonia. It may even result in death. Therefore, enhanced diagnosis and treatment of pneumonia is very crucial(*American Thoracic Society Journals*, n.d.).

However these programs do not work well when they are used in places that do not have a lot of resources like some hospitals in countries. This is because the machines that take pictures of lungs can be different and that can make it hard for the programs to work correctly. To fix this problem researchers are working on programs that can adapt to machines and pictures using things like transfer learning and special attention mechanisms.

It is also important to be able to tell what kind of pneumonia someone has like if it's caused by a virus, bacteria or fungus so that doctors can give the right treatment. Researchers are working on programs that can do this. They are also trying to automate the process of writing reports about patients conditions. They are using scoring systems like CO-RADS to measure how sick someones lungs are(Penha et al., 2021).

This information can help doctors decide who needs to be treated away and who is likely to get sicker. Researchers are also trying to combine types of computer programs like CNN and Transformer to get more information from pictures of lungs and to be able to segment or separate the parts of the lung that are infected even when there are not many pictures to look at(Khan et al., 2023).

Pneumonia diagnosis is getting better with these computer programs and pneumonia diagnosis is very important, for reducing the number of people who get sick around the world. Pneumonia diagnosis is critical for doctors to be able to give the treatment to patients.

2.2. AI-Based Imaging Interpretation

Pneumonia diagnosis and treatment have recently begun to have assistance of artificial intelligence or AI. AI systems have the potential to analyze images also such as the chest X-rays and CT scans known to be accurate.

These systems are trained picture-wise and thus, identify patterns which are associated with pneumonia like regions in the lungs. An example is Chex Net, a learning model that can even detect pneumonia on a chest X-ray, and better than experienced doctors(Rajpurkar et al., 2017b).

In hospitals AI tools are being used to help doctors. They are able to fasten-track X-rays. Highlight areas that might be infected. This can assist physicians to allocate more importance to patients and speed up diagnosis. This particularly comes in handy in emergency departments or even in specialist regions.

The severity of the pneumonia can also be determined with the help of AI. This is done by examining to what extent of the affected AI systems of the lung can be used to determine the amount of care that a particular patient requires. This involves making decisions on whether or not one should be admitted to the hospital(Ebrahimian et al., 2021).

Figure 2. Comparison between human interpretation and AI-assisted analysis of chest X-ray for pneumonia detection

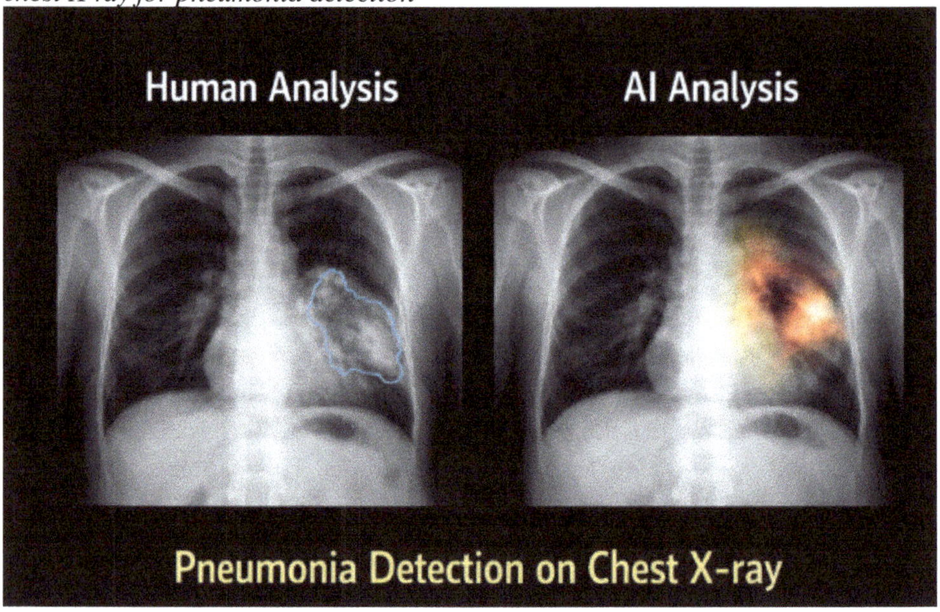

Source: Author-generated illustration based on AI-assisted imaging concepts.

AI is also being used with CT scans. It can aid in distinguishing between pneumonia and others. This can assist doctors to select the treatment and prevent unnecessary usage of antibiotics.

Doctors can use AI to assist them, rather than to replace them. Properly applied it can yield more accurate diagnoses, speed up efficiency and result in patient outcomes, with pneumonia.

AI-based interpretation of medical imaging will change the way modern radiologists will use today's technology to interpret complex medical imaging performed on different body parts, by utilizing a very precise digital assistant to help radiologists interpret these complex images that they will have to review. Today's advanced computer vision technologies, combined with advanced deep learning algorithms, make it possible for advanced computer systems to interpret complex diagnostic data (MRIs, CTs, X-rays, etc.) in an incredibly fast and accurate manner compared to the traditional way these types of complex images are interpreted(Rutsch et al., 2023). The intelligent algorithms used by the advanced computer system are not intended to displace human expertise, but instead are very good at detecting subtle changes in the structure of the body, detecting fine pathology and detecting micro-anomalies that the average exhausted radiologist would have trouble detecting. The above mentioned type of technology helps eliminate a number of tedious, time-consuming tasks that radiologists would typically perform prior to interpreting the final report and therefore alleviates the risk of diagnostic errors; enhances the speed at which a radiologist can complete his/her work; and allows the radiologist to concentrate on making the final diagnosis and providing quality direct patient care.

2.3. The Severity Prediction and ICU Triage

pneumonia is diagnosed, it's important to quickly figure out how bad it is. This is just as important as finding out they have pneumonia in the place. Systems that aid physicians in determining the severity of pneumonia are available such as the Pneumonia Severity Index and CURB-65(Jones et al., 2011; Parsonage et al., 2009). However these systems are not perfect. They will just only look at a things and not consider how such things interact with one another. They have been based also on information of patients in the past and this may not apply to patients nowadays.

An algorithm has been created to further predict the severity of pneumonia using machine learning. These models are based on various variables such as laboratory test results, vital signs, medical history and other health issues. They can even utilize the pictures of imaging tests. This will enable doctors know which patients are at risk and require to be in the intensive care unit. Certain machine learning programs such as gradient boosting algorithms, random forests and deep neural networks can extremely effectively predict which patients will require treatment(Krauss et al., 2017; Nhat-Duc & Van-Duc, 2023).

Early warning systems at hospitals are one of the potential applications of artificial intelligence. Such systems are an ongoing supervision of patients. Refreshing their risk scores when new information is available. This has the capability of assisting physicians to identify issues earlier, and preventing their escalation. Research has indicated that these systems have the potential to cause a decrease in the amount of transfers to the intensive care unit, decrease in-hospital deaths, and help in a better timing of relevant treatments.

The utilization of artificial intelligence (AI) in the field of respiratory medicine provides one of the greatest advantages for determining patients who will experience rapid deterioration leading to the need for intensive care. For example, AI models may have the ability to analyze results from clinical assessment, laboratory/diagnostic test results, and scan imaging results more quickly than standard bedside scoring systems permit, particularly in instances where patients present with severe pneumonia or other pulmonary -related infectious processes(*JMIR Bioinformatics and Biotechnology - Use of Artificial Intelligence in the Search for New Information Through Routine Laboratory Tests: Systematic Review*, n.d.; Lennerz et al., 2023). Therefore, this technology can provide an opportunity for the early stratification of at-risk patients, especially in those hospital settings where the need to make timely, life-saving decisions regarding ICU placements is essential due to overwhelming patient census. However, evidence supporting AI as an adjunct to clinician decision-making is much stronger than evidence supporting the use of AI as a means of replacing the clinician; therefore; clinicians should utilize existing AI models as a tool to aid decision-making until there is more definitive evidence supporting the use of AI independently, as studies indicate that most current models still lack generalizability, transparency, and external validation across the different healthcare settings.

3. AI IN TUBERCULOSIS DIAGNOSIS AND SCREENING

3.1. For a long time, tuberculosis has been a disease that spreads easily.

Although there have been good treatments more than sixty years, it remains a tremendous health concern across the globe. A lot of people are still killed by tuberculosis(Huang et al., 2022). The problem of tuberculosis is related to public health(Nguyen et al., 2026).

People all over the world are affected by the disease. In 2022, it claimed over a million and a half and infected ten million residents. The majority of them reside in the middle-income countries where it is difficult to diagnose tuberculosis. Doctors and laboratories are not available to test the disease as many people are not diagnosed in time(Qin et al., 2021).

The most prevalent method of screening with regards to tuberculosis is by use of a chest X-ray. One will however need a lot of expertise to interpret these X-rays. This knowledge is not common in other regions of the world. A community health worker or a nurse in an area cannot tell whether a person is at risk or not at a glance of their X-rays whether or not a person has tuberculosis. This is where AI can come in. In regions with limited doctors, AI can be used to analyze the X-rays of the chest and identify the presence of tuberculosis. This could be an important tool in the fight, against tuberculosis.

Figure 3. Chest X-ray demonstrating AI-identified features of pulmonary tuberculosis such as cavitary lesions and infiltrates

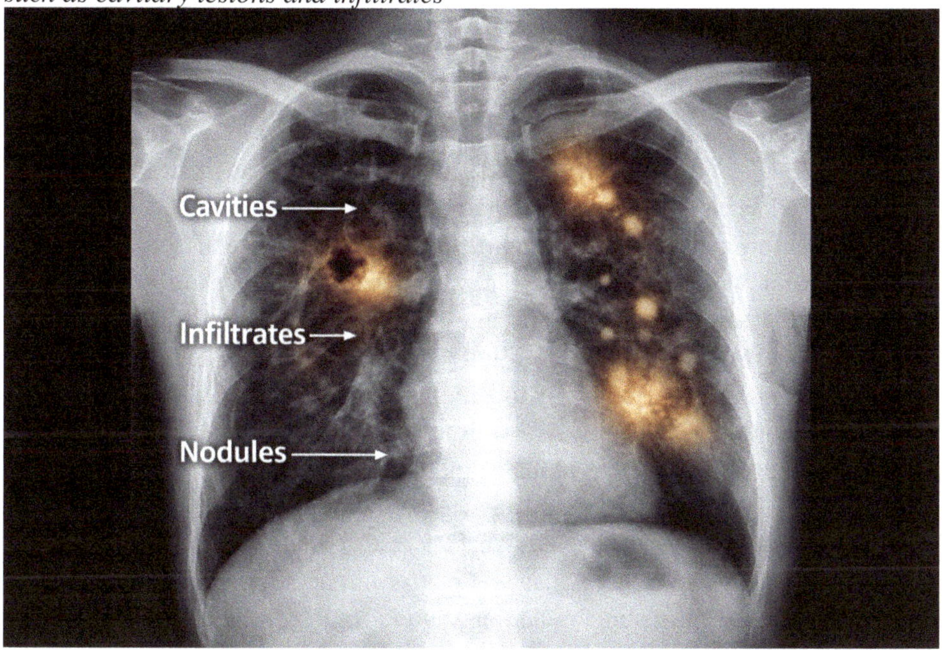

Source: Author-generated illustration based on typical radiographic features described in the literature.

Since tuberculosis (TB) is transmitted through the air and is typically found in poorly-resourced settings, it has been a major public health challenge for decades. Artificial intelligence (AI) is revolutionizing this by making TB screening more rapid, scalable, and accessible worldwide. A new way for health systems to use artificial intelligence is to use it to identify and prioritize high-risk patients for screening, and to assist in the diagnosis of TB patients in under-resourced areas, so that effective treatment for TB patients can be administered as soon as possible. In addition, because the transmission of TB is ongoing, the timing from exposure to diagnosis is critical to stopping the ongoing transmission of the disease in high-burden countries. Nevertheless, experts continue to emphasize that the best use of AI tools is in conjunction with local evaluation and as part of an overall diagnostic strategy rather than as a sole-source solution for diagnosing TB(Hwang et al., 2024; *Application of Artificial Intelligence in Diagnosis of Pulmonary Tuberculosis | Chinese Medical Journal*, n.d.).

3.2. AI-Powered Chest Radiograph Analysis for Tuberculosis

Tuberculosis can now be detected by using AI platforms, which can help interpret chest radiographs. Such sites CAD4TB, (Fehr et al., 2023)have been prototype tested in nations and have demonstrated success(Codlin et al., 2025; *Computer Aided Detection of Tuberculosis on Chest Radiographs: An Evaluation of the CAD4TB v6 System | Scientific Reports*, n.d.). They can detect tuberculosis in the chest radiographies as well as better or even else, than human readers.

These platforms have been utilized through research of thousands of patients in Africa, Asia and Latin America. These studies have been the result of. They demonstrate that such AI solutions are quite effective in the detection of tuberculosis.

In 2021, the World Health Organization stated that these AI systems can be implemented by human readers to inspect tuberculosis screening on the chest radiograph using AI. This was a win as it was first time when the World Health Organization officially claimed that the help in managing tuberculosis should be provided with the help of AI tool(Organization, 2024).

This decision was made by the World Health Organization since, as it was evidenced by numerous studies, these AI platforms can be used to recognize individuals who require the testing, including sputum testing or molecular diagnostics. This has the potential to aid identification of tuberculosis in large screening programmes(Bouderhem, 2022).

AI chest radiography analysis could not only tell whether the film was abnormal or not. It can create a report which declares how probable it is that the individual has tuberculosis, where the issue of how bad it is. It is also able to detect issues including fluid in the lungs or ruptured lung.

It can even come up with a list of causes of the problem which can guide the doctors in other cases. This is quite useful in the areas where the individual viewing the radiograph lacks information on the patient and cannot easily discuss with a doctor each case.

Chest X-ray analysis with AI has established itself as a practical step forward for tuberculosis (TB) screening. Today's computer-aided detection (CAD) systems can assess digital chest X-rays, assign a score of abnormality, and help identify individuals needing to have further testing done to confirm TB disease. This is particularly useful for sites with limited numbers of radiologists. At these remote locations, it is possible for AI to provide consistent triaging help to treat more patients in a shorter amount of time. The most recent studies show that many of these CAD systems have a high level of sensitivity; therefore, they have the potential to minimize the number of cases that are missed, while simultaneously decreasing the number of unnecessary confirmatory tests. However, there are no global thresholds that work across all patients, and the performance of the system may become less accurate when used with older individuals, those infected with HIV, or individuals with a history of prior TB. Therefore, it is critical to have a local calibration in place.

3.3. Molecular Diagnostics and AI

AI is not being applied in picture-looking only. It is also applied to aid in comprehending diagnostic information on tuberculosis. By viewing the genome of the tuberculosis bacteria, do a fair amount of discovery about which drugs it resists... To interpret such information, we require special computer programs.

It is possible to consider machine learning models that analyze databases of genomic information and identify the mutations that enable the bacteria to become drug resistant. This will provide us a list of which drugs the bacteria is resistant to using a single sputum sample and we will be able to get the list within two days.

This strategy has been. It is much quicker than the old method of operation that was extremely time consuming. It is currently in operation in national reference laboratories of countries where tuberculosis is a significant issue.

There is even the use of AI in assisting in microscopy a method of examining samples with equal aid under a microscope. Even though microscopy is facing the risk of being taken over by diagnostics, in most regions it remains the primary method of diagnosing tuberculosis in certain regions.

This can be aided by AI by analyzing slides and counting the bacteria. This implies that we do not require an individual to carry out this task and this may be done in areas that lack many lab technicians.

Introducing AI to help with contact tracing and screening is also being utilized. It is able to plan on areas where tuberculosis is likely spreading by analyzing where they are already happening, where people are traveling and other parameters. Where to concentrate screening efforts can be determined with the use of this information. The approach may allow detecting cases of tuberculosis and lower the screening cost.

The use of Artificial Intelligence (AI) coupled with molecular diagnostics is transforming how we treat TB, creating new possibilities in patient care. Presently, the existence of relatively rapid nucleic acid tests like Xpert MTB/RIF, line probe assays (LPAs), and newer genome sequencing methodologies allows for considerable time savings in the detection of M. TB and their mutation profiles, which are characteristics associated with drug resistance through traditional culture techniques. With the assistance of AI to assist with interpreting complex molecular pathways, identifying drug resistance signatures, and making decisions in the context of larger genomic datasets, we can expect that the application of AI will further enhance the capabilities of molecular diagnostic tools in the future and help clinicians establish appropriate treatment more promptly and confidently than ever before. Thus, AI will increase the clinical utility of molecular diagnostic testing.

4. THE FUNCTION OF AI IN COVID-19: IMAGING ANALYTICS, PROGNOSIS, AND PRIORITIZATION

4.1. AI as a Quick-Reaction Instrument in a Changing Epidemic

The COVID-19 epidemic led to the need to have rapid diagnostic and prognostic methods. A large number of patients with a new disease overcame healthcare systems all over the world during the months of 2020. Back then physicians were inexperienced with this disease and there were no effective instruments to be used to determine who was a high-risk patient. The researchers of Artificial Intelligence made rush attempts to implement their techniques in the vast number of COVID-19 data that was being obtained. The Artificial Intelligence systems that were in place were put to test by the pandemic. Provided us with lessons that will guide us to utilise and apply Artificial Intelligence tools in healthcare over the long run.

In the area of diagnosis Artificial Intelligence models that could detect COVID-19 pneumonia from chest CT and chest radiograph images were among the Artificial Intelligence applications to get a lot of attention. In 2020, many research groups released models that were able to detect COVID-19 pneumonia with high accuracy. These models could identify the trends of the images that are most characteristic of COVID-19 pneumonia. During the first outbreak some of these models were deployed in hospitals, and it was able to make the process of interpreting the images less time-consuming (from hours down to seconds). This enabled the doctors to commence treatment and isolation measures in a shorter time.

Nevertheless, even the COVID-19 pandemic indicated that there are some issues with the development of the Artificial Intelligence models. An examination of more than 200 Artificial Intelligence models created to diagnose and prognose COVID-19 revealed that the majority of them had certain shortcomings. These shortcomings consisted of utilizing the data that was not representative of the world having inadequate data and failure to test the models according to the standards. Not even many models were tested to determine whether they had a practical use in a clinical context. This served as a call to action of the discipline of Artificial Intelligence in healthcare. It gave rise to the attempts to establish more efficient criteria to design and assess Artificial Intelligence models.

When an epidemic is evolving, AI can become a rapid-response tool because speed is just as important as accuracy. AI-driven epidemic intelligence systems can conduct real-time scans of both structured and unstructured data sources (e.g., clinical reports, search behavior, news updates, and social media) to connect these disparate signals and enable earlier detection of abnormal disease activity, better forecasting of outbreaks, and faster triage planning in hospitals and emergency departments whenever a respiratory infection spreads rapidly throughout communities. Although these types of systems must still be closely supervised and have high-quality data input, they could represent a significant improvement in moving public health from a reactive mode of control to a proactive mode of prevention.

4.2. Prognostic Models for Disease Severity and Mortality

The COVID-19 pandemic has shown that artificial intelligence could be composed to forecast those who are most likely to get very sick or die. This is due to the fact that COVID-19 can produce a variety of symptoms, from minor to severe. Doctors needed tools to identify the patients who were at risk and those who could be treated at home. The ancient risk factors were age, diabetes, and heart disease, among others, and obesity. They could not be sufficient to enable predictions(Piccialli et al., 2021).

The combination of clinical, laboratory and imaging data, used as artificial intelligence models, was developed and tested. In these models it was established that there were a few laboratory tests that were very good predictors of the patients who were at risk; these included: C-reactive protein and D-dimer. An analysis of imaging data, such as CT scans, of imaging data using an artificial intelligence was also highly helpful. The percentage of lung involvement which can be measured using Artificial Intelligence was a predictor of which patients would need to be admitted to the intensive care unit.

There were some of the models that had been developed during the pandemic that were highly effective in predicting the patients who would fall so ill. Some hospitals used these models to assist doctors when deciding on patients to admit to the care unit and the ones that can be treated at home. This was to ensure that the care that the patients required was made available and it helped save lives. Artificial Intelligence has contributed to the response to the COVID-19 pandemic and it will remain a central part of healthcare, in the long-term.

Predictive models using artificial intelligence can be used to evaluate the severity of disease and risk of death in a patient. In TB patients, the predictive model uses imaging, clinical data, and sometimes microbiological data to identify patients who are at higher risk and may need to be monitored more closely or may need more aggressive treatment. New research has shown that AI determined measurements of imaging/in radiographic findings related to the extent of disease can predict success of treatment as well as predict whether or not the patient will quickly convert from positive to negative cultures; therefore, imaging has the ability to provide more than simply diagnosing disease. However, many AI-based predictive algorithms still have significant biases relating to the datasets from which they were derived, so while the promise of artificial intelligence being implemented in predictive algorithms exist, it is imperative that these algorithms be developed and improved prior to their routine use in clinical practice.

4.3. AI in Drug Repurposing and Treatment Response Monitoring

AI assisted in identifying applications of the available drugs and enhancing the response to COVID-19. Natural language processing tools were used to go through the large amount of research on SARS-CoV-2. This aided in finding solutions using the available medicines by correlating their established impacts with the novel realization of the virus mechanism. This did not result in the use of this treatment but helped researchers to narrow down to the most promising ones. It also informed important clinical trials.There was also the use of AI in monitoring the effectiveness of treatments in hospitalized patients. The CT scans given to the doctors would give an accurate idea of the extent to which the lungs were damaged by the virus in the long term by analyzing them using AI tools(*Applications of Artificial Intelligence in Drug Repurposing - Wan - 2025 - Advanced Science - Wiley Online Library*, n.d.).

This gave an accurate measure of response to treatment as opposed to clinical judgment. The use of AI-based imaging analysis provided a more objective and reliable measure of outcomes in trials of new therapies.This methodological benefit does not just apply to COVID-19. The pandemic led to the creation of a scale of clinical data that continues to be employed in creating AI models. Models trained and validated on the large clusters of patients that are gathered when the pandemic strikes have been applied to the COVID-19 pandemic and other respiratory infections. The amount of data available for current AI research has increased due to the quick uptake of telemedicine, digital health monitoring, and health records.

Artificial intelligence is transforming how tuberculosis (TB) patients are processed on their way through the TB treatment continuum. In research, it assists researchers in finding new applications for previously established medicines for TB, as well as tracking treatment response over time. For TB, re-purposing medicines for TB is advantageous because it is expensive and time-consuming to create new medications, and resistance to current medications is rapidly growing. AI has the ability to analyze large amounts of chemical and biological data to identify existing TB medications or predictors of immune function improvement in people with TB. In the clinical area, predicting outcomes of TB treatment (used to determine an individual patient's treatment success) and determining how closely an individual patient adhered to the prescribed treatment are two examples of how AI can assist in tracking TB treatment progress. By utilizing AI to provide treatment progress data across multiple points in the treatment process, rather than through limited and fixed-tracked progress measurements, TB patients receive more real-time and patient-centered care throughout the TB treatment continuum.

5. PREDICTIVE MODELS FOR ANTIMICROBIAL RESISTANCE IN PULMONARY INFECTIONS

5.1. The Respiratory Medicine Crisis of Antimicrobial Resistance

The use of predictive models for anti-microbial resistant organisms is growing in importance in patients with pulmonary infection. These models allow medical practitioners to make better decision making based on clinical criteria prior to receiving full laboratory susceptibility testing results. By utilizing past treatment history, electronic patient records, microbiological data, and demographic characteristics, machine learning algorithms are able to predict the probability of pathogen resistance to different classes of antibiotics. This improvement in antibiotic stewardship, the reduction of delays to appropriate therapy initiation and the potential to decrease the mortality associated with serious lung infections. However, these predictive models will only be successful if the underlying data is of good quality. If the data used for building the models contains inaccurate or missing information, or if there are discrepancies between the laboratory or hospital systems the predictive models are based on, their predictive ability will be adversely affected. Therefore, until local validation and clinical implementation of these models are performed across geographic regions, caution should be used(Guitor & Wright, 2018).

One of the threats to global health is resistance. Medicine is one of the areas where the situation is critical. Mortality rates of resistant bacteria resulting in hospital-acquired and ventilator-associated pneumonias in some intensive care units are higher than 50 percent. Pneumonias that are a result of drug use complicate the treatment of otherwise curable diseases. The emergence of M which is resistant to the fluoroquinolone. It can result in tuberculosis strains that can make the treatment regimens less successful.

The largest hurdle is time: results of microbiological culture require 48 to 72 hours to be obtained. Clinicians have to make therapeutic judgments in the absence of knowledge during this period. Treatment failure, increasing resistance, and needless exposure to broad-spectrum drugs might result from treatment that is not customized to the patient's needs.

5.2. Machine Learning for Resistance Prediction

The AI solutions to antimicrobial resistance work at two tiers: predicting resistance in individual patients and at the population level mobility. At individual level, models are based on microbiological and epidemiological characteristics to approximate the risk of infection with resistant organisms. Such models are based on the exposure to antibiotics, prior hospitalization and underlying immunosuppression. Research has revealed that machine learning algorithms are able to forecast antibiotic resistance with precision that can be valuable in clinical settings(*Machine Learning for Antimicrobial Resistance Prediction: Current Practice, Limitations, and Clinical Perspective | Clinical Microbiology Reviews*, n.d.).

For hospital-acquired pneumonia models have achieved levels of accuracy in predicting carbapenem-resistant Gram-negative infection. The models of community-acquired pneumonia have provided subgroups of patients that are vulnerable of infection by drug-resistant bacteria. The way forward of resistance prediction is genomic AI strategies(Sakagianni et al., 2023).

With increasingly accessible whole-genome sequencing machine learning models have the capability to predict resistance based on sequence information alone with high accuracy. Deep learning sequence models have shown very high accuracy, both in predicting resistance to various classes of antibiotics. The promise to get a genomic resistance profile within 24 hours of sample testing would be a radical change to the circuit of antibiotic therapy optimization.

As machine learning (ML) models have developed, there has been a greater increase in their use for predicting antimicrobial resistance via large datasets that include genomic sequence, microbiology laboratory results and patient clinical data. Algorithms (such as random forests, support vector machines, and deep learning) assist in identifying hidden resistant patterns and markers in these datasets so that resistant strains can be quickly identified, often before culture-based results become available. This aids in making more timely decisions, helping to support precision medicine, and assists with choosing the most effective antibiotic while minimizing trial-and-error prescribing(Sakagianni et al., 2023).

5.3. AI in Antibiotic Stewardship Programs

Antimicrobial rationing uses ai to improve the selection, dose, & duration of antibiotics by providing real-time clinical decision support systems (cdss). ai tools integrate data from a patient's electronic health records, microbiology lab test results, and local resistance patterns to produce evidence-based recommendations, reduce unnecessary use of antibiotics, and reduce over-prescribing of antibiotics. they also support the monitoring of prescribing trends, flagging inappropriate use, and improving compliance with antimicrobial rationing guidelines, ultimately leading to reduced resistance & improved patient outcomes(Harandi et al., 2025; Pinto-de-Sá et al., 2024).

Standard hospital programs to make use of antibiotics in a manner possible are the antibiotic stewardship programs. They want to lessen consumption and maintain the efficiency of the existing antibiotics. These programs are now implemented using AI to advise doctors on two issues; preceding and following the prescriptions of antibiotics.

The AI tools in these programs are used in systems where the physicians prescribe antibiotics. They cross-examine the prescription with the knowledge of the patients infection local resistance patterns, and treatment guidelines. In case of a mismatch between the prescription and the system provides warning to the doctor on time. Such AI applications can also assist physicians to prevent the use of antibiotics which are unnecessary. This is based on lab results. Condition of the patient. This is however not done adequately by doctors, who are usually busy treating patients.

When analyzed on medical records, AI can help in determining patients whose use of antibiotics is ambiguous too. This assists the stewardship in going through such cases. Based on machine learning, models can be used to forecast the quality of performance a patient will have on antibiotic treatments. These AI systems can detect disease outbreaks in advance as compared to the traditional methods. They also have the ability of recognizing patient groups with the resistant infection, which might be an indication that it is spreading.

Resistance tracking has been initiated in the use of AI in some countries. These systems provide up-to-date information on resistance patterns. This assists hospitals in decision making, when to use which antibiotics.

5.4. Implications

In the clinical, operational, and public health area, Artificial Intelligence's application within the management of pulmonary infectious diseases,.and antimicrobial resistance has huge affects. Clinically; AI-assisted tools can improve early diagnosis, predict the severity of disease, and allow for the use of personalized treatments for better patient outcomes and reduced mortality rates; this is particularly evident for conditions such as pneumonia and tuberculosis. The application of machine-learning technology to predict antimicrobial resistance also allows physicians the ability to begin targeted therapies sooner rather than later; thus minimizing inappropriate use of antibiotics and slowing down the emergence of antimicrobial resistance. From an operational standpoint; AI can increase the efficiency of health care systems (e.g., by providing automated image interpretation and optimizing ICU triage) by relieving the clinician's burden of completing numerous tasks as well as reducing their workload and improving resource utilization through better, real time decision-making. Lastly; through public health, AI can assist in undertaking widespread screening of populations, predicting outbreaks, as well as monitoring drug resistance; these benefits will be key in addressing the overall burden of global infectious diseases. There are numerous challenges associated with these applications, such as the dependency on data quality, ethical issues, biases in algorithms, and requiring robust validation (via clinical studies) to support widespread use.

5.5. Future Directions

The potential of AI in this area is considerable and changing. The development of genomics along with combining these two technologies will allow clinicians to have quick, real-time, resistance profiles through whole-genome sequencing, speeding up diagnosis from days to hours. Clinical decision support systems powered by AI will also continue to improve and become more sophisticated, using multiple data types (clinical, images, genomics, and real-time monitoring) to generate very accurate and personalized treatment options. Additionally, the impact of predictive epidemiology on using AI will allow for earlier detection of pandemics and to provide public health officials with guidance on how to proactively intervene. In areas with few health care providers, solutions using scalable AI may help reduce barriers to accessing health care services by helping with diagnosis and screening when there are not enough specialists. Future research will likely focus on improving the generalizability, explainability, and ethical use of the models created using AI and work on creating a seamless integration of AI in healthcare processes. Ultimately, AI is expected to become a core component rather than just an enhancement of intelligent, data-based decision making in healthcare.

6. SUMMARY

The use of intelligence in managing pulmonary infectious diseases is a big change. It is already assisting the patients in a number of ways and will keep on doing so as the technology improves. There are noteworthy considerations.

The first is that artificial intelligence is actually adept at doing things that are difficult to humans such as processing large amounts of data in a short time or any other activity that would consume a lot of attention. To illustrate, artificial intelligence can be applied to assist doctors in reading x-rays of the chest, track the level of sickness and anticipating whether a disorder will be incurable. In certain instances artificial intelligence can even out-perform doctors in these tasks.

Second, artificial intelligence might become a breakthrough in places in the world where tuberculosis is prevalent and there is a lack of doctors to detect and treat the disease. Artificial intelligence can assist in the analysis of chest x-ray.Diseases are sometimes not detected by doctors due to their rarity or mild manifestation, because they are rarer or display less severe symptoms for the first time, researchers made AI-based crisis computing a high priority. Scientists labored extremely hard in order to develop AI-based or crisis solutions. Nevertheless, it was sure that AI is not flawless. Otherwise, you might not construct it properly, things may get askew. AI should be fully tested and it should be capable of functioning in a manner that protects and benefits the patients.

Antibiotic Artificial intelligence is not made without errors in case it is not created attentively. Recreate past health inequalities. We need to make sure that artificial intelligence is transparent, fair and safe for patients.

Despite these challenges artificial intelligence is making an impact on pulmonary infectious diseases. The existing tools are already saving lives and the emerging tools may continue to revolutionize healthcare. Physicians should have an idea of the artificial intelligence functioning and practice the application of the technology. Artificial intelligence is not a substitute, to doctors but it is a tool that can assist doctors do their work in a better way. Pulmonary infectious diseases, artificial intelligence and human doctors can work together to provide the possible care for patients. A team that consists of artificial intelligence and pulmonary infectious diseases will be able to assist patients in the future.

KEY POINTS

- Some of these are: Artificial Intelligence deep learning models of chest radiograph interpretation can perform a task similar to expert radiologists and can indeed dramatically reduce the time spent in interpreting the chest radiograph in busy clinics.
- The machine learning models that consume large amounts of data such as clinical and laboratory data can predict the severity of a disease better than conventional approaches such as CURB-65 and PSI and can sort out patients in need of intensive care.
- In 2021 the World Health Organization said that Artificial Intelligence tools to analyze chest radiographs are good at detecting TB and they could assist in locations that lack radiologists.
- With whole-genome sequencing and machine learning we can readily discover which drugs will work against M. Tuberculosis and we can have the answer in 24 to 48 hours after we've got the sample.

- RTL - COVID-19 made us realize that Artificial Intelligence can be deployed rapidly during health crises. It also taught us that we should be cautious and ensure that our models are good and functioning well.
- The reasons why Artificial Intelligence can assist us in how we use antibiotics wisely is that it can provide advice in good time and also we can be able to observe antibiotic resistance which is a significant problem.
- We must be cautious about how we apply Artificial Intelligence to treating lung infections We must ensure fair models, transparent models and must observe them all the time to ensure they are working well to all patients.
- Machine learning provides accurate early prediction for antimicrobial resistance utilizing vast amounts of complex data.
- Artificial intelligence allows for more personalized antibiotic therapy while minimising error in empirical treatment.
- Integration with existing hospital data systems improves real-time clinical decision making.
- Hospital antibiotic stewardship programs can take advantage of artificial-intelligence-assisted monitoring and compliance tools.
- Overall benefits include reductions in levels of resistance, enhanced patient safety, and increased healthcare resource efficiency.

REFERENCES

American Thoracic Society Journals. (n.d.). OUP Academic. Retrieved May 28, 2026, from https://academic.oup.com/atsjournals/atsjournals

Application of artificial intelligence in diagnosis of pulmonary tuberculosis | Chinese Medical Journal. (n.d.). Retrieved May 28, 2026, from https://mednexus.org/doi/full/10.1097/CM9.0000000000003018

Applications of Artificial Intelligence in Drug Repurposing—Wan—2025—Advanced Science—Wiley Online Library. (n.d.). Retrieved May 28, 2026, from https://advanced.onlinelibrary.wiley.com/doi/full/10.1002/advs.202411325

Bouderhem, R. (2022). AI Regulation in Healthcare: New Paradigms for A Legally Binding Treaty Under the World Health Organization. *2022 14th International Conference on Computational Intelligence and Communication Networks (CICN)*, 277–281. DOI: 10.1109/CICN56167.2022.10008303

Codlin, A. J., Vo, L. N. Q., Dao, T. P., Forse, R. J., Dang, H. T. M., Nguyen, L. H., Nguyen, H. B., Dinh, L. V., Annerstedt, K. S., Lundin, J., & Lönnroth, K. (2025). Comparison of different Lunit INSIGHT CXR software versions when reading chest radiographs for tuberculosis. *PLOS Digital Health*, *4*(4), e0000813. DOI: 10.1371/journal.pdig.0000813 PMID: 40233023

Computer aided detection of tuberculosis on chest radiographs: An evaluation of the CAD4TB v6 system | Scientific Reports. (n.d.). Retrieved May 28, 2026, from https://www.nature.com/articles/s41598-020-62148-y

Ebrahimian, S., Homayounieh, F., Rockenbach, M. A. B. C., Putha, P., Raj, T., Dayan, I., Bizzo, B. C., Buch, V., Wu, D., Kim, K., Li, Q., Digumarthy, S. R., & Kalra, M. K. (2021). Artificial intelligence matches subjective severity assessment of pneumonia for prediction of patient outcome and need for mechanical ventilation: A cohort study. *Scientific Reports*, *11*(1), 858. DOI: 10.1038/s41598-020-79470-0 PMID: 33441578

Fehr, J., Gunda, R., Siedner, M. J., Hanekom, W., Ndung'u, T., Grant, A., Lippert, C., & Wong, E. B. (2023). CAD4TB software updates: Different triaging thresholds require caution by users and regulation by authorities. *The International Journal of Tuberculosis and Lung Disease : the Official Journal of the International Union against Tuberculosis and Lung Disease*, *27*(2), 157–160. DOI: 10.5588/ijtld.22.0437 PMID: 36853104

Guitor, A. K., & Wright, G. D. (2018). Antimicrobial Resistance and Respiratory Infections. *Chest, 154*(5), 1202–1212. DOI: 10.1016/j.chest.2018.06.019 PMID: 29959904

Harandi, H., Shafaati, M., Salehi, M., Roozbahani, M. M., Mohammadi, K., Akbarpour, S., Rahimnia, R., Hassanpour, G., Rahmani, Y., & Seifi, A. (2025). Artificial intelligence-driven approaches in antibiotic stewardship programs and optimizing prescription practices: A systematic review. *Artificial Intelligence in Medicine, 162*, 103089. DOI: 10.1016/j.artmed.2025.103089 PMID: 39955846

Huang, Y., Ai, L., Wang, X., Sun, Z., & Wang, F. (2022). Review and Updates on the Diagnosis of Tuberculosis. *Journal of Clinical Medicine, 11*(19), 5826. DOI: 10.3390/jcm11195826 PMID: 36233689

Hwang, E. J., Jeong, W. G., David, P. M., Arentz, M., Ruhwald, M., & Yoon, S. H. (2024). AI for detection of tuberculosis: implications for global health. Radiology: Artificial Intelligence, 6(2), e230327.

Integrative Physiology of Pneumonia | Physiological Reviews | American Physiological Society. (n.d.). Retrieved May 28, 2026, from https://journals.physiology.org/doi/full/10.1152/physrev.00032.2017

JMIR Bioinformatics and Biotechnology—Use of Artificial Intelligence in the Search for New Information Through Routine Laboratory Tests: Systematic Review. (n.d.). Retrieved May 28, 2026, from https://bioinform.jmir.org/2022/1/e40473

Jones, B. E., Jones, J., Bewick, T., Lim, W. S., Aronsky, D., Brown, S. M., Boersma, W. G., van der Eerden, M. M., & Dean, N. C. (2011). CURB-65 Pneumonia Severity Assessment Adapted for Electronic Decision Support. *Chest, 140*(1), 156–163. DOI: 10.1378/chest.10-1296 PMID: 21163875

Khan, A., Rauf, Z., Sohail, A., Khan, A. R., Asif, H., Asif, A., & Farooq, U. (2023). A survey of the vision transformers and their CNN-transformer based variants. *Artificial Intelligence Review, 56*(3), 2917–2970. DOI: 10.1007/s10462-023-10595-0

Krauss, C., Do, X. A., & Huck, N. (2017). Deep neural networks, gradient-boosted trees, random forests: Statistical arbitrage on the S&P 500. *European Journal of Operational Research, 259*(2), 689–702. DOI: 10.1016/j.ejor.2016.10.031

Lennerz, J. K., Salgado, R., Kim, G. E., Sirintrapun, S. J., Thierauf, J. C., Singh, A., Indave, I., Bard, A., Weissinger, S. E., Heher, Y. K., de Baca, M. E., Cree, I. A., Bennett, S., Carobene, A., Ozben, T., & Ritterhouse, L. L. (2023). Diagnostic quality model (DQM): An integrated framework for the assessment of diagnostic quality when using AI/ML. [CCLM]. *Clinical Chemistry and Laboratory Medicine*, *61*(4), 544–557. DOI: 10.1515/cclm-2022-1151 PMID: 36696602

Machine Learning for Antimicrobial Resistance Prediction: Current Practice, Limitations, and Clinical Perspective | Clinical Microbiology Reviews. (n.d.). Retrieved May 28, 2026, from https://journals.asm.org/doi/full/10.1128/cmr.00179-21

Michaud, C. M. (2009). Global Burden of Infectious Diseases. *Encyclopedia of Microbiology*, 444–454. DOI: 10.1016/B978-012373944-5.00185-1

Nguyen, H. T. T., Le-Quy, V., Dinh-Xuan, A. T., & Nguyen, L. N. (2026). Artificial Intelligence for Tuberculosis Screening and Detection: From Evidence to Policy and Implementation. *Diagnostics (Basel)*, *16*(8), 1127. DOI: 10.3390/diagnostics16081127 PMID: 42072753

Nhat-Duc, H., & Van-Duc, T. (2023). Comparison of histogram-based gradient boosting classification machine, random Forest, and deep convolutional neural network for pavement raveling severity classification. *Automation in Construction*, *148*, 104767. DOI: 10.1016/j.autcon.2023.104767

Organization, W. H. (2024). *Ethics and governance of artificial intelligence for health: Large multi-modal models. WHO guidance*. World Health Organization.

Parsonage, M., Nathwani, D., Davey, P., & Barlow, G. (2009). Evaluation of the performance of CURB-65 with increasing age. *Clinical Microbiology and Infection*, *15*(9), 858–864. DOI: 10.1111/j.1469-0691.2009.02908.x PMID: 19702590

Penha, D., Pinto, E. G., Matos, F., Hochhegger, B., Monaghan, C., Taborda-Barata, L., Irion, K., & Marchiori, E. (2021). CO-RADS: Coronavirus Classification Review. *Journal of Clinical Imaging Science*, *11*, 9. DOI: 10.25259/JCIS_192_2020 PMID: 33767901

Piccialli, F., di Cola, V. S., Giampaolo, F., & Cuomo, S. (2021). The Role of Artificial Intelligence in Fighting the COVID-19 Pandemic. *Information Systems Frontiers*, *23*(6), 1467–1497. DOI: 10.1007/s10796-021-10131-x PMID: 33935585

Pinto-de-Sá, R., Sousa-Pinto, B., & Costa-de-Oliveira, S. (2024). Brave New World of Artificial Intelligence: Its Use in Antimicrobial Stewardship—A Systematic Review. *Antibiotics (Basel, Switzerland)*, *13*(4), 307. DOI: 10.3390/antibiotics13040307 PMID: 38666983

Qin, Z. Z., Ahmed, S., Sarker, M. S., Paul, K., Adel, A. S. S., Naheyan, T., Barrett, R., Banu, S., & Creswell, J. (2021). Tuberculosis detection from chest x-rays for triaging in a high tuberculosis-burden setting: An evaluation of five artificial intelligence algorithms. *The Lancet. Digital Health*, *3*(9), e543–e554. DOI: 10.1016/S2589-7500(21)00116-3 PMID: 34446265

Rajpurkar, P., Irvin, J., Zhu, K., Yang, B., Mehta, H., Duan, T., Ding, D., Bagul, A., Langlotz, C., Shpanskaya, K., Lungren, M. P., & Ng, A. Y. (2017a). *CheXNet: Radiologist-Level Pneumonia Detection on Chest X-Rays with Deep Learning* (arXiv:1711.05225). arXiv. https://doi.org//arXiv.1711.05225DOI: 10.48550

Rajpurkar, P., Irvin, J., Zhu, K., Yang, B., Mehta, H., Duan, T., Ding, D., Bagul, A., Langlotz, C., Shpanskaya, K., Lungren, M. P., & Ng, A. Y. (2017b). *CheXNet: Radiologist-Level Pneumonia Detection on Chest X-Rays with Deep Learning* (arXiv:1711.05225). arXiv. https://doi.org//arXiv.1711.05225DOI: 10.48550

Revolutionizing healthcare: The role of artificial intelligence in clinical practice | BMC Medical Education | Springer Nature Link. (n.d.). Retrieved May 28, 2026, from https://link.springer.com/article/10.1186/s12909-023-04698-z

Rosenfeld, L. S., Goldmann, F., & Kaprio, L. A. (1957). Reasons for prolonged hospital stay: A study of need for hospital care. *Journal of Chronic Diseases*, *6*(2), 141–152. DOI: 10.1016/0021-9681(57)90048-6 PMID: 13449139

Rutsch, N., Amrein, P., Exadaktylos, A. K., Benneker, L. M., Schmaranzer, F., Müller, M., Albers, C. E., & Bigdon, S. F. (2023). Cervical spine trauma – Evaluating the diagnostic power of CT, MRI, X-Ray and LODOX. *Injury*, *54*(7), 110771. DOI: 10.1016/j.injury.2023.05.003 PMID: 37164902

Sakagianni, A., Koufopoulou, C., Feretzakis, G., Kalles, D., Verykios, V. S., Myrianthefs, P., & Fildisis, G. (2023). Using Machine Learning to Predict Antimicrobial Resistance—A Literature Review. *Antibiotics (Basel, Switzerland)*, *12*(3), 452. DOI: 10.3390/antibiotics12030452 PMID: 36978319

Sluimer, I., Schilham, A., Prokop, M., & van Ginneken, B. (2006). Computer analysis of computed tomography scans of the lung: A survey. *IEEE Transactions on Medical Imaging*, *25*(4), 385–405. DOI: 10.1109/TMI.2005.862753 PMID: 16608056

Vaishya, R., Javaid, M., Khan, I. H., & Haleem, A. (2020). Artificial Intelligence (AI) applications for COVID-19 pandemic. *Diabetes & Metabolic Syndrome*, *14*(4), 337–339. DOI: 10.1016/j.dsx.2020.04.012 PMID: 32305024

Chapter 4
AI in Critical Care and Mechanical Ventilation Predictive Models:
Closed-Loop Systems, ARDS Intelligence, and Multimodal ICU Decision Support

Astha Kamdar
Symbiosis International (Deemed to be) University, India

Vaishnavi Deshmukh
Symbiosis International (Deemed to be) University, India

Milind Chunkhare
http://orcid.org/0000-0001-9299-2075
Symbiosis International (Deemed to be) University, India

ABSTRACT

AI technology has changed the course of CC medicine both for mechanical ventilation and for respiratory failure in general, very quickly. This chapter will discuss four important aspects of AI in ICUs: 1) predicting early deterioration through predictive modelling; 2) automation to manage closed-loop ventilation systems (ventilators); 3) more accurate identification of patients with ARDS and identifying them by phenotype; and 4) integration of multimodal sources of data to support decision-making about treatment plan development. Our analysis will demonstrate that ML and DL algorithms are advancing from theoretical validation studies to 'in-practice' use at the bedside and, therefore, will help physicians decrease cognitive load during

DOI: 10.4018/979-8-3373-7759-9.ch004

patient assessment, ultimately leading to tailored treatment plans and improved patient outcomes. However, there are many challenges related to the heterogeneity of data, algorithmic bias, algorithm interpretability, and the ethical implications needed to ensure the safe use of AI in clinical practice.

1 INTRODUCTION

Today's Intensive Care Unit (ICU) is one of the most data-dense (and cognitively demanding) spaces in clinical care. Intensive care clinicians must often be able to make time- and high-stakes decisions regarding patients experiencing complex multi-organ failure, while integrating multiple streams of fragmented, high-velocity data, frequently exceeding human cognitive capacity for processing these data. Data ecology in the ICU is mind-bogglingly large and complex; a single critically ill patient can produce more than 100,000 patient-specific data points a day (Bellani et al., 2016) via appraising data in: structured electronic health record (EHR) data; 250Hz (Hz= cycles per second) high-frequency physiological waveforms / traces; breath-by-breath ventilator logs; high-resolution radiographic images; unstructured clinical free text notes, etc. Demographics and clinical data support the view that the contemporary "crisis in critical care" represents an aging population with higher levels of comorbidity; global shortages of intensivists / specialty physicians; and an explosion of physiological data that exists, remains underutilized (due to barriers related to interoperability and limits of human cognition) (Beil et al., 2019) via use of standard level of clinical practice, growing at rates exponential. In the environment described above, and beyond an example of a technologically-based "novelty," artificial intelligence (AI) has developed into a necessary way to scale the practice of critical care medicine and to enhance the provision of critical care in a manner that far exceeds that what humans alone can accomplish.

By integrating AI into the field of respiratory critical care, we can leverage unique capabilities available to us that will improve care delivered to patients. Many medical specialties consider the progression of illness over long periods of time (e.g., weeks to months). In the patient with progressive respiratory failure (< 30 days), however, the physiologic processes of respiration and gas exchange are time-sensitive and often occur within second to minute intervals around an event. The real-time physiologic feedback loop(s) of respiratory mechanics including the impact that the modification of PEEP (positive end-expiratory pressure) has on oxygen delivery and lung compliance are ideal for developing algorithms providing both predictive analysis and closed loop control. Finally, a mechanical ventilator is both a technological and therapeutic device enabling direct interaction with computational models (monitoring and automation).

For many years, the CDSS system in an ICU was based on a rules-based system. The initial CDSS were comprised of expert consensus rules (i.e., based on the group's opinion and agreement to use these rules as the basis for care) and applied a strict "if-then" framework. The original CDSS were helpful for providing protocolized care for simple patient clinical presentations, but they had significant limitations in the management of critically ill patients due to their unpredictability, non-linear course, and individualized care paths (Biesheuvel et al., 2025). Since that time, the medical informatics industry has seen rapid advancements, transitioning to a data-driven system as opposed to a rules-based system. This has allowed for the detection of non-linear relationships as well as subtle physiological markers that cannot be detected with the naked eye, providing greater accuracy in diagnosis and prognosis (Berkhout et al., 2025).

The use of AI technologies to support clinicians in managing care is becoming increasingly popular with the introduction of AI applications in the ICU. The three main areas of machine learning (ML), deep learning (DL), and reinforcement learning (RL) all provide their own unique challenges and methodologies. Traditional ML algorithms are commonly thought to include algorithms like random forests (RF), support vector machines (SVM), and extreme gradient boosting (XGBoost), each of which has been specifically designed to analyze large sets of tabular data and look for patterns to determine future outcomes without having been pre-programmed with specific rules by a person. As such, they are designed to operate without the assistance of an individual through manual/automated feature engineering, but rather by working with the data directly to derive the features it will ultimately need to generate the results it needs to provide the clinician with insights into care decisions. In this regard, the use of DL is the next logical evolution of the use of ML in the ICU; DL employs the use of multiple layers of artificial neural networks (e.g., convolutional neural networks [CNNs] and recurrent neural networks [RNNs]) to process large volumes of unstructured data (including high-resolution medical images and continuous physiological waveform telemetry) directly, without requiring the need for manual feature engineering. Use of RL in the ICU further adds a new dimension to the way that clinicians can leverage AI technology to treat patients. RL assigns the use of an agent-environment paradigm and enables an algorithm to learn how to perform a sequential series of actions to maximize a clinical reward over time (e.g., net positive clinical outcome) (Botta et al., 2021). RL has the potential to be used to make real-time clinical recommendations for optimizing the delivery of mechanical ventilation, but RL algorithms are also subject to extrapolation errors if the RL algorithm is applied inappropriately outside the realm of the safe application of the RL algorithm.

Table 1. Paradigms of artificial intelligence in respiratory critical care

AI Paradigm	Primary Algorithm Types	Optimal Data Modalities	Representative Clinical Application	Methodological Caveat
Machine Learning (ML)	XGBoost, Random Forest, SVM, Logistic Regression	Tabular EHR data, laboratory results, discrete vital signs	Predicting the onset of respiratory failure; ARDS sub-phenotyping	Requires intensive manual feature engineering; limited temporal awareness.
Deep Learning (DL)	CNNs, RNNs, LSTMs, Transformers	Unstructured text, medical imaging (CXR/CT), high-frequency waveforms	Automated lung CT segmentation; patient-ventilator asynchrony detection	High computational cost; significant "black-box" opacity requiring XAI tools.
Reinforcement Learning (RL)	Q-Learning, Batch-Constrained Deep Q-Learning (BCQ)	Sequential state-action-reward trajectories (MDP)	Optimizing dynamic ventilator settings (PEEP, FiO2); weaning protocols	Prone to extrapolation error; retrospective off-policy evaluation is mathematically complex.

In addition to these significant improvements in technology, there are also important methodological and ethical issues associated with the use of artificial intelligence (AI) in providing bedside critical care. With the increasing use of algorithm-based decision-making, there are many potential problems associated with "black box" opacity, shifting datasets, algorithmic disparities, and the continuing requirement for strong human oversight (Buess et al., 2025). Therefore, creating a partnership that promotes a collaborative and transparent partnership between human clinicians and AI systems is essential. This chapter will describe the current technical environment, evaluation criteria, and implementation challenges associated with using AI for providing respiratory critical care.

Section 4.2 specifically delves into predictive models for respiratory failure and ICU admissions, utilizing sophisticated algorithms designed to facilitate timely escalation of care. The employment of these models serves to ensure that patients receive appropriate interventions without unnecessary delays, thereby potentially improving outcomes significantly.

In Section 4.3, the discussion shifts to closed-loop ventilation management systems, tracing their evolution from basic feedback loops to advanced AI-controlled systems. These developments highlight the potential for continuous and automatic adjustments in patient ventilation, ultimately improving the patient's experience and clinical outcomes. Section 4.4 addresses the utility of AI in the context of ARDS, emphasizing early detection methodologies, sub-phenotyping patients, and improving prognostic assessments. Early identification of ARDS can lead to more tailored treatment approaches that enhance patient survival rates.

Finally, Section 4.5 articulates the forefront of multimodal data integration, exploring how disparate data types—such as electronic health records, medical imaging, and genomic data—can be synthesized to create a comprehensive understanding of the patient's care pathway. This holistic view paves the way for the implementation of precision medicine, ensuring that treatment plans are uniquely tailored to individual patient needs. Despite the immense potential of AI technology, significant challenges remain in successfully integrating these advancements into bedside healthcare practice, necessitating ongoing research and collaboration among healthcare professionals. Significant challenges include data quality, generalizability of the model, "black-box" opacity, and ethical accountability as they relate to AI analytics. Misseri et al. have stated that AI technology must enhance the clinical workflow (as opposed to disrupting it) with the clinician being the ultimate authority in decisions about patient treatment. This chapter will work to close the gap between the technical advancements of AI technology and its application within the clinical environment by providing a framework for the responsible introduction of AI into the delivery of care to patients in the ICU.

Figure 1. Taxonomy of AI applications in the ICU. The field is broadly categorized into predictive analytics, closed-loop control systems, disease-specific intelligence (e.g., ARDS), and multimodal clinical decision support.

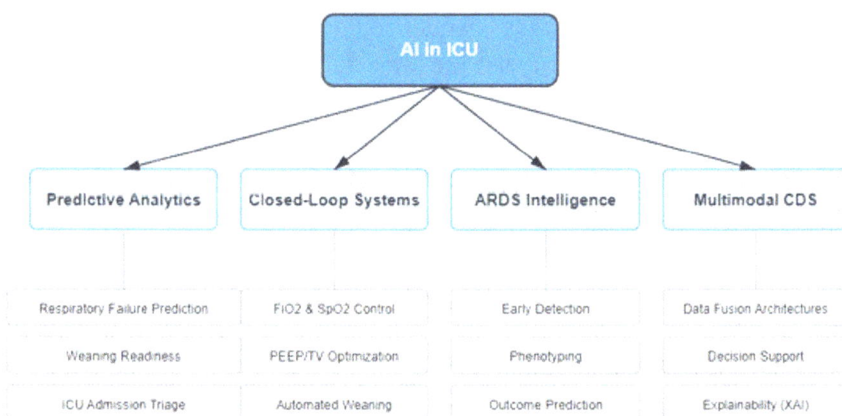

Source: Original diagram created by the authors for this chapter. Conceptual framework adapted from Misseri et al. (2024) and Hadweh et al. (2025).

2 PREDICTION OF RESPIRATORY FAILURE AND ICU ADMISSION

In the field of hospital medicine, one of the many challenges we face is recognizing patients at risk for rapid decline before irreversible decompensation occurs. There are many conditions that can be attributed to sudden onset (such as respiratory failure or cardiac arrest), yet these conditions typically have hours (if not days) of subtle physiological prodromal events prior to the actual manifestation of the acute event- a phenomenon that has been termed "failure to rescue" in the professional literature. Current models for evaluating patients (e.g., Modified Early Warning Score [MEWS], National Early Warning Score [NEWS]) make use of aggregate point scoring scores based on intermittent, manually recorded vital sign measurements. While these traditional heuristic models are frequently used, they have low positive predictive values and poor sensitivity/specificity trade-offs- which produce a high rate of false alarms resulting in the chronic alarm fatigue experienced by health care providers (Cecconi et al., 2025). In addition, these linear scoring systems do not account for the complex, non-linear and temporal nature of the many physiological parameters that are measured with such high frequency.

One of the main obstacles to predictive modeling in critical care is the issue of how to define the outcome (i.e., what the label will be). If you look at historical EHR data, it is hard to determine when someone has experienced respiratory failure from the data itself; there are many ways a model could define "respiratory failure" and not all sets of data will necessarily use the same definition. For example: whether a patient starts using mechanical ventilation, increasing levels of non-invasive oxygen (i.e., high-flow nasal cannula), dropping below a certain oxygen saturation level, or even being transferred to the intensive care unit (ICU) unexpectedly – these could all have different outcomes for the patient and require different ways of defining respiratory failure. Therefore, there are serious limitations to transportability and external validation of predictive algorithms due to the differences in how each study has labeled their data. Additionally, when choosing a time frame for prediction of respiratory failure, there is often a tradeoff: if we try to predict 10 minutes prior to intubation, the care team would be working on the patient already, but if we try to predict 48 hours ahead of time, we produce too many false positives.

These complex temporal factors necessitate a significant transformation of the paradigms adopted by data driven ML methodologies to remedy the situation. Continuous streams of EHR data provide an opportunity to detect slow/gradual deterioration (i.e., being able to see small deviations from normal/expected clinical conditions) prior to any overt (i.e., observable) clinical failure through the utilization of ML technologies (e.g., algorithms such as XGBoost and LSTM networks). Many studies have shown that errors are lower (i.e., predictive discrimination is higher) for patients who are being monitored using these data compared to those being monitored using conventional score based methods. In particular, LSTMs are specifically designed for sequential time series data and are highly effective at retaining and mapping historical context relating to physiological memory in order to provide insight into where a pt's current trajectory lies within the context of very large datasets associated with other historical patients and therefore inflection points being detected very early in a patient's interaction with the system (Chatburn & Mireles-Cabodevila, 2011).

An example of the use of this type of method is the FAST-PACE model, which uses gradient boosting type architectures to predict if a patient is at risk for acute respiratory failure and cardiac arrest. This prediction can take place up to six hours before the event occurs. The FAST-PACE model achieved an area under the ROC curve (AUROC) of 0.869 and 0.886 for respiratory failure and cardiac arrest, respectively (Chen et al., 2022). However, when evaluating these types of models the AUROC alone is not adequate because of the extreme class imbalance that typically occurs in critically ill populations (1% of the ward population or less may have an event, like an unplanned intubation). In these extremely imbalanced populations, the AUROC can provide a too optimistic view of the predictive capability of the models because the large number of true negatives is equally weighted. Therefore, in highly imbalanced situations, the area under the PR curve (AUPRC), the positive predictive value (PPV), and the negative predictive value (NPV) are mathematically more appropriate for determining the true medical utility of a tool and for preventing overestimation of predictive capability. In addition, rigorous calibration parameters, such as the Brier score, the calibration slope, and the Hosmer-Lemeshow statistic, are necessary to provide an accurate representation of true predictive capability. A model may have excellent discrimination (AUROC) but poor calibration, meaning it correctly ranks patients by risk but incorrectly estimates their absolute probability of deterioration, leading to misallocation of clinical resources.

Table 2. Common methodological pitfalls in predictive modeling for respiratory failure

Methodological Pitfall	Description	Consequence on Clinical Utility	Recommended Mitigation Strategy
Data/Temporal Leakage	Including features in the training data that would not logically be available at the time of prediction (e.g., using post-intubation ABG results to predict intubation).	Gross overestimation of model accuracy; immediate failure upon real-time bedside deployment.	Strict temporal masking; strict separation of feature-window, gap-window, and target-window.
Improper Missingness Handling	Dropping patients with missing labs or using mean-imputation improperly across time-series data.	Loss of informative missingness (the fact that a lab wasn't ordered is clinically relevant).	Last-Observation-Carried-Forward (LOCF), multivariate imputation, or missing-indicator variables.
Reliance Solely on AUROC	Evaluating a highly imbalanced dataset (e.g., 1% event rate) using only the ROC curve.	Obscures high false-positive rates, leading to severe alarm fatigue in practice.	Report Area Under Precision-Recall Curve (AUPRC), F1-score, and Net Benefit (Decision Curve Analysis).
Calibration Drift	Model probabilities become inaccurate over time as clinical practices or patient demographics change.	Clinicians lose trust as the absolute risk predictions no longer match observed realities.	Continuous post-deployment surveillance and periodic recalibration routines.

AI will continue to evolve and impact how to clinically make decisions regarding ventilatory transition points such as weaning or extubation. This decision ultimately involves determining when to liberate a patient from being mechanically ventilated, which involves high-risk stratification; if a patient is taken off the ventilator too early and needs to be put back on due to reintubation, the mortality rate associated with reintubation is known to be high, as well as the physiological stress associated with reintubation, whereas if the patient is left on the ventilator too long, there are known complications including increased risk of developing ventilator-associated pneumonia, ventilator-induced lung injury (VILI), or diaphragm atrophy. Traditional methods for determining readiness for extubation have limited physiologic usefulness (e.g., RSBI) because they use static measurements and have moderate predictive value. They also do not account for the dynamic and multisystemic nature of being ready for extubation. Current ability to analyze multiple variables within time-series analyses and utilize machine learning (ML) will allow clinicians to predict extubation success based on dynamic analysis of trends throughout the entire duration of ventilation.

There are predictive models which use continuous ventilator telemetry (like ventilatory time and tidal volume variability), in addition to hemodynamic parameters, sedation, and fluid balance, that help to estimate both the probability that SBTs will succeed and the amount of time that is appropriate for beginning an SBT after extubation. These models are transitioning from providing predictions based on static baselines to providing daily predictions. That is, they will recalculate how likely it is that a given patient will successfully be extubated every 24 hours. Algorithms driven by AI will assist with weaning protocols and reduce the amount of time patients are on mechanical ventilation and thus reduce resource utilization and improve patient morbidity by providing an objective set of guidelines for clinicians to address their own uncertainty (Gallifant et al., 2022).

Table 3. Comparison of conventional vs. AI-driven weaning and extubation prediction models

Approach / Metric	**Data Modalities Utilized**	**Analytical Methodology**	**Strengths**	**Limitations**
Conventional RSBI	Respiratory Rate, Tidal Volume	Static Point-in-time calculation (f/V_T)	Simple to calculate at the bedside; requires no computational infrastructure.	Low specificity; ignores cardiovascular reserve, sedation status, and secretional load.
Static ML Classifiers	Demographics, Labs, Pre-SBT vitals	Logistic Regression, Random Forest	Integrates multiple physiological domains; outperforms traditional single indices.	Does not account for temporal trends leading up to the extubation decision.
Dynamic Time-Series AI	Continuous waveforms, EHR sequences	RNNs, LSTMs, Temporal Transformers	Captures physiological reserve and dynamic trajectory; highly accurate.	Computationally expensive; highly sensitive to artifactual data and sensor disconnection.
RL-Driven Weaning	MDP state-action pairs	Off-policy Reinforcement Learning	Provides actionable recommendations for optimal timing of PSV reduction and extubation.	Difficult to prospectively validate; high risk of extrapolation error.

Figure 2. Flowchart: AI-driven respiratory failure prediction pipeline. The process moves from raw multimodal data acquisition through preprocessing and machine learning analysis to generate actionable risk scores that trigger clinical protocols.

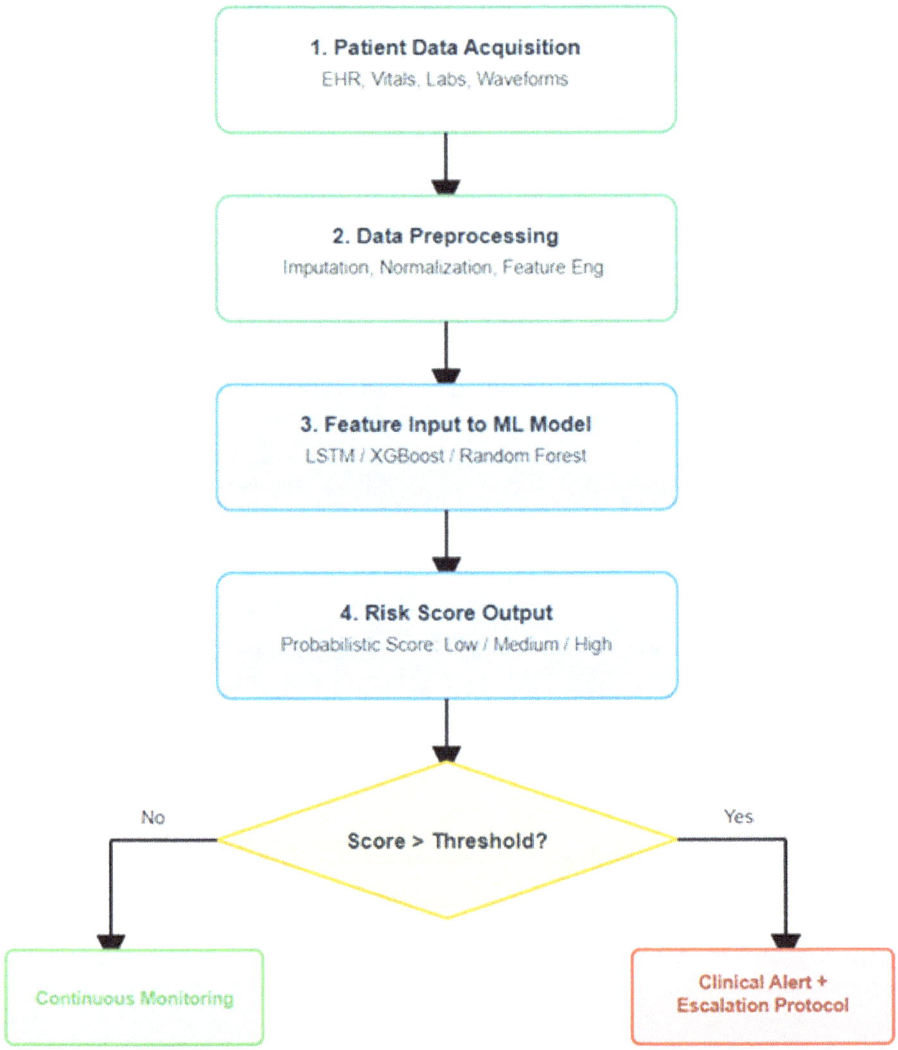

Source: Original flowchart created by the authors for this chapter. Pipeline design informed by: Misseri, et al. (2024), Liu et al. (2024), and Pinsky, et al. (2024)

3 CLOSED-LOOP VENTILATOR MANAGEMENT SYSTEMS

Mechanical ventilation has become a powerful life-saving tool. However, mechanical ventilation can be hazardous if not done correctly. For example, if a ventilator is used with an excessive driving pressure, with inappropriate positive end-expiratory pressure (PEEP), or if tidal volumes are not calibrated, these mistakes will ultimately cause lung injury due to ventilator induced lung injury (VILI). The mechanisms of VILI include volutrauma, barotrauma, atelectrauma, and biotrauma.

In the traditional management of patients on mechanical ventilation, an "open-loop" system is used. In an "open-loop" system, a clinician reacts to assess the patient's condition at predefined checkpoints, interprets intermittent physiological data, manually adjusts the mechanical actuator (ventilator) and lets the ventilator run at an established set of ventilator settings until the clinician assesses the patient again. This system is highly susceptible to lag time between changes in the mechanical properties of the patient's lungs (compliance and resistance) and the clinician's assessment of those properties. As a result, when the clinician evaluates the patient's condition, the patient's lungs may have been exposed to injurious pressure for a long time (Hadweh et al., 2025).

Control engineering principles have been used to design Physiologic Closed Loop Control (PCLC) systems to help reduce risk. A PCLC system is made up of multiple components: some type of sensor (flow sensor, pulse oximeter, capnometer), a control algorithm and some type of actuator (ventilator valves). The PCLC system continuously measures selected physiological variables and provides them as input to an algorithm controller (commonly using Proportional-Integral-Derivative logic) and makes adjustments to the output of the ventilator in real time based on a pre-set target. Development of these systems is tremendously complicated due to the existence of physiological cross-coupling; for instance, when there is an automated increase in respiratory rate for the purpose of clearing CO2, this leads to an indirect change in intrinsic PEEP and mean airway pressure, creating a requirement for changes to be coincidentally made to multiple variables to maintain patient safety. In addition, it is critical that PCLC systems are highly resilient to noise and artifact and that they can determine whether a sudden decrease in SpO2 is, in fact, a true desaturation, or simply due to the finger probe being disconnected, and if so, return control of the PCLC system back to the clinician via a fail-safe mechanism.

Today's technologically advanced commercial healthcare systems are employing new adaptive targeting methodologies that greatly increase the level of automation in delivering most aspects of healthcare. For example, using continuous data from SpO2 and etCO2, the automated closed-loop ventilator (INTELLiVENT-ASV by Hamilton Medical) continually titrates minute volume, PEEP and FiO2 to maintain patients at optimal physiological target zones. NAVA (Neurally Adjusted Ventilatory Assist) is one of several new advanced modes of mechanical ventilation that automate the process of helping to wean patients off ventilators by gradually decreasing pressure support according to their respiratory rates and tidal volume. All of these types of advanced technologies are very successful in maintaining optimal functioning for patients while also significantly reducing the cognitive and manual burden to ICU staff (Kim et al., 2023).

Table 4. Design choices and methodological constraints in RL for mechanical ventilation

RL Component	Design Consideration in Critical Care	Methodological Challenge
State Representation (S)	Selection of vital signs, lab values, demographic data, and ventilator telemetry to represent the patient.	Curse of dimensionality; too many variables dilute learning, too few fail to capture physiological complexity.
Action Discretization (A)	Converting continuous ventilator settings (e.g., PEEP 0-24) into discrete bins (e.g., Low, Med, High).	Coarse bins lose precision; fine bins drastically increase the computational action space.
Reward Engineering (R)	Defining what constitutes a "good" outcome (e.g., +100 for 90-day survival, -10 for barotrauma).	Reward sparsity (survival is only known at the end); difficulty in balancing competing short-term physiological goals.
Policy Constraints	Ensuring the algorithm does not suggest medically lethal exploratory actions.	Requires algorithms like BCQ to restrict outputs to the distribution of human clinician behavior

Whereas commercial PCLC systems use deterministic control systems and extensive rule-based frameworks created by experts, automated ventilation's future development lies predominantly in using Reinforcement Learning (RL). Rules-based controllers minimize immediate physiological goal state (e.g. SpO2 at 94%) while RL algorithms are designed to (statistically) identify (mathematically) long-term cumulative reward (e.g. maximize 90-day survival while minimizing cumulative lung injury). RL conceptualizes the clinical environment as defined by a Markov Decision Process (MDP) that has defined states S, actions A (such as precise changes to PEEP or FiO2), transition probability P and reward function R (Li et al., 2025).

The VentAI algorithm and comparable algorithms serve as flagship instances of reinforcement learning (RL) applied to intensive care medicine. Typically, RL algorithms are constrained by limited training samples that do not generalize well to rare patient care scenarios. To address this limitation, many RL algorithms exploit archival databases such as MIMIC-IV to train algorithms via batch-constrained deep Q-learning (BCQ). The motivation behind these models is to eliminate extrapolation error—that is, the tendency of conventional off-policy RL algorithms to recommend unsafe and/or untested treatments when an observation does not correspond with any previous experiences. BCQ achieves this objective by constraining the RL algorithm with an additional clinician-policy regularization term, which ensures that the RL algorithm's recommended therapeutic continuations are mathematically close to the historical actions taken by a clinician. In this manner, BCQ not only guarantees safe therapy recommendations but also allows for the precise titration of therapy within those safety limits (Misseri et al., 2024).

Opportunistic evaluation (evaluation of experienced models) of those models demonstrates when historic practices for clinician behaviours occurred in retrospect, the clinical recommendations of the [RL agent] retrospectively could reduce or prevent deaths. Researchers have often used methods of evaluating potential outcomes using mathematical procedures including [inverse probability weighting (IPW)] or [consistent weighted per-decision importance sampling (CWPDIS)] when attempting to estimate potential outcomes if the AI policy [RL agent] were to be followed. However, the retrospective evaluation has inherent limitations. It relies on the assumption that every factor affecting the clinician's decision is included in the data set. This is almost never true in ICU settings, as visual data (e.g., patient sight/diaphoresis, respiratory effort) is not recorded. Therefore, the assumption of superior outcomes from retrospective evaluations does not imply the same for bedside practice; thus prospective evaluation studies (i.e., randomised evaluation studies) should be done before RL agent outputs are assumed to be safe (Parreco et al., 2018).

A concurrent application area of artificial intelligence in the area of ventilation is the development of automated detection methods that can automatically detect patient-ventilator asynchrony. Types of asynchrony include double triggering, ineffective triggering, and flow starvation; asynchrony occurs when the output from the ventilator does not match the neural respiratory demand of the patient, resulting in severe dysfunction of the diaphragm, increased need for sedation, and poorer clinical outcomes. Many clinicians do not have good visual detection of asynchrony by looking at ventilator waveforms which results in many cases being missed. Deep learning frameworks, most commonly convolution neural networks (CNNs) that are trained on annotated waveforms of pressure-time and flow-time, will have very high sensitivity and specificity values when detecting these subtle asynchronies automatically. However, the performance of these models will ultimately be limited by the quality of the clinician's annotations that were used during the training process, so it is important to have highly curated datasets that have been built via consensus by multiple experts.

Figure 3. Closed-Loop Ventilator Control System (PCLC). A continuous feedback loop where patient physiological data drives ventilator adjustments via an AI controller, with provisions for clinician override

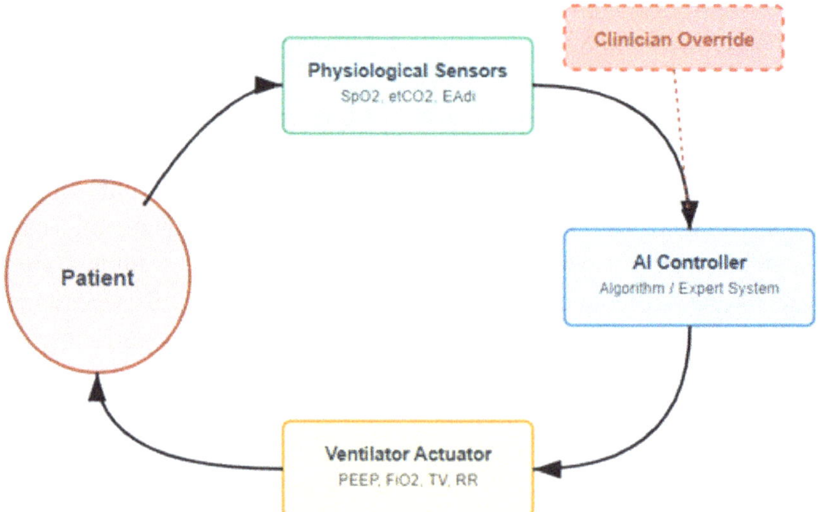

Source: Original diagram created by the authors for this chapter. Architecture based on: Von Platen, P., et al. (2020). The dawn of physiological closed-loop ventilation—a review. Critical Care, 24, 161. DOI: 10.1186/s13054-020-2810-1; Chatburn, R. L., & Mireles-Cabodevila, E. (2011). Closed-loop control of mechanical ventilation. Respiratory Care, 56(1), 85–102. DOI: 10.4187/respcare. 00967; and Botta et al. (2021). Effectiveness, safety, and efficacy of INTELLiVENT–ASV. Expert Review of Medical Devices. DOI: 10.1080/17476348.2021.1933450

4 AI FOR ARDS RECOGNITION AND PROGNOSIS

Acute respiratory distress syndrome (ARDS) is one of the deadliest and most difficult syndromes to diagnose within the intensive care unit (ICU). Mortality rates in ARDS often exceed 35-40% (Peine et al., 2021). The reason for this prevalence is that ARDS is not a singular biological disease entity; but rather it represents a heterogeneous clinical syndrome. Currently, ARDS should be diagnosed according to the criteria established by the Berlin Definition. These include: (1) the acute onset of ARDS must occur within 1 week of an identified clinical insult; (2) bilateral opacities must be present on chest imaging; (3) the partial pressure of arterial oxygen (PaO2) / fractional inspired oxygen (FiO2) ratio must be < 300mmHg ; and (4) respiratory failure must not be fully accounted for by congestive heart failure (CHF) or fluid overload. Manual application of the Berlin criteria is often subjectively delayed or missed due to the inherent inter-rater variability in chest x-ray interpretations. In addition, many units sample arterial blood gases (ABGs) intermittently, further complicating the diagnosis process. Several artificial intelligence (AI) methodologies are currently being developed to address the diagnostic bottlenecks caused by the subjective nature of the aforementioned criteria and the varied techniques used to interpret chest x-rays.

Deep learning architectures have been trained for the purpose of automating the segmentation and classification of bilateral opacities on chest X-rays (CXRs) and computer tomography (CT) scans. Current automated CT segmentation pipelines are designed to perform much more than basic detection, as they are capable of volumetrically quantifying lost lung aeration and providing highly accurate measures of normal lung aeration, poor lung aeration, and fully consolidated lung aeration. The ability to accurately volumetrically quantify lung aeration directly correlates with the severity of ARDS and the recruitability of the lung (Moons et al., 2025). When traditional computer vision algorithms generating these advanced volumetric measures of aerated volume are merged with natural language processing (NLP) algorithms to analyze free-text reports of radiology (as well as clinical notes stored within electronic health records), the resulting multi-modal pipelines have pooled sensitivities and specificities significantly greater than conventional clinical forms of monitoring (Pinsky et al., 2024).

An application of AI technology in ARDS research is to identify biological subphenotypes within ARDS patients. Retrospective research performed using Latent Class Analysis (LCA) on prospective ARDS clinical trial data has shown that there are two distinct ARDS phenotypes: hyper-inflammatory and hypo-inflammatory. The hyper-inflammatory phenotype has more elevated plasma levels of inflammatory biomarkers such as interleukin (IL-6), soluble tumor necrosis factor receptor-1 (sTNFr-1). It is also more likely to be associated with requiring vasopressor support, metabolic acidosis, and increased overall mortality. Additionally, the phenotypes respond differently to standard therapy with true treatment-effect heterogeneity. For example, hyper-inflammatory patients may achieve improved outcomes with increased PEEP and fluid restriction versus hypo-inflammatory patients who will not receive any benefit or may have an adverse response to similar interventions (Liu et al., 2024).

Due to being challenged mathematically coupled with historically having to wait an extended time and large cost to have multiplex, biomarkcrs; LCA cannot be run effectively at bedside. Supervised machine learning classifiers (i.e., XGBoost, Random Forest) have been developed to bridge this gap from research to practice as parsimonious bedside classifiers that allow clinicians to accurately predict the phenotype derived from an individual's LCA at the time of ICU admission using only immediate and easily accessed clinical variables (i.e., vital signs, basic metabolic panel, vasoactive medication dosages) within hours post admission to the ICU. As such, clinicians can apply and realize the promise of precision medicine to the ICU bedside by being able to stratify ARDS patients for specific interventions(THE) on an ongoing basis (Sinha et al., 2020).

Table 5. Methodological approaches to ARDS phenotyping and prognosis

Methodological Approach	**Primary Goal**	**Algorithms Utilized**	**Clinical Application & Limitations**
Latent Class Analysis (LCA)	Discover hidden biological sub-phenotypes.	Unsupervised probabilistic modeling	Identifies hyper/hypo-inflammatory states; relies on delayed biomarker data making it unsuitable for real-time use.
Parsimonious Bedside Classifiers	Real-time assignment of phenotype.	XGBoost, Random Forest, SVM	Uses standard EHR data to predict LCA class; requires rigorous external validation across different hospital systems.
Mortality/VFD Prediction	Forecast 28-day survival and Ventilator-Free Days.	Deep Neural Networks, Ensemble models	Outperforms traditional SOFA scores; highly sensitive to dataset shift and variations in end-of-life care practices.
Automated CT Segmentation	Quantify lung aeration and recruitability.	UNETR, 3D CNNs	Provides exact morphological data for PEEP titration; limited by the risk of transporting unstable patients to the CT scanner.

Figure 4. ARDS AI detection and phenotyping pipeline. Multimodal data is processed to detect ARDS and classify patients into phenotypes (e.g., hyperinflammatory vs. hypoinflammatory) to guide personalized therapy

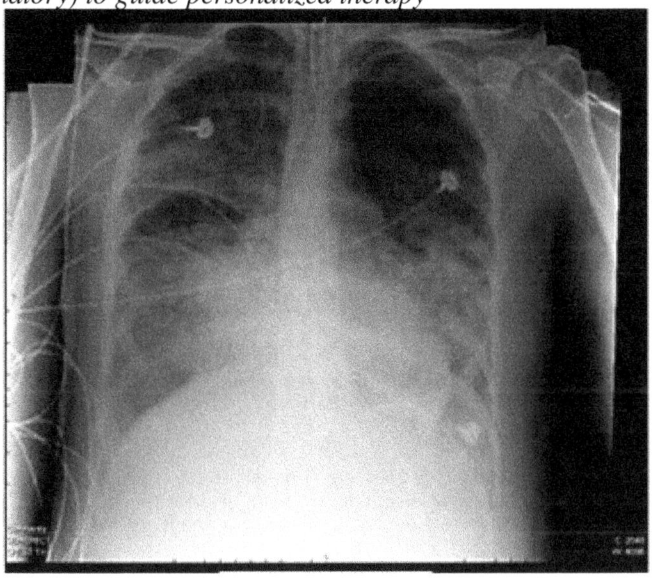

Source: Original flowchart created by the authors for this chapter. Pipeline informed by: Li, et al. (2025) and Tran et al. (2024)

Increasingly, AI-based models are also being used to create prognostic models for ARDS, predicting outcomes for 28-day mortality, length of stay, and number of ventilator-free days with accuracy better than traditional ICU scoring systems (APACHE II/SOFA). However, there are many limitations to external validation of prognostic models because mortality rates from ARDS vary greatly depending on variable institutional practice patterns concerning withdrawal of life-sustaining therapies.

In the future, the combination of these predictive models based on data with mechanistic/deterministic physiological equations will lead to "Digital Twins." A digital twin is a virtual replica of each patient's precise cardiopulmonary mechanics that exists in an assistive technology environment and is computed by utilizing a set of differential equations that characterize a patient's lung compliance and airway resistance. Using AI solvers to run various PEEP titration strategies against the digital twin allows clinicians to predict the mechanical effect (e.g., overdistension vs. recruitment of alveoli) on the biological patient without having to subject the patient to the trauma of the trial and error involved with adjusting ventilator therapy in actual practice. Digital twin technologies are promising scientifically but are still primarily experimental in nature; significant computational resources and bedside limitations will need to be overcome to achieve routine clinical applicability.

Figure 5. Chest X-ray demonstrating the characteristic bilateral opacities of Acute Respiratory Distress Syndrome (ARDS). AI-based convolutional neural networks are trained on such images to automate early ARDS detection and severity classification

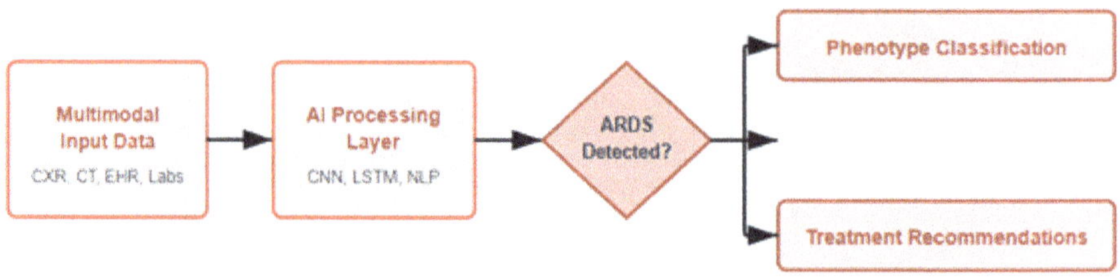

Source: "ARDS X-Ray.jpg" — Wikimedia Commons. Available at: https://commons.wikimedia.org/wiki/File:ARDS_X-Ray.jpg. License: Public Domain. See also: Battaglini, D., et al. (2025). Imaging and pulmonary function techniques in ARDS diagnosis and management. Critical Care. DOI: 10.1186/s13054-025-05520-6.

5 INTEGRATION OF MULTIMODAL ICU DATA FOR CLINICAL DECISION SUPPORT

Modern-day ICUs have created an extremely diverse and fast-paced data ecosystem. The data that can be collected in ICUs are continuous physiological waveforms, intermittent laboratory test results, high-resolution images, and unstructured clinical text. Historically, in medicine, most AI applications have been unimodal in nature (e.g., CNNs only analysing one picture such as a chest X-ray or LSTMs only analysing vital signs without reference to any CXRs). The reality is that to make appropriate clinical decisions, many data types must be integrated to make a single cognitive decision as the intensivist does when he/she takes a chest X-ray opacity, the current PaO2/FiO2 ratio, inflammatory markers, and information from the patient's clinical history and uses those data to establish a treatment plan. MMAI seeks to mathematically reproduce and scale this cognitive abstraction process by integrating varying data types into one predictive modelling framework (Soenksen et al., 2022).

There are three main architectural approaches to MMAI, which are differentiated by how the different data streams are combined. The first approach is called "early fusion," where raw data from each of the various types of input modalities is concatenated together at the input layer. The problem with this method is that it is simple to understand; however, statistical issues arise because the dimensionality and sampling rates of each data type are so vastly different (e.g., daily blood pressure readings compared to 12-lead ECG readings). The next approach is known as "late fusion," where separate unimodal networks are trained on their own and combined at the end of this process using an ensemble method based on their respective statistical predictions, which does not provide the network with any information about complex cross-modal interactions. The final architectural approach is described as "intermediate fusion," which is currently regarded as the most advanced MMAI architectural approach and employs neural network architectures of various types (often transformer-based foundation models) to first learn the deep feature representations of each data modality independently and to then combine them at the hidden layers. In this case, the model's attention mechanism (i.e., the way in which the model learns how to identify cross-modal interactions) is dynamic—the model learns that a specific pattern of data on the ECG is only strongly predictive of deterioration when it is examined in conjunction with a finding in a specific radiology report. The HAIM framework has established that for a number of healthcare applications, intermediate fusion has consistently outperformed unimodal standard benchmarks (Tran et al., 2024).

Since two years ago, LLMs and Multimodal Foundation Models have emerged to help researchers integrate unstructured text with structured physiological data much more quickly than before. The groundbreaking capabilities of LLMs in natural language processing allow them to summarize large volumes of patient history, identify structured phenotypes located within disorganized clinical notes, and serve as a conversational support for decision-making.

Nevertheless, the use of LLMs in critical care is still in its early stages. They are still subject to "hallucinations," lack reliable reasoning ability when evaluating hypothetical clinical situations, and create potential data privacy issues associated with using third-party APIs (Vasey et al., 2022).

MMAI systems have made it difficult (if not impossible) for healthcare providers to adequately understand why an alert was generated. For MMAI to be trusted and acted on by healthcare providers, they need to know the underlying rationale of how the algorithm works when creating alerts (i.e., how would the practitioner know that an algorithm used a recent 15% drop in mean arterial pressure and a concurrent increase in lactate level as part of this reasoning) – this is referred to as "explainable AI" (Yang et al., 2025). As such, XAI systems have become an essential part of clinical implementation of MMAI systems. For example, if an XAI system generated an alert for sepsis, and the XAI system displays a visual representation of how the alert was generated in a dashboard displaying the 15% drop in mean arterial pressure, the growing lactate level, and a shift in wording (i.e., changing from "patient" to "patient's" in the nursing notes) based on the last week, then the clinician would have the necessary information to determine whether or not to act on the alert (and to act on it appropriately). One limitation with some XAI systems is that they can be computationally intensive to run in real-time, and another limitation is that some XAI systems generate explanations that are mathematically accurate but not medically accurate (e.g., "the model created an explanation that uses a 1% increase in heart rate." When written mathematically, the explanation is correct. However, when considered from the clinician's perspective, it does not register as physiologically true.

Table 6. Reporting and governance frameworks for healthcare AI

Framework / Guideline	Primary Focus	Application in ICU AI Deployment
DECIDE-AI (Vasey et al., 2022)	Early-stage clinical evaluation and live deployment.	Guides the reporting of human factors, usability, and safety when a model is first introduced to a live ICU environment.
TRIPOD+AI (BMJ, 2024)	Transparent reporting of prediction models.	Ensures that researchers clearly report data handling, missingness, and internal validation metrics for ML models.
PROBAST+AI (BMJ, 2025)	Risk of bias and applicability assessment.	Used to critically appraise AI studies to determine if the predictive model suffers from temporal leakage or selection bias.

As well as a mathematical architecture, the successful operation of AI in clinical practice will require strict compliance with ethical governance, fair algorithmic design, and stringent quality control measures. A recent thorough literature review of the use of AI in the ICU setting revealed a consistent pattern of transition problems from retrospective internal validation to externally validated, highly controlled prospective trials for AI interventions (Von Platen et al., 2020). Dataset shift, or the failure of an AI model when deployed in a new clinical demographic or time period compared with the original training dataset, is a serious risk to our patients' safety and will continue to cause an increase in model drift over time. Additionally, fair algorithmic performance for AI models should be actively monitored through subgroup analysis of clinical performance to identify instances of modeling underperformance and rectify the issue prior to deployment to achieve fair outcomes for all patients, including those from marginalised groups (such as darkly pigmented skin when using pulse oximetry derived from optical sensor data).

Regulatory agencies and academic organizations promote uniform reporting standards to help mitigate the bottlenecks associated with the deployment of AI systems for health care. The DECIDE-AI guidelines outline an organized approach to the initial clinical evaluation of AI-based decision support systems, while stressing human factors, usability, and the monitoring of safety in live clinical practice (Vasey et al, 2022). In addition, two other guidelines have been created, TRIPOD+AI and PROBAST+AI, which seek to provide a common structure for transparent reporting of ML-based predictive models and thorough assessments regarding the risk of bias. Moving forward, the AI implementation science will need to prioritize the completion of prospective "silent trials" (where the model is active in the background without affecting care) prior to completing full randomized controlled trials. Ongoing post-deployment surveillance is critical to identify inaccurate calibration as soon as possible and to avoid harm to patients (Cecconi et al, 2025).

Table 7. Deployment barriers and mitigation strategies in the ICU

Deployment Barrier	Impact on Clinical Workflow	Implementation Strategy
Alert Fatigue	Clinicians ignore AI warnings due to excessive false positives.	Optimize AUPRC over AUROC; implement tiered alert thresholds based on clinical severity.
Workflow Disruption	System requires manual data entry or exists on a separate, non-EHR screen.	Seamless API integration directly into existing EHR dashboards via FHIR standards.
Lack of Clinician Trust	Opaque "black-box" predictions are dismissed by skeptical intensivists.	Integrate XAI (e.g., SHAP visualizations) to provide physiological justification for alerts.
Calibration Drift	Model accuracy degrades as hospital protocols or patient demographics change.	Establish an AI governance committee for continuous post-market surveillance and automated recalibration pipelines.

Figure 6. Multimodal ICU Data Integration Architecture. A layered approach where diverse raw data sources are harmonized, fused via advanced transformer-based AI models, and converted into actionable clinical insights including risk scores, treatment recommendations, and smart alerts

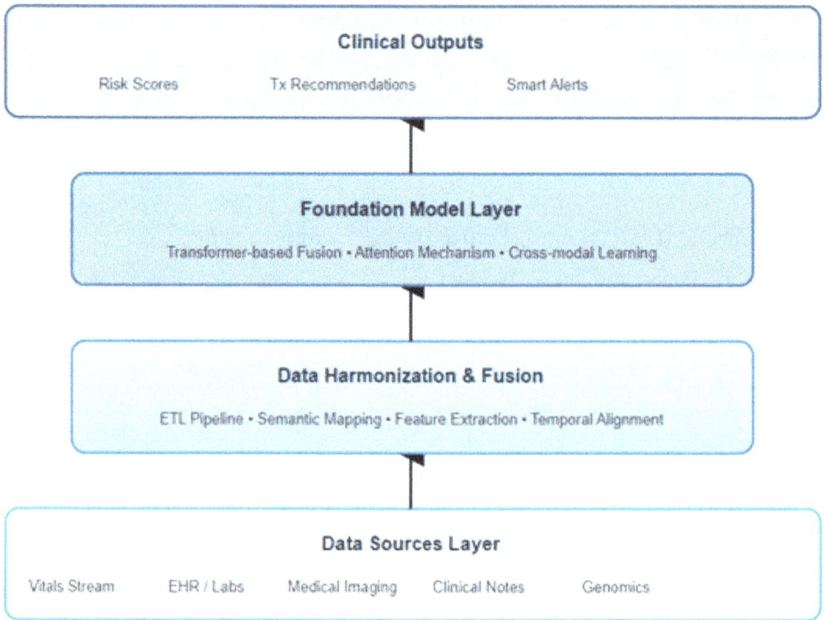

Source: Original architecture diagram created by the authors for this chapter. Design informed by Soenksen et al. (2022), Yang et al. (2025), and Wang et al. (2025)

6 SUMMARY

In the field of respiratory critical care, Artificial Intelligence (AI) is producing a vital and necessary transformation in the fundamental way we practice. By going beyond the limits of human cognitive bandwidth and rigid, rules-based heuristics, sophisticated data-driven algorithms are providing us the opportunity to optimally influence patient trajectories in an incredibly data-rich, high-stake, high-risk environment. As has been described throughout this chapter, predictive machine learning (ML) models utilizing continuous data streams are able to identify undetectable physiological deterioration and respiratory failure hours before clinical collapse occurs, creating a critical opportunity to intervene early. Advanced reinforcement learning and physiologic closed-loop control (PCLC) systems are actively redefining mechanical ventilation from a static and open-loop intervention to a highly dynamic and personalized therapeutic process that minimizes the risk for ventilator-induced lung injury. Additionally, the use of deep learning in the recognition of acute respiratory distress syndrome (ARDS) and the fusion of multimodal data will ultimately lead us to the long-sought goal of precision medicine by allowing us to tailor our therapy to specific biological sub-phenotypes that have been derived algorithmically.

There still remains a significant translational gap from compelling computational benchmarks using retrospective data to safe, operationalized integration of those algorithms at the bedside. The path from retroactively demonstrating superiority through algorithms to proving their clinical efficacy once deployed presents considerable methodological, ethical, and systemic challenges. Algorithms that are accurate retroactively may not be accurate once in practice due to data leakage, extrapolation errors, or dataset shift problems. In order to realize the incredible potential of AI in critical care safely, we need to shift from proliferating isolated algorithms toward implementation science. We must therefore prioritize the use of prospective, multicenter randomized controlled trials designed to assess predictive accuracy, clinical outcomes, human-computer interaction, and workflow integration with respect to the implementation of new algorithms.

To build trust and ensure safety for patients using algorithms in healthcare, it is vital to perform thorough subgroup audit procedures, ensure a reliable external validation process, and employ open and transparent XAI tools (Explainable Artificial Intelligence). Additionally, researchers in this area should focus on achieving interoperability of data and developing standardised structures for electronic health records (EHRs) to facilitate the ability for AI models to be used across multiple hospital systems. While the use of AI in the intensive care unit will not be autonomous or replace the physician, it will augment human intelligence; i.e., a "human-in-the-loop" model that combines computational power with the physician's experience to derive greater precision, safety, and compassion for patients receiving respiratory critical care.

REFERENCES

Beil, M., Proft, I., van Heerden, D., Sviri, S., & van Heerden, P. V. (2019). Ethical considerations about artificial intelligence for prognostication in intensive care. *Intensive Care Medicine Experimental*, *7*(1), 70. Advance online publication. DOI: 10.1186/s40635-019-0286-6 PMID: 31823128

Bellani, G., Laffey, J. G., Pham, T., Fan, E., Brochard, L., Esteban, A., Gattinoni, L., van Haren, F., Larsson, A., McAuley, D. F., Ranieri, M., Rubenfeld, G., Thompson, B. T., Wrigge, H., Slutsky, A. S., & Pesenti, A.LUNG SAFE Investigators and the ESICM Trials Group. (2016). Epidemiology, patterns of care, and mortality for patients with acute respiratory distress syndrome in intensive care units in 50 countries. *Journal of the American Medical Association*, *315*(8), 788–800. DOI: 10.1001/jama.2016.0291 PMID: 26903337

Berkhout, W. E. M., van Wijngaarden, J. J., Workum, J. D., van de Sande, D., Hilling, D. E., Jung, C., Meyfroidt, G., Gommers, D., Buijsman, S. N. R., & van Genderen, M. E. (2025). Operationalization of artificial intelligence applications in the intensive care unit. *JAMA Network Open*, *8*(7), e2522866. DOI: 10.1001/jamanetworkopen.2025.22866 PMID: 40699572

Biesheuvel, L. A., van Workum, J. D., & Reuland, M.. (2025). Large language models in critical care. *Journal of Intensive Medicine*, *5*(2), 113–118. Advance online publication. DOI: 10.1016/j.jointm.2024.12.001 PMID: 40241839

Botta, M., Wenstedt, E. F. E., Tsonas, A. M., Buiteman-Kruizinga, L. A., van Meenen, D. M. P., Korsten, H. H. M., Horn, J., Paulus, F., Bindels, A. G. J. H., Schultz, M. J., & De Bie, A. J. R. (2021). Effectiveness, safety and efficacy of INTELLiVENT–adaptive support ventilation, a closed-loop ventilation mode for use in ICU patients: A systematic review. *Expert Review of Respiratory Medicine*, *15*(11), 1403–1413. DOI: 10.1080/17476348.2021.1933450 PMID: 34047244

Buess, L., Keicher, M., Navab, N., & Maier, A. (2025). From large language models to multimodal AI: A scoping review on the potential of generative AI in medicine. Biomedical Engineering / Biomedizinische Technik. Advance online publication.

Cecconi, M., Greco, M., Shickel, B., Angus, D. C., Bailey, H., Bignami, E., Calandra, T., Celi, L. A., Einav, S., Elbers, P., Ercole, A., Gómez, H., Gong, M. N., Komorowski, M., Liu, V., Park, S., Sarwal, A., Seymour, C. W., Zampieri, F. G., & Bihorac, A. (2025). Implementing artificial intelligence in critical care medicine: A consensus of 22. *Critical Care*, *29*(1), 29. Advance online publication. DOI: 10.1186/s13054-025-05532-2 PMID: 40629428

Chatburn, R. L., & Mireles-Cabodevila, E. (2011). Closed-loop control of mechanical ventilation: Description and classification of targeting schemes. *Respiratory Care*, *56*(1), 85–102. DOI: 10.4187/respcare.00967 PMID: 21235841

Chen, C., Hung, C.-M., Ko, S.-C., Cheng, K.-C., Chao, C., Sung, M.-I., Hsing, S., Wang, J.-J., Chen, C., Lai, C., Chen, C., & Chiu, C. (2022). An artificial intelligence system to predict the optimal timing for mechanical ventilation weaning for intensive care unit patients: A two-stage prediction approach. *Frontiers in Medicine*, *9*, 935366. Advance online publication. DOI: 10.3389/fmed.2022.935366 PMID: 36465940

Gallifant, J., Zhang, J., del Pilar Arias Lopez, M., Zhu, T., Camporota, L., Celi, L. A., & Formenti, F. (2022). Artificial intelligence for mechanical ventilation: Systematic review of design, reporting standards, and bias. *British Journal of Anaesthesia*, *128*(2), 343–351. DOI: 10.1016/j.bja.2021.09.025 PMID: 34772497

Hadweh, P., Niset, A., Salvagno, M., Al Barajraji, M., El Hadwe, S., Taccone, F. S., & Barrit, S. (2025). Machine learning and artificial intelligence in intensive care medicine: Critical recalibrations from rule-based systems to frontier models. *Journal of Clinical Medicine*, *14*(12), 4026. DOI: 10.3390/jcm14124026 PMID: 40565770

Kim, Y., Kim, H., Choi, J., Cho, K., Yoo, D., Lee, Y., Park, S. J., Jeong, M. H., Jeong, S. H., Park, K. H., Byun, S.-Y., Kim, T., Ahn, S.-H., Cho, W. H., & Lee, N. (2023). Early prediction of need for invasive mechanical ventilation in the neonatal intensive care unit using artificial intelligence and electronic health records: A clinical study. *BMC Pediatrics*, *23*(1), 525. Advance online publication. DOI: 10.1186/s12887-023-04350-1 PMID: 37872515

Li, S., Yue, R., Lu, S., Luo, J., Wu, X., Zhang, Z., Liu, M., Fan, Y., Zhang, Y., Pan, C., Huang, X., & He, H. (2025). Artificial intelligence and machine learning in acute respiratory distress syndrome management: Recent advances. *Frontiers in Medicine*, *12*, 1597556. DOI: 10.3389/fmed.2025.1597556 PMID: 40740956

Liu, S., Xu, Q., Xu, Z., Liu, Z., Sun, X., Xie, G., Feng, M., & See, K. C. (2024). Reinforcement learning to optimize ventilator settings for patients on invasive mechanical ventilation: Retrospective study. *Journal of Medical Internet Research*, *26*, e44494. DOI: 10.2196/44494 PMID: 39219230

Misseri, G., Piattoli, M., Cuttone, G., Gregoretti, C., & Bignami, E. G. (2024). Artificial intelligence for mechanical ventilation: A transformative shift in critical care. *Therapeutic Advances in Pulmonary and Critical Care Medicine*, *19*, 29768675241298918. Advance online publication. DOI: 10.1177/29768675241298918 PMID: 39534716

Parreco, J., Hidalgo, A., Parks, J. J., Kozol, R., & Rattan, R. (2018). Using artificial intelligence to predict prolonged mechanical ventilation and tracheostomy placement. *The Journal of Surgical Research*, *228*, 179–187. DOI: 10.1016/j.jss.2018.03.028 PMID: 29907209

Peine, A., Hallawa, A., Bickenbach, J., Dartmann, G., Fazlic, L. B., Schmeink, A., Ascheid, G., Thiemermann, C., Schuppert, A., Kindle, R., Celi, L., Marx, G., & Martin, L. (2021). Development and validation of a reinforcement learning algorithm to dynamically optimize mechanical ventilation in critical care. *NPJ Digital Medicine*, *4*(1), 32. DOI: 10.1038/s41746-021-00388-6 PMID: 33608661

Pinsky, M. R., Bedoya, A., Bihorac, A., Celi, L., Churpek, M., Economou-Zavlanos, N. J., Elbers, P., Saria, S., Liu, V., Lyons, P. G., Shickel, B., Toral, P., Tscholl, D., & Clermont, G. (2024). Use of artificial intelligence in critical care: Opportunities and obstacles. *Critical Care*, *28*(1), 113. DOI: 10.1186/s13054-024-04860-z PMID: 38589940

Sinha, P., Calfee, C. S., & Delucchi, K. L. (2020). Practitioner's guide to latent class analysis: Methodological considerations and common pitfalls. *Critical Care Medicine*, *49*(1), e63–e79. DOI: 10.1097/CCM.0000000000004710 PMID: 33165028

Soenksen, L. R., Ma, Y., Zeng, C., Boussioux, L., Villalobos Carballo, K., Na, L., Wiberg, H. M., Li, M. L., Fuentes, I., & Bertsimas, D. (2022). Integrated multimodal artificial intelligence framework for healthcare applications. npj. *Digital Medicine*, *5*(1), 149. Advance online publication. DOI: 10.1038/s41746-022-00689-4 PMID: 36127417

Tran, T. K., Tran, M. C., Joseph, A., Phan, P. A., Grau, V., & Farmery, A. D. (2024). A systematic review of machine learning models for management, prediction and classification of ARDS. *Respiratory Research*, *25*(1), 232. Advance online publication. DOI: 10.1186/s12931-024-02834-x PMID: 38834976

Vasey, B., Nagendran, M., Campbell, B., Clifton, D. A., Collins, G. S., Denaxas, S., ... & McCulloch, P. (2022). Reporting guideline for the early stage clinical evaluation of decision support systems driven by artificial intelligence: DECIDE-AI. *bmj, 377*.

Von Platen, P., Pomprapa, A., Lachmann, B., & Leonhardt, S. (2020). The dawn of physiological closed-loop ventilation—A review. *Critical Care*, *24*(1), 121. DOI: 10.1186/s13054-020-2810-1 PMID: 32223754

Yang, J., Zeng, S., Cui, S., Zheng, J., & Wang, H. (2025). Predictive modeling of acute respiratory distress syndrome using machine learning: Systematic review and meta-analysis. *Journal of Medical Internet Research*, *27*, e66615. DOI: 10.2196/66615 PMID: 40359510

Chapter 5

AI-Powered Approaches in Lung Cancer Diagnosis and Treatment

S. Harini
http://orcid.org/0009-0008-0300-5081
Department of Microbiology, Sacred Heart College, India

B. Lokeshwari
http://orcid.org/0009-0005-6612-5134
Department of Microbiology, Sacred Heart College, India

P. Saranraj
http://orcid.org/0000-0002-5052-6532
Department of Microbiology, Sacred Heart College, India

Mukesh Kumar Dharmalingam Jothinathan
Saveetha Medical College and Hospital, Saveetha Institute of Medical and Technical Sciences, Saveetha University, Chennai, India.

T. Elavarasi
http://orcid.org/0009-0003-0792-4484
Department of Microbiology, Sacred Heart College, India

P. Gowtham
Department of Microbiology, Sacred Heart College, India

ABSTRACT

Lung cancer accounts for the majority of deaths due to malignancies owing to late diagnosis and high degree of heterogeneity within tumours. Artificial intelligence (AI) has been noted as a game-changer in the field of pulmonary oncology by providing innovative solutions throughout the entire cycle of patient management. This paper aims at reviewing comprehensively the use of AI technologies in the radiomic analysis, pathology, detection, and personalised lung cancer treatment. The principles of AI and theranostics, we will further consider their possible role in imaging and early detection of cancers. Analysis of the theoretical concepts and practices of radiomics will reveal the possibilities of using the technology in

DOI: 10.4018/979-8-3373-7759-9.ch005

extraction of images biomarkers for cancer diagnosis, treatment, and prognosis. Further, the discussion will focus on targeted drugs and personalised treatment approaches through prediction of biomarkers (EGFR, PD-L1), prognosis, response to treatment, and surgical decisions.

1. INTRODUCTION

Cancer that leads to death is lung cancer, which causes 1.8 million deaths per year. The number of deaths caused by lung cancer continues to be significant despite some advancements in treating lung cancer, including the use of immunotherapy and tailored drugs (Sung et al., 2021). The ultimate level of cancer identification and complexity hampers the chances of curing cancer. In general, the theranostic field is dynamic due to the need for enhancing medical interventions. The emergence of artificial intelligence and its innovative applications in the field of theranostics has witnessed a paradigm shift in precision medicine. Artificial intelligence has the potential of addressing many of the challenges in the treatment of lung cancer. Studies show that artificial intelligence has been proven to provide enhanced accuracy in diagnosis, predicting discoveries of genetic markers, and in helping in decision-making processes related to treatment options. These software algorithms might detect trends that cannot be detected by humans (Akter et al., 2025). For example, artificial intelligence-based tumour characterization including automated image analysis, precise tumor localization, robust features extraction, and the prediction of high-risk lesions has significantly boosted the diagnostic process. Through providing a comprehensive assessment based on the uniqueness of each patient, artificial intelligence algorithms are expected to significantly enhance patient risk stratification, thus improving the match of patient requirements and therapeutic interventions. Unveiling possible biological elements that are imperceptible to humans, for example, differences in the sensitivity of tumors to radiation or molecular changes, artificial intelligence-based software algorithms have the potential to revolutionize heterogeneity response predictions (Bilgin et al., 2024).

Utilization of artificial intelligence technology has played a crucial role in transforming the healthcare industry, especially oncology. One thing that seems clear from current trends is that the utilization of precision medicine plays a pivotal role in diagnosing and treatment of different types of cancer. Hence precision oncology will be transformed by using artificial intelligence technologies. This can be regarded as a paradigm shift in the existing practice of oncology as the utilization of precision medicine is sure to lead to better and more precise diagnostic and treatment approaches (Pesapane et al., 2021). In such cases, machine learning and deep learning algorithms come in handy as they have the ability to process highly complex and extensive amounts of data that cannot be done using conventional techniques. Machine learning and deep learning algorithms are best placed in extracting complex patterns from imaging, genomics, and clinical data which ultimately contribute towards improving accuracy and early diagnosis of malignancies. In turn, this makes it possible to intervene in time leading to increased survival rate of patients.

The impact of AI in pulmonary oncology goes beyond diagnosis and imaging to the personalization of therapy protocols. One of the strengths of AI in healthcare is its capacity to analyze multidimensional data that includes genomics, tumor markers, pathologic results, and treatment history in order to build advanced prediction models for patient responses to different therapeutic approaches (Swanson et al., 2023). This becomes even more important in the modern era of targeted therapy and immunotherapy, when the response to therapy is largely dependent on the patient's molecular profile. Through personalization of treatment approaches, the medical field can come up with more efficient approaches without exposing patients to needless toxicity and harm. In spite of these impressive achievements, the first use of artificial intelligence in the field of oncology was met with much skepticism because of several reasonable doubts about its reliability, transparency, and risks associated with possible diagnostic errors. Initially, artificial intelligence applications were confined to conducting elementary image analyses using simplistic machine learning algorithms that necessitated considerable human supervision.

There have been many promising developments in this area, surprisingly little has been done to incorporate artificial intelligence into standard oncological practice. Some of the obstacles that exist in relation to this include those having to do with the problems of generalizability, transparency, and external validity of the models being used. Further, the complexity of the molecular structure of lung cancer makes the development of accurate prediction models particularly difficult. The opacity of some of the deep learning algorithms used in AI systems, often referred to as black box methods, has also proven to be problematic. Furthermore, the majority of these models are built on extremely filtered data sets, which may not be sufficiently representative of the diverse population of patients seen in practice. For instance, if a training data set includes only large and well-defined tumors, the machine learning algorithm could potentially struggle to detect small and less obvious lesions, and therefore fail to detect them altogether. Most published research papers lack an independent validation of the trained model on an external data set, thus contributing to the problem of overfitting (Aberle et al., 2019).

This lack of standardisation for validation procedures, along with variations in performance in diverse clinical environments, only serves to hinder the adoption process in practice. Issues around the ethics of data protection, discrimination, and clinical liability must also be taken into account to promote the safe and ethical use of artificial intelligence systems. As an illustration of the problem in Europe, the regulation for protecting personal data means that data cannot be transferred easily between countries, making it difficult to develop artificial intelligence technology collaboratively. Financial factors also form another major obstacle to AI implementation. While AI technology can offer significant savings in certain medical situations, cost-benefit analysis is still lacking, and many health care institutions do not have the necessary finances and personnel to support AI applications. The objective of this literature review is to give an in-depth evaluation of the current situation regarding the use of artificial intelligence applications in the study and clinical management of lung cancer, specifically considering areas such as diagnosis and therapy (Baumann et al., 2016). In-depth evaluation of the pathological and molecular characteristics of lung cancer to lay the foundation for the subsequent analysis of clinical applicability of artificial intelligence interventions in treating this disease. After that, Artificial Intelligence applications in various areas including screening, disease sub-typing, prediction of response to therapy, and prognosis will be discussed, and current limitations and potential future research directions for these areas explored. Through an in-depth examination of the current status and projection of future developments in the application of artificial intelligence interventions in the management of lung cancer, this review hopes to provide an insight into the revolutionary impact of artificial intelligence in pulmonary oncology research and clinical care.

2. LUNG CANCER FUNDAMENTALS

2.1. Lung Cancer Definition

According to World Health Organization (WHO), lung cancer remains the leading cause of cancer-related death nationwide. Cigarette smoke, environmental contaminants, and occupational carcinogens are the main causes of the disorder, which results in the growth of respiratory systems epithelial cells (Thandra et al., 2021). Lung cancer is often divided into two main categories based on histology. These are small cell lung cancer (SCLC) and non-small cell lung cancer (NSCLC). The two primary types of non-small cell lung cancer, which account for 85% of lung tumours cases, are squamous cell carcinoma and adenocarcinoma. A commonly occurring kind of NSCLC is adenocarcinoma, which is more common in nonsmokers and female patients. It occurs at the periphery of the lungs and originates from glandular epithelial cells (Sartor et al., 2021). Squamous cell carcinoma, on the other hand, is a centrally located subtype near the bronchial airways, thus having an association with cigarette smoking. Another subtype of NSCLC is large cell carcinoma, which is highly aggressive (Sartor et al., 2021).

2.2. Tumor Histology

Lung cancer can be divided into nine forms based on the 2015 WHO histological classification. Postoperative pathological sections are the only way to gather pathology data when CT-guided needle biopsy is not practical (Wu et al., 2016). There is currently no non-invasive way to classify pathology prior to surgery or biopsy. Radiological evaluation employing AI's massive databases provides a preoperative opportunity to classify various forms of pathology, and CT is less costly and non-invasive than pathology. In patients with lung cancer, oncologists are always searching for segments of cancer cells (Haga et al., 2018). Haga et al. classified early-stage NSCLC subtypes among numerous observers using the quantity useful approach.

The AUC for distinguishing lung adenocarcinoma (ADC) from squamous cell carcinoma (SCC) in validation cohorts was 0.893. In a multiphasic CECT study, radiomics models identified ADC and SCC in the unaffected, arterial, and venous phases, with AUC values of 0.857, 0.855, and 0.864, respectively (Chen et al., 2020).

3. AI AND THERANOSTICS: FOUNDATIONAL CONCEPTS

3.1. AI in Theranostics

A lot of imaging data is produced by contemporary molecular imaging techniques. In the end, complex automated techniques and software systems are needed for these data. Since the introduction of initially FDA-approved AI-supported clinical instrument in 1995, artificial intelligence has been incorporated into numerous facets of healthcare procedures. Over 520 AI/ML algorithms have been authorised, most of which fall under radiological and oncological applications (Brosch-Lenz et al., 2021)

3.2. Tumor Dosimetry

The quantity of ionizing radioactive material administered for each unit mass or voxel of organs or tissues is measured by interior rays dosage. Dosimetry-based evaluations offer essential information regarding the goal-based evaluation regarding a therapy's security and effectiveness of every individual through predicting and estimating radiation absorption doses by the target, organ-affected, as well as normal tissue (Bilgin et al., 2024). Though being widely used for radiotherapy clinics, interior dose monitoring is seldom carried out within nuclear-associated therapeutic settings. The intricate fluctuations in radioactive materials inside an organism as well as a laborious procedures involved using standard dosimeter methods were the main causes for this discrepancy. In theranostics, radioactivity frequently comes as a set action dosage or modified according to each individual's weight. Because the absorbed dose is influenced by several well-known external and internal variables, such as physiological half-life, the kind of radium released, biological distributions and ejection rate, tissues weighing parameters, and patient and tumour properties, personalised dosimetry methods are essential (Willegaignon et al., 2023).

These radiation-related destruction of normal cells are generally considered insignificant since diagnostic investigations only employ very small levels of radioactivity. This challenge can be addressed by artificial intelligence-powered learning methods, including reconstructed image neural systems. As an example, DL framework SPECT net, which creates high-quality, noise-free pictures from unprocessed projected information. Using a large dataset of 2D phantoms and an innovative two-step training process, the research shows that their DL-model can generate more clear SPECT pictures in less than a second when compared to conventional reconstruction techniques (Shao et al., 2021). The accuracy and efficiency of dosimetry investigations for theranostics could be greatly improved by using AI-based techniques. It is still necessary to confirm their efficacy and incorporate them into standard clinical procedures.

4. AI IN CANCER IMAGING AND EARLY DETECTION

4.1. Applications of AI in Cancer Imaging

Within the realm of imaging techniques for cancer treatment, AI has become a disruptive technology within this industry due to its ability to develop advanced analysis capabilities that significantly increase the accuracy of image interpretation and enhance predictive models (Ahmad et al., 2024). One of the most promising inventions within the scope of AI technologies applied in the area of imaging techniques in cancer includes radiomics and deep learning algorithms that can provide a much more detailed analysis of tumor characteristics compared to traditional radiology methods. The key idea behind the rapidly evolving science of medical imaging called radiomics is to obtain high-dimensional information based on traditional imaging techniques like CT, MRI, and PET scans. Such features can include different parameters related to shape, texture, intensity, and correlation in space and provide valuable data about the heterogeneity of the tumors.

There is a huge potential in this radiomics research to be applied clinically, particularly in the planning of treatments and prognosis. According to recent research, characteristics taken from CT (computed tomography) scans can reliably forecast the risk of lung metastasis in children with osteosarcoma at diagnosis. Improved decision-making for patient management would lead to better patient outcomes due to the early detection of possible risks, which might lead to better decisions by clinicians (Lee et al., 2020). Besides focusing on modality-specific approaches in medical imaging, AI is providing opportunities for multimodal imaging techniques involving the fusion of anatomic and functional imaging modalities, which would increase accuracy and precision in diagnosing diseases. AI-enhanced PET and MRI have proved to be much more accurate in detecting complex cancer types such as pediatric lymphoma. Minor variations in the tumor size, shape, or density, which could indicate successful treatment or disease relapse, can be spotted through algorithms based on pre- and post-treatment images. The use of AI in cancer imaging is a revolutionary development in the field of oncology (Ardila et al., 2019). AI is revolutionizing the field of diagnostic radiology by enhancing the abilities of radiologists, increasing image quality, and offering predictive information through radiomics and deep learning. This technology can bring about great improvements in cancer detection, treatment planning, and even patient survival in the long run.

4.2. AI in Lung Cancer Diagnosis

The development of AI technology has been groundbreaking in the diagnosis of lung cancer. By tackling important issues related to early diagnosis, medical imaging, and decision-making processes, It might possess a big effect (Lee et al., 2020). A great deal of research evaluating artificial intelligence systems upon CT pictures have mostly focused towards the detection and classification of cancers from radiography, CT, MRI, as well as PET scans. When it involves nodules detection, both mechanical learning and deep learning-based artificial intelligence (AI) algorithms exhibit accuracy on par with or better than radiologists. Because DL algorithms perform better than traditional ML algorithms, most research now focuses on them. Regarding radiologic image comprehension, convolutional neural network models (CNNs) and its variants (DCNN, U-net, 3D-CNNS) are very useful. Excellent sensitivity and specificity enabling the identification for nodule-like on chest CT imaging could be attained by CNN-based simulations learned using sizable imaging databases, especially these coming from the National Lung Screening Trial (NLST). By spotting small lesions that could go unnoticed during manual interpretation, these models allow for early identification and action (Ahmad et al., 2024). As comparing with different CNN-based techniques, deep convolutional neural networks (DCNN) had the greatest effectiveness towards lung tumour diagnosis.

For accurate plans for therapy, involving operative excision as well as radiation administration, AI-powered automatic tumours separation improves diagnosis of the cancer and related physiology. DL-driven classification algorithms were demonstrated to be more accurate and efficient than conventional methods. GANS and U-nets is frequently used within this software. Regarding cancer segmenting,

U-nets along with their variants exhibit remarkable performance (Meeradevi et al., 2025). Crucially, the imaging modalities (X-ray, CT, MRI) can affect how well AI algorithms function. For instance, CNNs which employed acquire knowledge methods performed very well within tumour classification within X-ray scan pictures, whereas U-net derivatives as well as the building of 3D CNNs perform exceptionally well in volume imaging including CT and MRI. Particularly useful is generative AI's ability to produce 3D tumour reconstructions. Excessive computational cost as well as unreliable information represent two drawbacks of generated artificial intelligence. According to recent research, AI may be able to differentiate between histological subgroups of NSCLC based solely on image data. The automated examination of histologic specimens in pathology has been made easier by the combination of DL models and AI-powered whole slide imaging (WSI). These instruments have proven to be able to speed up histological assessments, improve uniformity, and decrease diagnostic variability (Gould et al., 2021).

4.3. AI Application in CT Imaging for Precision Treatment

In addition to predicting the microscopic appearance of tumour lesions, AI can evaluate patients' gene mutations, molecular expression, and prognosis, giving lung cancer patients individualised treatment recommendations (Wang et al., 2022).

5. RADIOMICS IN LUNG CANCER

5.1. Applications of Radiomics in Diagnosis and Treatment of Oncology

Since radiomics was first proposed, a growing number of radiomic research have been published to enhance cancer detection and treatment. An increasing number of research show how valuable radiomic characteristics are as an additional tool for physicians' decision-making. These clinical problems that occur during the whole diagnosis and treatment process in several common cancers, including brain cancer, cervical cancer, cancer of the breast, lung, prostate carcinoma, colon cancer, hepatic cancer, and gastrointestinal cancer (Lambin et al., 2012).

5.2. Overall Procedure for Radiomic Analysis

A comprehensive radiomic analysis process to identify prognostic markers that may be used to forecast patient outcomes. The prognosis characteristic is vector made up of elements that represent important characteristics (Aerts et al., 2014).

This process is comparable to several medical scans (such as CT, MRI, along with PET images of individual tumour patients whom had similar therapy) is first constructed in compliance with radiomic analysis rules. Second, to extract an abundance unique picture characteristics (for example, more than 400), including texture features, medical photographs are divided manually, semi-automatically, or automatically. Third, radiomic characteristics were chosen based on how they have contributed to stabilisation (e.g., test-retest) as well as prognosis (including a the Coxnet-based approach). Fourth, basic thresholding or clustering methods are used to divide the patients into multiple patient subtypes. The averages about a picture's attributes often serve as criteria settings. Lastly, survival studies are used to forecast patient outcomes; important characteristics that indicate prognoses are selected as signatures. Two patients categories separated by a radiomic characteristic may respond differently to the same treatment if their survival curves differ statistically significantly. Thus, there may be a connection between the radiomic traits of the patients and their survival times (Gillies et al., 2016).

5.3. AI in Radiomics of Lung Cancer

Radiology is a computational approach that emphasises obtaining several aspects, including texture, appearance, radiance, along with wave qualities, through clinical images. An in-depth analysis of such features provides specific data upon pulmonary tumours, thereby making identification, prognosis prediction, along with therapy result evaluations easier. The numerous uses of artificial intelligence (AI) towards pulmonary tumour radiation significantly increase the automated nature and quality of image processing (Zhou et al., 2023). One of the primary applications of artificial intelligence within lung cancer-related radiology is controlled segmented images. AI can precisely separate tumour spots within lung pictures with the aid of deep learning techniques, especially convolutional neural networks, which lowers the likelihood of errors and saves time. Medical image segmentation frequently uses structures like U-net and Mask R-CNN, that both show excellent performance in distinguishing cancer boundaries from adjacent tissue features.

The ML techniques are very important for feature selection and extraction. The high dimensional imaging features like shapes, textures, and wavelets are automatically selected using the ML technique and it is done on the basis of the features which have the highest level of importance from diagnostic and predictive purposes (He et al., 2020). The commonly used methods for feature selection are random forest, SVM, and PCA. With the help of AI-based diagnostic support tools and CAD, we can identify the abnormal regions of CT images and can provide areas of interest to the physicians.

The importance of the implementation of AI into medical practice is seen through some popular AI tools, including the systems such as IBM Watson Health and the DeepMind system owned by Google, both having offered solutions contributing to the rapid identification of lung cancer. Prognosis prediction tools based on AI algorithms, including deep learning algorithms, can be used to predict patients' outcomes in relation to the probability of survival, progression, and effectiveness of treatment. For instance, individualized forecasts can be made to facilitate appropriate decision making, which involves combining survival analysis models with imaging data. The role of AI in developing and evaluating personalized treatment strategies cannot be ignored (Zhong et al., 2022).

AI leverages distributed computing and cloud computing technology to deal with the large volume of radiomic data. Scalable tools for analyzing huge amounts of medical imaging data are provided by cloud computing solutions such as Google Cloud and Amazon Web Services (AWS). Being able to detect lymph node metastases within initial stages of non-small cell lung cancer (NSCLC) as well as to improve the precision and effectiveness of lungs nodules identification along with diagnostics through routine scans, AI-driven radiology is crucial (Zhong et al., 2022). Studies utilising artificial intelligence (AI) together combined CT/ PET scans is significantly helping the diagnosis and assessment of non-small cell lung cancer (NSCLC), especially in the identification for unseen metastatic growths in lymph nodes and the prediction of treatment outcomes based on radiomic features.

5.4. Potential of Radiomics for Avoiding Undesirable Complications Caused by Biopsy

Unfavourable biopsy-related outcomes can be avoided with radiomics. Depending on where the tumour is located, a craniotomy or stereotactic biopsy may cause hemiparesis and intracerebral haemorrhage. Fearing a pneumothorax, some patients would decline a biopsy to remove cells underlying a potential pulmonary malignancy (Lucia et al., 2018). Sometimes, as opposed to using an examination to determine a patient's course of therapy, doctors will use the radiomics results. Pancreatic-specific antigens (PSA) testing reduced prostatic malignancy deaths, according to the European Randomised Study of Screening for Prostate Cancer (ERSPC) (Chiu et al., 2017). However, this also significantly raised the number of needless biopsy procedures, that led to unfavourable consequences including fever, haematuria, and hematospermia. Additionally, Fukugai's study discovered that after taking into account the initial biopsy tumour grade supplied by nine different pathologists, there was less agreement between the biopsy and prostatectomy outcomes. Radiomics data can therefore benefit radiologists and pathologists by increasing biopsy accuracy or reducing unnecessary biopsies.

5.5. Perspectives of Radiomics in Radiation Therapy

By classifying patients into many variations, including EGFR as well as non-EGFR instances, through multiple imaging biomarkers, radiology were equipped to rapidly, affordably, and non-invasively forecast patient prognosis depending on detailed data regarding the tumours. Effective radiomics for groupings of patients and biomarker identification may depend on artificial intelligence (Baumann et al., 2016). To characterise carcinoma morphologies or signatures and identify the best course of action when making decisions at each stage of radiotherapy (diagnostic, therapy scheduling, treatments implementation, as well as monitoring), statistical picture-feature modelling for indicators should be developed. The predictive powers of radiomics may be enhanced by AI, particularly machine learning (Peeken et al., 2017). The third-generation wave of artificial intelligence may represent the real-world tasks stage in application of artificial intelligence within radiotherapy because many forms of algorithmic learning technologies were freely available and straightforward to radiotherapy oncologist professionals to utilise. By forecasting radiation outcomes through therapy and toxicity for specific patients, radiological techniques might possess a useful application in accurate medicine.

5.6. Clinical Outcome Prediction

It is difficult to predict the prognosis or response to treatment for lung malignancies. The prospects of those with lung carcinoma receiving standard radiotherapy, surgery, as well specific treatments were effectively predicted using radiology. Distant metastasis and local recurrence are important prognostic variables. Predicting risk variables for these outcomes accurately is crucial (Baumann et al., 2016).

5.6.1. Radiotherapy

Predicting radiation-induced damage and assessing irradiation sensitivity are key components of tailored therapy plans for lung cancer patients. According to Huynh's research, certain prior therapy CT radiographic characteristics may be more accurate than conventional CT indicators in predicting the effectiveness of stereotactic radiotherapy for patients with phases I–II non-small cell lung cancer. Thus, decrease adverse reactions as well as therapy times, using radiological variables for estimating the implications of conventional radiation within stages I to II non-small cells malignancies (Peeken et al., 2017).

Lung cancer patients can receive tailored radiation guidance, improving the security during their treatment, by developing pertinent therapeutic models utilising CT radiometric information. SABR is the recommended therapy to superficially localised stage-1 NSCLC among individuals that aren't suitable applicants to operation. Hypofractionated radiation treatment with an elevated level biological comparable dose is recommended whether SABR is unavailable. The recommended radiotherapy for pulmonary cancer is stereotactic bodies radiotherapy (SBRT), especially for small local tumours in individuals who are incurable. Regarding individuals receiving SBRT, radiologic characteristics have proven to be able to estimate results which could be less achievable using traditional imaging methods. Accurately predicting a range of clinical endpoints, such as survival as a whole disease-free surviving, and local control, has been the focus of numerous investigations (Lucia et al., 2018). For NSCLC treated with SBRT, CT deep computing features have shown promise in predicting therapy failure and directing dose decrease. A classifier comprising nine radiomic features, including initial-order characteristics as well as gray-scale levels co-occurrence matrices (GLCM) texture features, demonstrated a thorough dose-effect interaction in various times following SBRT to distinguish between radiation-caused lung injury (RILI) and local failures. Considering the AUROC, of 0.905, PET-CT radiological characteristics including PET IC2 and CT flatness have also been connected to tumour recurrence following SBRT as well as been shown to be indicative of cancer persistence in exterior confirmation.

5.6.2. Chemotherapy

The RECIST standard, which uses CT imaging, is the main basis for evaluating the effectiveness of chemotherapy for lung cancer. Early chemotherapeutic effects might not be adequately captured by RECIST alone. Based on the amount of remaining tumour tissue, the pathological response following chemotherapy is a better indicator of the treatment's effectiveness and can be used to forecast lung cancer patients' chances of survival. Radiomics can be used to predict treatment results for patients experiencing non-small cell lung cancer (NSCLC), according to several studies (Hellmann et al., 2014). Radiology assessment of thorax main tumours and lymph nodes was used to predict pathologic comprehensive response (pCR) following neoadjuvant chemotherapy-based radiation therapy in 84 individuals with recurrent localised progressed (stage II–III) NSCLC. It was discovered that image-realistic parameters, which describe characteristics like homogeneous of lymphatic nodes and spherical structure of the primary tumour, significantly foresee PCR. Furthermore, compared to radiation parameters underlying a primary tumour, lymph node phenotypic data showed a greater capacity to predict pathology recurrence.

TP compared the tumour pathological response following surgery with the CT imaging characteristics of patients with stage II to III NSCLC prior to neoadjuvant chemoradiotherapy. Total pathological residual lesions were shown to be significantly correlated with a number of distinctive feature (Hellmann et al., 2014). Customised chemotherapy techniques can be guided by the strong association between CT imaging characteristics and the extent of pulmonary cancer individuals' pathologic reaction to treatment. For instance, in patients with limited-stage small cell lung cancer (SCLC) after chemoradiotherapy, the maximum tridimensional tumour thickness were substantially correlated to regional recurrent cancer, distant metastatic growth, and long-term survival. Survival was predicted using CT volumetric characteristics.

The combination of features from peritumoral areas of different distances improved the accuracy of chemotherapeutic responder prediction for patients including non-small cell lung cancer, attaining an AUROC of 0.85. With an AUROC of 0.673, CT-based radiomics, namely the percentage of GLSZM (gray-level size zone matrix) area, showed promise in predicting disease recurrence in patients undergoing radiation therapy within two years after treatment. The AUROC rose to 0.738 when clinical features were added (Cherezov et al., 2019). Additionally, an AUROC of 0.797 for the estimation of effectiveness in small cell lung cancer (SCLC) after chemotherapy was obtained utilising a radiation signature generated from CT scans collected before and following two sessions of chemotherapeutic exceeding predictions using existing clinical characteristics.

5.6.3. Targeted Therapy

Personalised therapy is now an essential therapy option for individuals suffering from lung cancer having driving gene alterations. Radiology assessment of CT images indicates promise for identifying the efficacy of specific therapy for these individuals (Wang et al., 2022). NSCLC patients prior to and following gefitinib-based therapy. From images of 47 individuals who have advanced non-small cell lung cancer, they extracted a number of imaging as well as volume characteristics. An investigation demonstrated that radiomics characteristics at baseline and the minor variations within traits among two examinations might be used to predict EGFR mutation status. This gradual shifts among such features had the best predicting significance, having a region beneath the curves (AUC) ranging from 0.75–0.92.

This study highlighted a correlation among image characteristics as well as cancer manifestations by examining variations in image characteristics before and after targeted treatment in NSCLC patients with different EGFR mutation statuses. In a different trial, the effectiveness of crizotinib therapy among patients with ALK rearrangement NSCLC was predicted using CT imaging characteristics (Mok ct al., 2019). In this study, 481 imaging features were produced by analysing the CT images of 63-stage IV patients. In the end, a test model for PFS prediction was constructed using three imaging features. The model indicates that it is feasible to predict the effectiveness of targeted therapy based on CT images, with an AUC value of 0.824 for progression-free survival (PFS). Lung-related cancer affected individuals and driver gene mutations, CT imaging characteristics may be able to predict the results of tailored targeted therapy. These findings suggest that developing tailored targeted medicines for patients with lung cancer may benefit greatly from CT-based radiomics analysis (Safarian et al., 2025).

5.6.4. Immunotherapy

NSCLC individuals undergoing PD-1 inhibitor therapy for the radiologic evaluation of image characteristics can provide important insights into immunotherapy's efficacy (Meissner et al., 2023). In order to differentiate between immunological inflammation and immune desert tumour immune subtypes, that may detect local CD8+ T cell infiltration in NSCLC patients. With an AUC of 0.76, the framework had a correlation with ORR as well as OS for individuals undergoing immunotherapy with immunologic checkpoint inhibitors. This illustrates how radiomics may be used to assess the localised tumour micro-environment as well as forecast treatment efficacy. In a different study including sixty-eight people associated malignant cancers undergoing combined therapies with palizumab as well as stereotactic radiotherapy (SBRT), low RS tumours were associated with greater rates of local tumour control failure and worse sensitivity to SBRT. Consequently, those with lower RS tumours had lower median OS and PFS (Tunali et al., 2019).

This suggests that RS can assist doctors in predicting those who would gain advantages through combination treatment while preventing immunotherapy adverse effects. Patients receiving ICI for non-small cell lung cancer as well as developed cancerous melanoma provided results to a machine learning classification system for identifying a treatment response utilising radiation characteristic obtained through preliminary treatment improved CT imaging of lesion (Mok et al., 2019). The 1-year survival rates of respondents and non-responding individuals varied, and the model's AUC value for estimating responses to therapy in NSCLC lesion were 0.83. In a previous study, from 228 NSCLC patients in an attempt to predict the onset of high-progressive disease (HPD). According to image characteristics of the tumour core as well as surrounding areas, they created an HPD forecasting system with an AUC of 0.843. The AUC rose to 0.865 when clinical factors were included. In order to identify the internal and peritumoral components of the tumour on 109 NSCLC patients (Liu et al., 2017b).

This HPD predicting framework, that achieved AUC levels of 0.85 as well as 0.96 in the simulated and evaluation datasets, subsequently confirmed how useful from basic radiology indicators for detecting people under possibility of HPD. CT scans, as well as CT/ PET combination images of 195 individuals who had advanced non-small cell lung cancer (NSCLC) in order to distinguish among durable clinical benefit (DCB) as well as no durable clinical benefit (NDB) based on PFS (Mok et al., 2019). The model's AUC values were 0.86, 0.83, and 0.81 in the instruction collection, retrospectively evaluation set, and prospective testing collection, correspondingly. When taken as a whole, these studies demonstrate the value of radiologic assessment for recognising individuals in danger of complications through pulmonary cancer immunotherapy, estimating therapeutic response, and finding immune microenvironment features.

5.7. Treatment Evaluation and Prognosis in Lung Cancer

Evaluation of therapy response is important in lung cancer because it influences treatment choices (Aerts et al., 2014). According to the radiomic signals may be able to predict if lung cancer will return following stereotactic ablative radiation therapy (SART). For individuals who had stage three non-small cell lung cancer. According to their findings, changes in radiomic characteristics brought on by radiation therapy may serve as markers of cancer response. CT radiologic parameters might indicate a pathology recovery after neoadjuvant chemoradiation for individuals featuring sophisticated non-small cell lung cancer (Huang et al., 2016). According to pre-treatment CT radiomic characteristic is linked to gefitinib response and can predict the EGFR mutation status in NSCLC. Numerous radiomic investigations have concentrated on prognosis in addition to therapy responses (Gillies et al., 2016).

6. AI-DRIVEN TARGETED THERAPIES IN ONCOLOGY

6.1. Advancements and Challenges in AI-Driven Targeted Therapies in Oncology

Targeted treatments have become an essential component of precision oncology, with therapeutic alternatives that specifically target the molecular pathways involved in the genesis and spread of cancer (Mondal et al., 2024). Compared to traditional methods like radiation and chemotherapy, these medicines offer improved efficacy and fewer adverse side effects by targeting specific genetic or molecular abnormalities. However, its widespread application in medical facilities is hindered by a number of issues. The adoption of precision medicine is hindered by the inconsistency between patients' genomics and available pharmaceuticals. Many prescription drugs are not optimally utilised due to the lack of connection to genetic biomarkers, stringent qualifications for administration, and poor insurance coverage. In addition, the intricate nature of tumour biology limits the ability to accurately identify targets and formulate therapies, making it difficult to create new drugs. The full potential of precision therapy can only be realised through advancements in drug development and the association between molecular diagnosis and therapeutic interventions. The application of artificial intelligence (AI) is transforming the way such problems are solved by facilitating the synthesis and interpretation of extensive and diverse health information (Mondal et al., 2025a).

The use of AI models to improve patients stratification, accelerate drug discovery, and provide personalized therapy options is increasing. Multi-omics profiling, which includes data from proteomics, transcriptomics, and genomics, is employed by novel techniques such as scTherapy and REFLECT to find therapies that are unique to each individual's tumor biology (Bhuiyan et al., 2025). Furthermore, AI is facilitating the creation of personalized cancer vaccines by predicting the immune response and enhancing vaccine composition, including potent adjuvants for increased immunogenicity. AI also enables tailored treatment plans based on predictive analytics to predict treatment success and possible adverse effects on patients. AI evaluates multiple factors in patients, including imaging, molecular changes, and medical history, to help physicians make better choices regarding medication and decrease toxicity levels. Such progress constitutes a huge leap forward in providing personalized medicine services that adjust to cancer development throughout the disease's life cycle (Tufael & Sunny, 2022). AI applications in oncology face multiple obstacles related to practice, ethics, and technology that need to be overcome. The availability and quality of molecular data matter. Restrictions and legal and ethical boundaries prevent organizations from sharing and implementing patient data even in light of legislation, such as GDPR requirements for privacy in Europe. AI's implementation is complicated by a fragmented system of data labeling and storage.

It is important to maintain privacy as well as allow the benefits of sharing data in science to occur, while at the same time managing patient authorization procedures effectively. Interpretability and transparency of AI systems also matter. It is difficult for patients and doctors to place their trust in results generated by an AI system, mainly because most deep learning algorithms are ambiguous in nature. The explainability of such AI systems must be improved so that the results produced are intelligible to even a layman. This enables one to make wise decisions, leading to greater use of AI-based technology in the clinics. For this purpose, the efforts of AI engineers, cognitive scientists, ethicists, and clinicians must come together to produce better results (Tufael & Sunny, 2022). UQ is another critical issue when using AI in medicine. AI systems can generate high confidence predictions even when there is a mistake in their functioning or training process, which can lead to mistakes during diagnosis and treatments. Quality control of UQ techniques is thus important to determine when to recheck recommendations generated by such algorithms.

In spite of the constant evolution of technology, there may still be structural inequalities and economic pressures that will hinder access to more advanced diagnostics and therapies. More researchers and policymakers have started to call for a change in emphasis from safeguarding the confidentiality of patient data to ensuring that costs and accessibility are equal for AI-powered cancer treatment. One other obstacle that needs to be overcome is the integration of AI functionalities within existing medical processes. While these innovations can enhance decision-making and efficiency, their adoption frequently involves radical modifications to existing procedures. Finally, regulatory barriers make the role more challenging (Bhuiyan et al., 2025). The strict and inconsistently implemented GDPR significantly hinders cross-border data interchange and collaborative AI development in Europe. Stakeholders are calling for new legal frameworks that enhance collaboration while ensuring patient safety and data privacy.

7. AI IN PERSONALIZED THERAPY

Nowadays, the majority of non-small cell lung cancer (NSCLC) treatment focuses on tailored care, which depends on precise patient characterisation to direct particular therapy methods (Wang et al., 2022). The application of AI (artificial intelligence) for estimating genetic alterations, indicator activity, as well as treatment efficacy has been the subject of numerous studies. Immunotherapy and tailored drugs have revolutionised the treatment of lung cancer. AI has important uses in NSCLC tailored care, including prognosis, treatment response, and biomarker prediction.

7.1. AI for Biomarker Prediction

One important indicator used to detect individuals who are expected to gain advantages through immune therapy is the presence of programmed death-ligand 1 (PD-L1). Test results may be enhanced by quick and precise PD-L1 status predictions. AI algorithms have made it possible to assess PD-L1 expression in NSCLC patients non-invasively. These models used controlled learning classifications based upon collected histopathology characteristics using full-slide pictures, including random forest, support vector machines, as well as gradient boosting. To reduce dimensions as well as increase the generalisability of outcomes, choosing features were refined. The use of deep learning process employed logistic regression for feature sorting and a ResNet-50 based baseline for feature extraction. Differentiating among teams was rendered simpler by combining several data sources, such as patient information as well as disease stage (Wang et al., 2022). Biomarker prediction using artificial intelligence for personalized lung cancer therapy. The upper part shows the pipeline of artificial intelligence for biomarker prediction from multicenter patient datasets. The table at the bottom left side shows the performance measures (area under curve, accuracy, and F1 score) for PD-L1 expression, EGFR mutation, ALK rearrangement, KRAS mutation, and BRAF mutation prediction. ROC, precision recall curves, and calibration curves show the ability of the models to discriminate between different classes and their reliability (Safarian et al., 2025).

Additional research using PET/CT-based deep computing radiation has yielded area under the curve (AUC) values ranging from 0.6 to 0.96. The therapeutic utility of AI-driven PD-L1 predictions as a possible additional or replacement instrument to immunohistochemical within therapy choice-making is demonstrated by the fact that multifunctional systems combining the two radiologic as well as medical variables typically beat radiology-only techniques. Status of EGFR Mutations (Felfli et al., 2023). EGFR mutations are another important focus on the therapy of non-small cell lung cancer, and AI has demonstrated encouraging results in identifying their status. Excellent accuracy in prediction has been continuously shown in numerous further investigations, however more validation as well as optimisation are still required (Mok et al., 2019). Figure 1 depicts the role of Artificial Intelligence in predicting biomarkers for personalized lung cancer therapy through the analysis of genomic, imaging, and clinical data. It demonstrates how AI models assist in identifying predictive biomarkers, enabling targeted treatments, early intervention, and improved therapeutic outcomes for patients.

Figure 1. AI-driven biomarker prediction for personalized lung cancer therapy

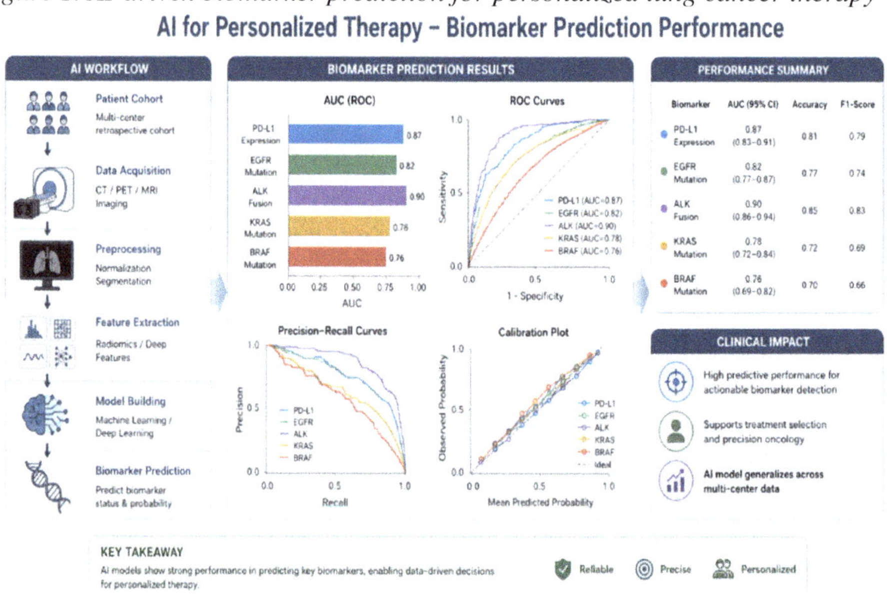

7.2. AI in Predicting Treatment Response

Other models have shown promising results by predicting therapy efficacy using metabolomics, protein biomarkers, H&E-stained slides, and clinical factors. Additional studies have evaluated AI's capacity to predict the responses to induction therapy in locally advanced non-small cell lung cancer as well as pathologically full reaction to neoadjuvant chemoimmunotherapy. These include one-slice as well as full-tumor ROIs were used for histogram analysis (Hellmann et al., 2014). The full-tumor method fared better than one-slice analysis, highlighting the importance of volume evaluation in identifying intrauterine inconsistency as well as facilitating precise, non-disruptive chemoimmunotherapy reaction predictions (Mondal et al., 2025b).

7.3. AI for Surgical and Radiotherapy Decision-Making

AI is increasingly being used to help with difficult clinical decisions about radiation and surgery. Neural networks to predict long-term survival as well as disease development among individuals undergoing stereotactic body radiation therapy (SBRT) to early-onset non-small cell lung cancer (NSCLC) (Zhong et al., 2022; Baumann et al., 2016). Multilabel deep neural networks are being developed to tailor radiation dosages and assess failed therapy hazards based on CT images and clinical data.

8. AI IN MULTI-OMICS

8.1. AI in Lung Cancer Metabolomics

Metabolomics in lung cancer studies have seen great applications of AI, resulting in significant improvements in methodologies used. In this case, the study and analysis of changes in metabolism in people suffering from lung cancer or lung cancer metabolomics need effective management of huge and intricate databases that come from advanced technology such as nuclear magnetic resonance spectroscopy and mass spectrometry (Mondal et al., 2024). This is necessary because the initial database is usually characterized by high levels of noise and complexity. AI has been instrumental in ensuring high quality results through automated data cleansing and denoising. It develops an expansive database by collecting data from various sources, which include urine, tissue, and blood samples. For instance, through the use of autoencoders in machine learning, one can detect important metabolic features and nonlinear differences in patients with cancer compared to healthy individuals, thus increasing the efficiency of data analysis. AI has helped in the detection of biomarkers that play an important role in diagnosis and monitoring treatment. AI detects molecules that have strong links with lung cancers through the application of pattern recognition techniques such as neural networks, SVM, and random forests.

The use of AI through DL models to identify automatically lung cancer subtypes, as well as precancerous conditions, using metabolomics data contributes significantly to both classification and personalized diagnosis. Just like CNN, the accuracy that comes with the use of DL models makes it possible to come up with customized treatment protocols that take into account the metabolism information of patients. Besides, AI is helpful in predicting prognoses from the use of metabolomics data to provide patient outcomes and disease progression forecasts. Prognosis markers are identified, and predictions made concerning the survival time and likelihood of disease relapse (Bhuiyan et al., 2025). This way, AI plays a vital role in aiding customized therapeutic decisions through survival analysis, for example, via Cox regression models. Lastly, AI enhances drug discovery and repurposing through metabolomics to discover target proteins and enzymes, predict drug effectiveness, and explore novel pharmaceutical applications.

9. CASE STUDIES AND CLINICAL APPLICATIONS OF AI IN ONCOLOGY

The application of AI and ML in oncology cannot be ignored since it has affected diagnosis and treatment of cancer, as well as clinical research to a great extent. In fact, the introduction of AI and ML into clinical trials and practice has transformed patient recruitment process, trial design, analysis of data, and even individualized therapy. With the help of such technologies, we will improve precision oncology by making it easier to gain valuable information from complex sets of data, detecting the disease earlier, predicting its course more precisely, and developing customized treatment regimens. Predictive analytics belongs to the important aspects of using AI for oncology (Ardila et al., 2019). The thing is that predictive algorithms can predict therapy response, the course of illness, and patient outcome based on the information about previous clinical cases. Oncologists will be able to develop personalized therapy more confidently (Coudray et al., 2018). In the field of diagnosis, ML-based algorithms proved themselves to be quite efficient when it comes to classification of bone and soft tissue cancers using radiology images. Such skills become highly useful in pediatrics, as tumor manifestations often overlap in children.

MRI sequence analysis using AI has improved diagnostic accuracy to a significant extent, and now healthcare practitioners can handle complex and rare cases with greater ease. Radiomics analysis through the use of artificial intelligence is one more breakthrough as it allows for better early diagnosis owing to the quantitative analysis of medical images (Wang et al., 2022). In the instance of individuals with lung cancer during the earliest stages of the illness, AI-based methods proven to be quite effective in identifying imaging biomarkers indicating the existence of malignancies after analysing radiomic characteristics in CT images. Speaking about detection rates, our algorithm outperformed the traditional interpretations of imaging diagnostics. AI-based systems analyzing mammograms have provided results that can compete with experienced radiologists in detecting breast cancers.

In addition, AI is experiencing rapid advancements in genomic data analysis, thus facilitating the process of therapy selection and personalization. Genetic mutations and markers, which indicate susceptibility or resistance to certain types of drugs, can be determined by advanced AI tools (Zhong et al., 2022). The ability is particularly valuable in the context of clinical trials since therapeutic outcomes might heavily depend on patients' precise matching to targeted drugs. For example, patient response to targeted medications has been positively associated with the guidance of therapy by the AI analysis of genetic profiling. In more than 90 percent of cases, the AI tool was able to offer cancer treatment plans for breast cancer, which aligned with the judgment of experts from tumor boards in a pioneering study based on the use of IBM Watson for Oncology.

The implementation of AI technology significantly enhances the process of recruiting patients because AI uses advanced algorithms to identify suitable patient populations from large databases of electronic health records while analyzing criteria of eligibility. Moreover, AI plays an instrumental role in supporting adaptive trials by analyzing interim trends in the collected data and recommending necessary changes without jeopardizing the scientific integrity of the trial (Zhong et al., 2022). For instance, AI can recommend modifications in drug dosage or terminate the study because of toxic effects. Lastly, AI reveals subpopulation-specific reactions, which are usually unnoticed by traditional statistical methods, during post-study analyses. However, there are several challenges associated with AI integration into clinical oncology.

Another challenge is the data heterogeneity problem. There will always be variation in the format, quality, and completeness of the data sets used in clinical studies, and this could affect model training and generalization. Another concern would be the transparency of AI models. The majority of deep learning systems operate as black box systems, making it difficult for doctors to understand how the system generated its output. Dimensionality reduction techniques must be performed to strengthen the robustness of the models. Collaboration between institutions will be critical in future work to develop large and diverse datasets (Coudray et al., 2018). The use of AI in the field of oncology can only escalate due to efforts by researchers aimed at improving the process and formulating policies to regulate the use (Ardila et al., 2019). This way, the success of the treatment processes will be improved, and its cost-effectiveness guaranteed. A major breakthrough in efforts to make cancer treatment processes more effective involves the use of AI and ML in oncology case studies.

10. CHALLENGES AND OPPORTUNITIES

AI has great possibilities for development, yet several critical barriers stand in the way of its practical application in lung cancer care (Bilgin et al., 2024). The models often go through very limited validation outside the developing laboratory, with poor model generalisability due to variations in imaging modality, patient cohort, and data quality. Problems with robustness were highlighted in some replications, such as the failed replication of a PD-L1 prediction model based on PET/CT radiomics. As many models lack transparency, the "black box" nature of deep learning reduces the confidence physicians have in AI, slowing down the adoption process. There is also an algorithmic bias – models trained on a very specific dataset are unlikely to work adequately in various different populations, especially underprivileged ones. Practical barriers include ethical and legal barriers (such as GDPR restrictions on data exchange and the issue of legal responsibility), as well as availability issues in resource-poor medical care because of the high cost of implementation (Mondal et al., 2024).

Multimodal combination of imaging, genetic and clinical information increases the precision and identifies novel therapeutic targets. With AI, it becomes possible to predict the presence of EGFR mutations and PD-L1 expression using CT and PET/CT scans without performing a biopsy (Baumann et al., 2016). By using techniques such as SHAP and Grad-CAM, explainable AI models can be designed to build the trust of clinicians for better-informed decision-making. Digital twins, as an innovative approach, enable real-time and adaptive therapy customization. Privacy-preserving algorithms such as federated learning not only enhance the generalization capability but also protect the confidentiality of patients' data without any need for centralized data sharing among multiple centers. In the end, through reducing the efforts required for selecting targets, virtual screening, and designing clinical trials, AI helps accelerate the drug discovery process (Felfli et al., 2023).

11. CONCLUSION

AI offers great promise for enhancing lung cancer care through radiomics, personalized therapy, and early detection. Current literature presents favorable results in lung cancer diagnostics, prognosis, treatment efficacy assessment, and biomarker prediction (such as EGFR mutations and PD-L1 positivity). There are still a number of issues that must be resolved, such as inconsistent data, insufficient external validation, poor interpretability, algorithmic biases, regulatory gaps, and excessive expenses. To address current obstacles, cooperation between several centers, standardised procedures, thorough prospective validation, and adherence to reporting requirements like CONSORT-AI and TRIPOD are crucial. In order to support clinical practice, the models must also be comprehensible, multimodal (incorporating data from imaging, clinicopathological, and genetic sources), and intended to support doctors rather than replace them. AI provides the ability to enhance patients' well-being and standard living conditions in tailored lung cancer treatment through proper validation and safe application.

REFERENCES

Aberle, D. R., Black, W. C., Chiles, C., Church, T. R., Gareen, I. F., Gierada, D. S., Mahon, I., Miller, E. A., Pinsky, P. F., & Sicks, J. D. (2019). Lung cancer incidence and mortality with extended follow-up in the National Lung Screening Trial. *Journal of Thoracic Oncology*, *14*(10), 1732–1742. DOI: 10.1016/j.jtho.2019.05.044 PMID: 31260833

Aerts, H. J. W. L., Velazquez, E. R., Leijenaar, R. T. H., Parmar, C., Grossmann, P., Carvalho, S., Bussink, J., Monshouwer, R., Haibe-Kains, B., Rietveld, D., Hoebers, F., Rietbergen, M. M., Leemans, C. R., Dekker, A., Quackenbush, J., Gillies, R. J., & Lambin, P. (2014). Decoding tumour phenotype by noninvasive imaging using a quantitative radiomics approach. *Nature Communications*, *5*(1), 4006. DOI: 10.1038/ncomms5006 PMID: 24892406

Ahmad, P., Xu, H., Nasir, M., & Shen, L. (2024). Deep learning for lung cancer detection: A review. *Artificial Intelligence Review*, *57*(12), 3345–3390. DOI: 10.1007/s10462-024-10807-1

Akter, L., Mondal, R. S., & Bhuiyan, M. N. A. (2025). Artificial intelligence application in public health: Advancement and associated challenges. *Journal of Primeasia*, *6*(1), 1–10. DOI: 10.25163/primeasia.6110325

Ardila, D., Kiraly, A. P., Bharadwaj, S., Choi, B., Reicher, J. J., Peng, L., Tse, D., Etemadi, M., Ye, W., Corrado, G., Naidich, D. P., & Shetty, S. (2019). End-to-end lung cancer screening with three-dimensional deep learning on low-dose chest computed tomography. *Nature Medicine*, *25*(6), 954–961. DOI: 10.1038/s41591-019-0447-x PMID: 31110349

Baumann, M., Krause, M., Overgaard, J., Debus, J., Bentzen, S. M., Daartz, J., Richter, C., Zips, D., & Bortfeld, T. (2016). Radiation oncology in the era of precision medicine. *Nature Reviews. Cancer*, *16*(4), 234–249. DOI: 10.1038/nrc.2016.18 PMID: 27009394

Bhuiyan, M. N. A., Mondal, R. S., & Akter, L. (2025). Advancing cancer imaging with artificial intelligence: Clinical application and challenges. *Journal of Primeasia*, *6*(1), 1–11. DOI: 10.25163/primeasia.6110322

Bilgin, G. B., Bilgin, C., Burkett, B. J., Orme, J. J., Childs, D. S., Thorpe, M. P., Halfdanarson, T. R., Johnson, G. B., Kendi, A. T., & Sartor, O. (2024). Theranostics and artificial intelligence: New frontiers in personalized medicine. *Theranostics*, *14*(6), 2367–2378. DOI: 10.7150/thno.94788 PMID: 38646652

Brosch-Lenz, J., Yousefirizi, F., Zukotynski, K., Beauregard, J. M., Gaudet, V., Saboury, B., Rahmim, A., & Uribe, C. (2021). Role of artificial intelligence in theranostics: Toward routine personalized radiopharmaceutical therapies. *PET Clinics*, *16*(4), 627–641. DOI: 10.1016/j.cpet.2021.06.002 PMID: 34537133

Chen, B. T., Chen, Z., Ye, N., Mambetsariev, I., Fricke, J., Daniel, E., Wang, T., Wong, C. W., Rockne, R. C., Colen, R. R., Nasser, M. W., Batra, S. K., Holodny, A. I., Sampath, S., & Salgia, R. (2020). Differentiating peripherally-located small cell lung cancer from non-small cell lung cancer using a CT radiomic approach. *Frontiers in Oncology*, *10*, 593. DOI: 10.3389/fonc.2020.00593 PMID: 32391274

Cherezov, D., Goldgof, D., Hall, L., Gillies, R., Schabath, M., Muller, H., & Gu, Y. (2019). Revealing tumor habitats from texture heterogeneity analysis for classification of lung cancer malignancy and aggressiveness. *Scientific Reports*, *9*(1), 4500. DOI: 10.1038/s41598-019-38831-0 PMID: 30872600

Chiu, P. K., Alberts, A. R., Venderbos, L. D. F., Bangma, C. H., Roobol, M. J., & Ng, C. F. (2017). Additional benefit of using a risk-based selection for prostate biopsy: An analysis of biopsy complications in the Rotterdam section of the European Randomized Study of Screening for Prostate Cancer. *BJU International*, *120*(3), 394–400. DOI: 10.1111/bju.13913 PMID: 28498624

Coudray, N., Ocampo, P. S., Sakellaropoulos, T., Narula, N., Snuderl, M., Fenyö, D., Moreira, A. L., Razavian, N., & Tsirigos, A. (2018). Classification and mutation prediction from non-small cell lung cancer histopathology images using deep learning. *Nature Medicine*, *24*(10), 1559–1567. DOI: 10.1038/s41591-018-0177-5 PMID: 30224757

Felfli, M., Liu, Y., Zerka, F., Voyton, C., Thinnes, A., Jacques, S., Iannessi, A., & Bodard, S. (2023). Systematic review, meta-analysis and radiomics quality score assessment of CT radiomics-based models predicting tumor EGFR mutation status in patients with non-small-cell lung cancer. *International Journal of Molecular Sciences*, *24*(14), 11433. DOI: 10.3390/ijms241411433 PMID: 37511192

Gillies, R. J., Kinahan, P. E., & Hricak, H. (2016). Radiomics: Images are more than pictures, they are data. *Radiology*, *278*(2), 563–577. DOI: 10.1148/radiol.2015151169 PMID: 26579733

Gould, M. K., Huang, B. Z., Tammemagi, M. C., Kinar, Y., & Shiff, R. (2021). Machine learning for early lung cancer identification using routine clinical and laboratory data. *American Journal of Respiratory and Critical Care Medicine*, *204*(4), 445–453. DOI: 10.1164/rccm.202007-2791OC PMID: 33823116

Haga, A., Takahashi, W., Aoki, S., Nawa, K., Yamashita, H., Abe, O., & Nakagawa, K. (2018). Classification of early stage non-small cell lung cancers on computed tomographic images into histological types using radiomic features: Interobserver delineation variability analysis. *Radiological Physics and Technology*, *11*(1), 27–35. DOI: 10.1007/s12194-017-0433-2 PMID: 29209915

He, K., Gkioxari, G., Dollár, P., & Girshick, R. (2020). Mask R-CNN. *IEEE Transactions on Pattern Analysis and Machine Intelligence*, *42*(2), 386–397. DOI: 10.1109/TPAMI.2018.2844175 PMID: 29994331

Hellmann, M. D., Chaft, J. E., William, W. N.Jr, Rusch, V., Pisters, K. M., Kalhor, N., Pataer, A., Travis, W. D., Swisher, S. G., & Kris, M. G. (2014). Pathological response after neoadjuvant chemotherapy in resectable non-small-cell lung cancer: Proposal for the use of major pathological response as a surrogate endpoint. *The Lancet. Oncology*, *15*(1), e42–e50. DOI: 10.1016/S1470-2045(13)70334-6 PMID: 24384493

Huang, Y. Q., Liang, C. H., He, L., Tian, J., Liang, C. S., Chen, X., Ma, Z. L., & Liu, Z. Y. (2016). Development and validation of a radiomics nomogram for preoperative prediction of lymph node metastasis in colorectal cancer. *Journal of Clinical Oncology*, *34*(18), 2157–2164. DOI: 10.1200/JCO.2015.65.9128 PMID: 27138577

Lambin, P., Rios-Velazquez, E., Leijenaar, R., Carvalho, S., van Stiphout, R. G., Granton, P., Zegers, C. M., Gillies, R., Boellard, R., Dekker, A., & Aerts, H. J. (2012). Radiomics: Extracting more information from medical images using advanced feature analysis. *European Journal of Cancer*, *48*(4), 441–446. DOI: 10.1016/j.ejca.2011.11.036 PMID: 22257792

Lee, J. H., Sun, H. Y., Park, S., Kim, H., Hwang, E. J., Goo, J. M., & Park, C. M. (2020). Performance of a deep learning algorithm compared with radiologic interpretation for lung cancer detection on chest radiographs in a health screening population. *Radiology*, *297*(3), 687–696. DOI: 10.1148/radiol.2020201240 PMID: 32960729

Liu, Y., Stojadinovic, S., Hrycushko, B., Wardak, Z., Lau, S., Lu, W., Yan, Y., Jiang, S. B., Jia, X., Wang, X., & Gu, X. (2017). A deep convolutional neural network-based automatic delineation strategy for multiple brain metastases stereotactic radiosurgery. *PLoS One*, *12*(10), e0185844. DOI: 10.1371/journal.pone.0185844 PMID: 28985229

Liu, Z. Y., Zhang, X. Y., Shi, Y. J., Wang, L., Zhu, H. T., Tang, Z. C., Wang, S., Li, X. T., Tian, J., & Sun, Y. S. (2017). Radiomics analysis for evaluation of pathological complete response to neoadjuvant chemoradiotherapy in locally advanced rectal cancer. *Clinical Cancer Research*, *23*(23), 7253–7262. DOI: 10.1158/1078-0432.CCR-17-1038 PMID: 28939744

Lucia, F., Visvikis, D., Desseroit, M. C., Miranda, O., Malhaire, J. P., Robin, P., Pradier, O., Hatt, M., & Schick, U. (2018). Prediction of outcome using pretreatment 18F-FDG PET/CT and MRI radiomics in locally advanced cervical cancer treated with chemoradiotherapy. *European Journal of Nuclear Medicine and Molecular Imaging*, *45*(5), 768–786. DOI: 10.1007/s00259-017-3898-7 PMID: 29222685

Meeradevi, T., Sasikala, S., Murali, L., Manikandan, N., & Ramaswamy, K. (2025). Lung cancer detection with machine learning classifiers with multi-attribute decision-making system and deep learning model. *Scientific Reports*, *15*(1), 8565. DOI: 10.1038/s41598-025-88188-w PMID: 40075131

Meissner, A. K., Gutsche, R., Galldiks, N., Kocher, M., Junger, S. T., Eich, M. L., Kessing, M., Ruge, M. I., Goldbrunner, R., & Lohmann, P. (2023). Radiomics for the non-invasive prediction of PD-L1 expression in patients with brain metastases secondary to non-small cell lung cancer. *Journal of Neuro-Oncology*, *163*(3), 597–605. DOI: 10.1007/s11060-023-04367-7 PMID: 37382806

Mok, T. S. K., Wu, Y. L., Kudaba, I., Kowalski, D. M., Cho, B. C., Turna, H. Z., Castro, G.Jr, Srimuninnimit, V., Laktionov, K. K., Bondarenko, I., Kubota, K., Lubiniecki, G. M., Zhang, J., Kush, D., Lopes, G., Adamchuk, G., Ahn, M.-J., Alexandru, A., Altundag, O., & Zippelius, A.KEYNOTE-042 Investigators. (2019). Pembrolizumab versus chemotherapy for previously untreated, PD-L1-expressing, locally advanced or metastatic non-small-cell lung cancer (KEYNOTE-042): A randomised, open-label, controlled, phase 3 trial. *Lancet*, *393*(10183), 1819–1830. DOI: 10.1016/S0140-6736(18)32409-7 PMID: 30955977

Mondal, R. S., Akter, L., & Bhuiyan, M. N. A. (2024). Artificial intelligence in drug development and delivery: Opportunities, challenges, and future directions. *Journal of Angiotherapy*, *8*(1), 1–10. DOI: 10.25163/angiotherapy.8810326

Mondal, R. S., Bhuiyan, M. N. A., & Akter, L. (2025). AI-driven innovations in cancer research and personalized healthcare. [Journal of Angiotherapy]. *Integrative Biomedical Research*, *9*(1), 1–10. DOI: 10.25163/angiotherapy.9110321

Peeken, J. C., Nüsslin, F., & Combs, S. E. (2017). "Radio-oncomics": The potential of radiomics in radiation oncology. *Strahlentherapie und Onkologie*, *193*(10), 767–779. DOI: 10.1007/s00066-017-1175-0 PMID: 28687979

Pesapane, F., Codari, M., & Sardanelli, F. (2021). Artificial intelligence and machine learning for medical imaging: A technology review. *Physica Medica*, *83*, 242–256. DOI: 10.1016/j.ejmp.2021.04.016 PMID: 33979715

Safarian, A., Mirshahvalad, S. A., Nasrollahi, H., Jung, T., Pirich, C., Arabi, H., & Beheshti, M. (2025). Impact of [18F]FDG PET/CT radiomics and artificial intelligence in clinical decision making in lung cancer: Its current role. *Seminars in Nuclear Medicine*, *55*(2), 156–166. DOI: 10.1053/j.semnuclmed.2025.02.006 PMID: 40050131

Sartor, O., de Bono, J., Chi, K. N., Fizazi, K., Herrmann, K., Rahbar, K., Tagawa, S. T., Nordquist, L. T., Vaishampayan, N., El-Haddad, G., Park, C. H., Beer, T. M., Armour, A., Pérez-Contreras, W. J., DeSilvio, M., Kpamegan, E., Gericke, G., Messmann, R. A., Morris, M. J., & Krause, B. J. (2021). Lutetium-177–PSMA-617 for metastatic castration-resistant prostate cancer. *The New England Journal of Medicine*, *385*(12), 1091–1103. DOI: 10.1056/NEJMoa2107322 PMID: 34161051

Shao, W., Rowe, S. P., & Du, Y. (2021). SPECTnet: A deep learning neural network for SPECT image reconstruction. *Annals of Translational Medicine*, *9*(9), 819. DOI: 10.21037/atm-20-3345 PMID: 34268432

Sung, H., Ferlay, J., Siegel, R. L., Laversanne, M., Soerjomataram, I., Jemal, A., & Bray, F. (2021). Global cancer statistics 2020: GLOBOCAN estimates of incidence and mortality worldwide for 36 cancers in 185 countries. *CA: a Cancer Journal for Clinicians*, *71*(3), 209–249. DOI: 10.3322/caac.21660 PMID: 33538338

Swanson, K., Wu, E., Zhang, A., Alizadeh, A. A., & Zou, J. (2023). From patterns to patients: Advances in clinical machine learning for cancer diagnosis, prognosis, and treatment. *Cell*, *186*(8), 1772–1791. DOI: 10.1016/j.cell.2023.01.035 PMID: 36905928

Thandra, K. C., Barsouk, A., Saginala, K., Aluru, J. S., & Barsouk, A. (2021). Epidemiology of lung cancer. *Contemporary Oncology = Współczesna Onkologia*, *25*(1), 45–52. DOI: 10.5114/wo.2021.103829 PMID: 33911981

Tufael, A. R. S., & Sunny, A. R. (2022). Transforming healthcare with artificial intelligence: Innovations, applications, and future challenges. *Journal of Primeasia*, *3*(1), 1–6.

Tunali, I., Gray, J. E., Qi, J. D., Abdalah, M., Jeong, D. K., Guvenis, A., Gillies, R. J., & Schabath, M. B. (2019). Novel clinical and radiomic predictors of rapid disease progression phenotypes among lung cancer patients treated with immunotherapy: An early report. *Lung Cancer (Amsterdam, Netherlands)*, *129*, 75–79. DOI: 10.1016/j.lungcan.2019.01.010 PMID: 30797495

Wang, S., Yu, H., Gan, Y., Wu, Z., Li, E., Li, X., Chen, J., Liu, S., Zhang, L., Lang, J., Tian, J., Liang, C., & Liu, Z. (2022). Mining whole-lung information by artificial intelligence for predicting EGFR genotype and targeted therapy response in lung cancer: A multicohort study. *The Lancet. Digital Health*, *4*(5), e309–e319. DOI: 10.1016/S2589-7500(22)00024-3 PMID: 35341713

Willegaignon, J., Fernandes, S. C. P., Pelissoni, R. A., Coura-Filho, G. B., Sapienza, M. T., & Buchpiguel, C. A. (2023). Radiation safety measures in diagnostic nuclear medicine, based on the potential radiation dose emitted by radioactive patients. *Radiologia Brasileira*, *56*(1), 13–20. DOI: 10.1590/0100-3984.2022.0064 PMID: 36926359

Wu, W., Parmar, C., Grossmann, P., Quackenbush, J., Lambin, P., Bussink, J., & Aerts, H. J. W. L. (2016). Exploratory study to identify radiomics classifiers for lung cancer histology. *Frontiers in Oncology*, *6*, 71. DOI: 10.3389/fonc.2016.00071 PMID: 27064691

Zhong, Y., She, Y., Deng, J., Chen, S., Wang, T., Yang, M., Ma, M., Song, Y., Qi, H., Wang, Y., Chen, J., Ye, X., Chen, C., & Xie, D. (2022). Deep learning for prediction of N2 metastasis and survival for clinical stage I non-small cell lung cancer. *Radiology*, *302*(1), 200–211. DOI: 10.1148/radiol.2021210902 PMID: 34698568

Zhou, J., Hu, B., Feng, W., Zhang, Z., Fu, X., Shao, H., Chen, W., Li, W., & Yu, H. (2023). An ensemble deep learning model for risk stratification of invasive lung adenocarcinoma using thin-slice CT. *NPJ Digital Medicine*, *6*(1), 119. DOI: 10.1038/s41746-023-00866-z PMID: 37407729

Chapter 6

AI in Pulmonary Oncology:

Early Detection, Personalized Therapy, and Radiomics

B. Lokeshwari
http://orcid.org/0009-0005-6612-5134
Department of Microbiology, Sacred Heart College, India

P. Saranraj
http://orcid.org/0000-0002-5052-6532
Department of Microbiology, Sacred Heart College, India

Prithiviraj Nagarajan
Aarupadai Veedu Medical College and Hospital, Vinayaka Mission's Research Foundation (Deemed to be University), Puducherry, India

A. Vidhya
Department of Microbiology, D.K.M. College for Women, Vellore, India

J. Reshma
Department of Biochemistry, Sacred Heart College, India

S. Kanshiya
Department of Biochemistry, Sacred Heart College, India

ABSTRACT

Artificial Intelligence (AI) is drastically reshaping pulmonary oncology with its capability of delivering precise, efficient, and tailored solutions to manage lung cancer cases. AI plays an important role in achieving precision medicine solutions, which involves optimizing treatment and managing immunotherapy and radiation therapy planning, as well as prognosis and survival prediction and treatment monitoring. Despite these advancements, challenges such as data quality, interpretability, ethical concerns, and regulatory issues remain significant barriers to clinical implementation. Emerging technologies including explainable AI, federated learning, and

DOI: 10.4018/979-8-3373-7759-9.ch006

AI-driven digital twins are expected to further revolutionize pulmonary oncology. This chapter shows that AI has the potential to significantly enhance early detection, improve diagnostic accuracy, enable personalized therapy, and ultimately transform clinical outcomes in lung cancer management.

1. INTRODUCTION

Despite the progress made in diagnostic and therapeutic modalities, lung cancer continues to be among the main contributors to cancer-associated deaths in the world. The heterogeneity, late-stage presentation, and inconsistent treatment responses to therapy have resulted in poor prognoses and outcomes associated with this type of cancer (Saul et al., 2020). The traditional means of diagnosing and assessing lung cancer include imaging and histopathology-based approaches, which are hindered by their low specificity, sensitivity, and limited scalability. Therefore, new solutions that can help detect, diagnose, and provide treatment plans for patients with this cancer are urgently needed. Artificial Intelligence (AI) technologies have gained momentum in the medical field owing to their potential to solve the existing challenges associated with pulmonary oncology (Siegel et al., 2019).

The term Artificial Intelligence refers to several types of computational methods that allow for simulating human cognitive functions such as learning, reasoning, and decision-making. Recently, the development of AI in the health care sector experienced impressive advancements with oncology serving as a good example. Namely, huge amounts of data can be generated with the help of different imaging, genomics, and electronic health records and thus analyzed (Shafiq-Ul-Hassan et al., 2018). ML and DL in particular are known to provide amazing performance when it comes to pattern identification and automation of specific activities. They are perfect for treating lung cancer because they involve early diagnosis through imaging, proper tumor classification, and individualized treatment.

This chapter provides a comprehensive overview of the applications of AI in pulmonary oncology, spanning the entire continuum of care from early detection to treatment monitoring and prognosis. It explores the fundamental concepts of AI in healthcare, the role of big data, and the integration of advanced computational techniques in lung cancer diagnosis and treatment. (She et al., 2018) Additionally, it highlights emerging trends such as radiomics, multi-omics integration, and AI-driven personalized medicine, while addressing the ethical, regulatory, and technical challenges associated with clinical implementation. Through this discussion, the chapter aims to demonstrate how AI can transform lung cancer management and contribute to improved patient survival and quality of life (Souza et al., 2023).

2. FUNDAMENTALS OF ARTIFICIAL INTELLIGENCE IN HEALTHCARE

AI in healthcare can be referred to as algorithms and models that can analyze complex health data, find patterns, and help with clinical decision-making. Due to the increased volume of electronic health data, images, and omics data, it has become necessary to develop new approaches in data processing and analysis as the process cannot be completed by using statistical models only. AI brings the necessary technology for the data processing and analysis and becomes quite important in enhancing patient care services. Artificial intelligence has gained greater importance in pulmonary oncology as the field is characterized by complex and voluminous data on lung cancer (Sujit et al., 2024).

The purpose of artificial intelligence software in the medical field is to develop and learn according to analysis and improve its skills based on experience and not necessarily by programming. The development of artificial intelligence in the oncology domain becomes possible thanks to increased computational ability, the availability of large data sets with descriptions, and better algorithms. Artificial Intelligence applications in the treatment of lung cancer can involve image analysis, detection of tumor existence, prediction of risks, and evaluation of therapy (Tunali et al., 2019). By using such technologies, one can not only avoid mistakes and save time but also improve work processes in clinics. Artificial Intelligence makes it possible to obtain and analyze large amounts of information and combine multiple data sources, such as radiographic images, microscopic slices, genetic analysis results, and case histories. In other words, this approach integrates tumor and patient data, which is a critical stage on the way to creating a personalized medicine policy for all patients (Vaid et al., 2021).

2.1 Types of Artificial Intelligence

The Artificial Intelligence technique can be grouped into various kinds depending on its operational capabilities. The common kinds applied in the healthcare industry are machine learning, deep learning, and neural networks. While these techniques differ in their technical details, they all contribute immensely to the development of AI in healthcare. Machine Learning, which falls under the group of AI, is an algorithm that learns from a supplied dataset and uses the information to make predictions and decisions. There are numerous ways of doing this in machine learning, such as regression, classification, clustering, and ensemble. In the case of lung cancer research, Machine Learning is applied as a prediction and classification technique (Wang et al., 2021).

Such models demand well-structured data and feature engineering where proper features need to be selected and engineered so that the algorithm performs well. On the other hand, deep learning can be seen as the evolution of machine learning because deep learning employs multilayered neural networks. It has been proven that convolutional neural network models in deep learning have produced remarkable results for tasks related to computer vision such as the identification of objects and their localization in medical images. In particular, deep convolutional neural networks perform excellently when it comes to detecting and segmenting lung nodules in CT images. Unlike traditional machine learning models, no feature engineering is required for deep learning.

2.2 Key AI Techniques Used in Oncology

The use of AI technology in the domain of oncology includes the application of diverse learning algorithms which have the capability of dealing with different types of data to deal with clinical issues. One of the common techniques in the application of AI in oncology includes supervised learning whereby machine learning algorithms are trained using labeled data sets in order to identify relationships between input and output data (Xu et al., 2019). This learning algorithm is useful in tumor classification through the use of labeled image or histopathology data sets in teaching machines about the differentiation between benign and malignant tumors. Another type of learning algorithm is unsupervised learning which does not require labeled data in identifying patterns within data sets.

Unsupervised learning will be helpful in discovering previously unknown relationships in the data and hence help develop a greater appreciation of the heterogeneity of the tumor and its process of formation. Reinforcement learning is another technique in artificial intelligence in which models are trained on how to act based on feedback from interactions with the environment and the feedback being positive or negative. In cancer studies, reinforcement learning has been used to discover the appropriate sequence for administering drugs or radiation treatments (Yu et al., 2018).

2.3 Role of Big Data in Cancer Research

Big data has been critical in improving the role of artificial intelligence in research on cancer. The term big data in medicine refers to large and complex data collected from various sources such as electronic health record, imaging modalities, genomics, and wearable devices (Zhang et al., 2021). Big data provides a useful source of information for optimizing cancer detection, treatment, and prevention. For example, regarding lung cancer studies, big data helps to acquire multi-dimensional information that allows researchers to examine the relationships between changes in genetic information and imaging information. However, the use of big data algorithms will solve such a challenge because the algorithm can provide information that cannot easily be achieved using the traditional method of collecting information. Specifically, analysis of radiological information and genomic information will lead to identification of certain biomarkers, which arise as a result of genetic changes. Despite being associated with many benefits, the use of big data has various challenges, including heterogeneous nature of big data, data privacy, and standardization of data (Tizhoosh and Pantanowitz, 2018).

3. AI IN EARLY DETECTION OF LUNG CANCER

The early detection of lung cancer is a crucial factor contributing to the increase in the number of people surviving after being diagnosed with this disease. The sooner the condition is identified, the better are the chances of positive outcomes during treatment. However, early-stage lung cancer does not have any symptoms that can be used for its recognition through traditional methods. One of the effective ways to address the discussed challenge is the use of AI for lung cancer early diagnosis. AI assists in attaining this purpose by analyzing the results of imaging tests and finding out specific signs that indicate lung cancer (Topol, 2019). Advanced techniques for imaging, particularly computed tomography and low-dose computed tomography, facilitate obtaining high-quality pictures and detecting nodules in them. The second solution is related to the creation of predictive risk models which identify people at high risk of contracting this type of cancer. The process of making predictions with the help of such models involves the consideration of various parameters such as demographic, clinical, and lifestyle factors (Subramanian and Simon, 2010).

3.1 AI-Based Imaging Techniques

The use of AI to aid in imaging is among the greatest breakthroughs in the early detection of lung cancer. Such technologies employ machine learning and deep learning techniques to perform image analysis to help detect abnormalities accurately. Computerized tomography (CT) scan and low-dose computerized tomography (LDCT) scans are common in lung cancer screening since they can create an image of the structure of the lung and help identify any nodule. Studies show that deep learning technologies, especially convolutional neural networks, have shown remarkable success in performing image analysis such as nodule detection, classification, and segmentation (Silva et al., 2018). Convolutional neural networks allow automatic feature learning from raw medical images, thus avoiding manual feature engineering. Such deep learning models allow for more accurate and consistent analysis of medical images than conventional methods. Not only are such algorithms able to detect abnormalities in the lungs, but they are also capable of performing image assessments to determine the characteristics of lung nodules like size and texture to predict the possibility of malignancy (Smeltzer et al., 2020).

3.1.1 Role of CT scans and Low-Dose CT (LDCT)

The importance of computed tomography (CT) examinations cannot be understated in the early detection and assessment of lung cancer as it provides high-quality cross-sectional images of the thoracic cavity. The use of CT examinations is highly valuable for detecting early signs of lung cancer since CT scanning allows observing detailed images of lung parenchyma, airways, and vessels. As a result, the possibility of diagnosing small pulmonary nodules, which can indicate a malignancy at an early stage of its development, becomes real. Thus, CT scanning has contributed significantly to improving sensitivity for lung cancer detection. Nevertheless, one of the main disadvantages of using CT examination is its high radiation dosage (Singh et al., 2020). Consequently, routine use of this method in population screening is limited due to the increased risk associated with excessive radiation exposure. For instance, CT examination is not recommended for people without symptoms of the disease to avoid adverse side effects. Low-dose computed tomography (LDCT) has become a preferred method for assessing lung cancer due to low radiation dosage used in this technique (Sollini et al., 2017).

Various large clinical studies have proved that the use of low-dose CT screenings results in a lower rate of deaths caused by lung cancer because the earlier diagnosis allows treating this type of malignancy on the early stages. However, although LDCT screenings have many benefits, they also pose several problems for healthcare professionals and patients. For example, the main disadvantage of the technique is the identification of numerous indeterminate nodules resulting in the need for additional tests and even treatment for non-malignant lesions. Artificial intelligence algorithms based on deep learning can successfully analyze CT images and identify nodules. Thus, this innovation helps radiologists to decrease the time required to interpret the scans, as well as minimize the potential human errors in the analysis process. Moreover, AI algorithms are able to measure different characteristics of nodules such as shape, size, and density (Saba et al., 2019).

3.1.2 AI Algorithms for Nodule Detection and Classification

The use of AI algorithms in lung nodule detection and classification has played a pivotal role in improving the sensitivity and specificity of detecting nodules in an individual, thereby addressing one of the major challenges encountered while diagnosing lung cancers. The traditional radiologic evaluation of patients is hampered by the observer variability and inability to identify smaller and less obvious nodules in a high-throughput manner (Sun et al., 2016). The use of AI algorithms based on deep learning models makes the detection and classification of nodules possible, with high sensitivity and specificity. Such algorithms are trained using datasets consisting of CT scans from thousands of patients and hence are capable of recognizing subtle patterns indicative of malignant and benign nodules. The convolutional neural network models have been found to be highly sensitive when compared to other models owing to their ability to extract spatial hierarchy information (Wang and Summers, 2012; Villaruz and Socinski, 2013).

3.1.3 Computer-Aided Detection (CAD) Systems

Computer-Aided Detection (CAD) stands out as one of the first AI applications within the field of radiology that has been undergoing constant development thanks to advanced machine learning technologies. The key feature of CAD is the automatic detection of suspicious spots on imaging tests, such as lung nodules. In essence, CAD can be seen as a second set of eyes that helps detect anomalies that could otherwise go unnoticed. Modern CAD tools employ advanced deep learning algorithms that allow for the accurate detection of any lung anomalies (Wang et al., 2021). Furthermore, CAD technologies possess the capability to classify patients in terms of their risk groups, thus helping radiologists focus their attention on patients at the highest risk. Despite the numerous advantages of CAD, some challenges remain, such as the possibility of false positives and interoperability issues with other medical equipment. However, the ongoing advancements in AI technology help address these challenges. With continued improvements in CAD performance, these tools are expected to become a necessary part of lung cancer screening and diagnosis processes in the near future (Wu and Hicks, 2021).

3.1.4 Deep Learning Models for Image Segmentation

The process of image segmentation is crucial when it comes to interpreting images since it requires detecting the outlines of different organs and diseases. Deep learning techniques have proved to be particularly helpful in segmenting images with incredible precision, and FCNs and U-Nets have demonstrated exceptional performance in this regard. It is important to note that the method used by the mentioned algorithms entails assigning a special label to each pixel of the picture, which helps the machine recognize the tumor tissue from its healthy surroundings (Xu et al., 2019). Besides, image segmentation is an important step in preparing a patient for treatment since it allows doctors to accurately detect and treat tumors without causing damage to healthy tissues through radiotherapy. Moreover, segmentation becomes possible due to deep learning algorithms saves much time and effort that would otherwise have been required to manually mark images, which is often an onerous task that might differ across physicians. Yet another benefit associated with the implementation of AI in segmentation refers to the possibility of conducting a quantitative assessment of tumors in terms of their size and growth rates (Yip and Aerts, 2016).

3.2 Screening and Risk Prediction Models

The implementation of artificial intelligence for screening and predicting risks has changed the methodology of preventive measures and early detection of lung cancer because of the introduction of customized predictive models. Conventional methods of screening may employ general indicators, like age and smoking history, to predict risk levels, but there are limitations to this strategy since the individual characteristics are overlooked. The use of AI in risk prediction takes into consideration various aspects, such as clinical factors, imaging features, genetics, and lifestyle behaviors, to make more accurate predictions of potential risks. The use of machine learning algorithms helps in analyzing extensive data sets and detecting any patterns linked to lung cancer development (Yu et al., 2018). This kind of an approach ensures that the right people are intervened upon without having to go through all sorts of unnecessary procedures. Another benefit of using AI-based screening techniques is that they may also be used in public health initiatives that would ensure optimal resource utilization. With the help of AI screening tools, those patients who will greatly benefit from screening will be identified and appropriate action will be taken on their cases. With the advancement of technology, it is very likely that AI will have a prominent role in screening protocols in the future (Zhang et al., 2021).

3.2.1 AI-Based Risk Stratification Tools

The role of risk stratification in lung cancer screening cannot be underestimated as it allows classifying patients according to their risks of suffering from the disease. AI applications in this area involve the use of algorithms aimed at analyzing data sets and creating personalized risk scores. This type of tool accounts for a variety of elements that include demographic data, environmental factors, genetics, imaging.

Logistic regression, random forests, and gradient boosting are some of the machine learning models applied to build predictive models of lung cancer risks. It helps health care providers provide customized screening and preventive care for each patient. This helps the predictions made by these tools stay accurate at all times. Finally, the use of AI tools in risk stratification allows moving toward precision medicine (Zhao et al., 2018).

3.2.2 Predictive Models for High-Risk Populations

Models that have been specifically developed for high-risk populations are key elements in predicting and preventing lung cancer in patients. Such models concentrate on pinpointing those patients who have high chances of developing lung cancer due to certain factors that include smoking, carcinogenic exposures at the workplace, and a history of cancer in their family. Predictive tools based on artificial intelligence have been successful in incorporating these factors with other relevant information to produce predictions about the onset of cancer among high-risk populations. The identification of high-risk individuals will enable medical personnel to undertake various interventions that include regular screening and changes in lifestyle to lower the burden of disease in the community. Predictive models will also enable the evaluation of screening interventions to support evidence-based decision making. The analysis of data from populations using AI technologies will help in developing optimal screening strategies for maximum benefit. As these models develop further, they will become important in lowering the rate of lung cancers (Tizhoosh and Pantanowitz, 2018).

3.3 Liquid Biopsy and Biomarker Detection

Liquid biopsy is an innovative diagnostic technique for detecting cancer without surgical intervention, which is based on testing biological substances in the patient's blood and other fluids. Artificial intelligence has contributed greatly to the development of liquid biopsy technology, allowing for the examination of complicated molecular data and making early-stage lung cancer detection more efficient. There are multiple benefits of this method compared to conventional tissue biopsy, such as lower risks, the possibility of repeated analysis, and identification of the genetic differences of the malignant tumors. AI algorithms help researchers analyze liquid biopsy results and interpret molecular changes in ctDNA, CTCs, and other markers of cancer. With the help of AI that incorporates data from liquid biopsies along with images and other clinical factors, one can have a comprehensive way of diagnosing lung cancer. Also, the use of artificial intelligence in biomarker discovery could result in the identification of new markers for lung cancer. Liquid biopsy techniques, in particular, will become even more critical in the future (Topol, 2019).

3.3.1 AI in Circulating Tumor DNA (ctDNA) Analysis

One of the key components of liquid biopsy is the analysis of circulating tumour DNA (ctDNA), which aids in comprehending the genetic modifications associated with lung cancer. It contains genes from the cancerous tumour which have been excreted into the blood stream. Artificial intelligence is vital for the interpretation of ctDNA since it usually involves complicated and noisy data. The DNA pattern recognition method aids in identifying patterns in the DNA sequence and separates normal noise from cancer-related DNA changes. Such models could detect rare mutations that could be potential markers for early stage cancers, thus enhancing the accuracy of screening. In addition, AI technology can also monitor any changes in the ctDNA, helping understand the evolution of tumors and their responses to different treatments. Moreover, AI applications to ctDNA analysis can also be used to create predictive models that can be used to forecast disease progression and treatment outcomes (Subramanian and Simon, 2010).

3.3.2 Early Detection Through Blood-Based Biomarkers

The use of blood-based biomarkers is an exciting new opportunity in the early diagnosis of lung cancer, particularly when combined with AI technology. These markers include proteins, metabolites and nucleic acids that play a role in the development of cancer disease. Using machine learning algorithms, data from the biomarkers can be analyzed to look for disparities between patients and healthy individuals. The machine learning approach to the data analysis allows for a more accurate diagnosis based on multiple marker signatures, not on a single biomarker. Combining the data from different sources through AI makes it possible to enhance both sensitivity and specificity. This factor is crucial in detecting cancer disease at an early stage because even small molecular changes can be hardly diagnosed using traditional techniques. Moreover, the use of biomarkers examined via machine learning can help develop non-invasive screening tests (Silva et al., 2018).

3.3.3 Integration of Omics Data

The combination of omics data like genomics and proteomics is a valuable method that will help understand lung cancer at the molecular level. This type of research provides us with a more comprehensive understanding of the development of tumors and how they can be treated on an individual basis. Proteomics is the study of proteins and genomics the study of genetics and mutations, and how they are expressed. Such algorithms will help identify biomarkers and pathways that lead to the development of lung cancer. Furthermore, this technology could result in identification of new treatment modalities and a better knowledge of the disease's mechanism. By integrating all the data acquired from omics research, clinical and imaging data, a comprehensive strategy can be created for lung cancer diagnosis, treatment, and monitoring disease progression. With further development of the techniques used in omics studies, their synergy with artificial intelligence will produce groundbreaking results in the field of pulmonology (Smeltzer et al., 2020).

3.4 Challenges in Early Detection

While significant advances have been made with AI-driven early detection tools, there are still challenges to be addressed when it comes to clinical application. The first challenge to implementing AI technology has to do with the collection of large amounts of high-quality data that will be used as input in the training of the model. The predictive capacity and validity of AI algorithms could be affected by variations in patient demographics and differences in image acquisition protocols. In addition, there is always the possibility of overdiagnoses and misinterpretations of the results, resulting in unnecessary treatment procedures and financial losses. Artificial intelligence algorithms have improved the predictive power of prediction models to a great extent, but reliability and consistency (Singh et al., 2020) play an important part. The integration of AI-based systems into the existing workflow process is another challenge that needs to be addressed in order to implement AI successfully. Usability and interoperability should be considered while creating new diagnostic tools since it will facilitate future adoption. Moreover, ethical and privacy issues also need to be considered while implementing artificial intelligence in medicine. Data security and confidentiality should be ensured while applying AI solutions to diagnose lung cancer (Sollini et al., 2017).

4. AI IN DIAGNOSIS AND TUMOR CLASSIFICATION

Accurate diagnosis and classification of lung cancer are crucial in the selection of appropriate treatment methods and to achieve optimal outcomes. The traditional diagnostic methods rely on imaging tests, pathological tests and molecular tests, which are very efficient but require a certain amount of time to complete and may give divergent results in different doctors. Artificial Intelligence technology proves extremely useful when aiming at increasing the accuracy of diagnosing because it helps automatize the process and avoid mistakes made by a person (Saba et al.,

2019). They can be especially useful in differentiating the various histological types of lung cancer, including adenocarcinoma, squamous cell carcinoma, and small cell lung cancer. AI can aid in more precise classification to facilitate personalized treatment planning and clinical decision-making.AI can help with better classification, which can lead to more personalized treatment plans and improved clinical decision-making. In addition, AI-powered diagnostic tools can help streamline clinical workflows by automating repetitive tasks, like image analysis and report generation. This will help to ease the workload of health care providers while, at the same time, providing consistency and reproducibility for diagnostic results. With the ongoing development of AI technologies, their application in clinical practice is anticipated to greatly enhance the efficiency and accuracy of lung cancer diagnosis (Sun et al., 2016). Figure 1 illustrates the application of Artificial Intelligence in lung cancer diagnosis and tumor classification, highlighting how AI algorithms analyze medical imaging and clinical data to detect abnormalities with high accuracy. It also demonstrates the role of machine learning and deep learning techniques in differentiating tumor types, enabling early diagnosis, precise classification, and improved decision-making in personalized cancer treatment.

Figure 1. Artificial intelligence in lung cancer diagnosis and tumor classification

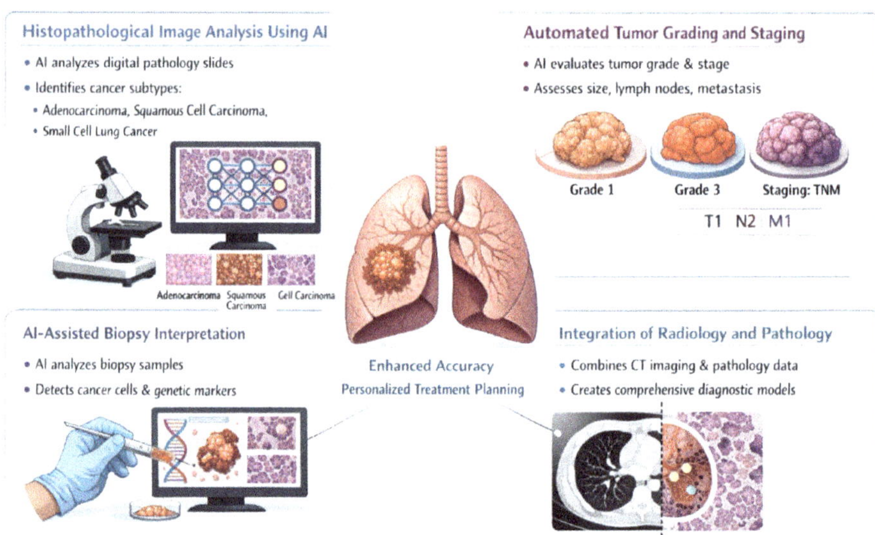

4.1 Histopathological Image Analysis Using AI

Histopathology remains the gold standard diagnostic tool when it comes to the diagnosis of cancers and provides useful insights into the physical characteristics of tumors and cells. However, the traditional method of examining histopathology slides is laborious and can be subject to inter-observer variability. In the field of medical science, AI has made a significant impact by automating the analysis of images captured using digital pathology, thereby enabling faster and more accurate diagnoses. Deep learning algorithms, especially convolutional neural networks, are extensively applied in analyzing histopathology images. The deep learning algorithm can identify certain cellular characteristics, such as the presence of nuclear atypia, mitosis, and architectural patterns, that are important to cancer diagnosis. AI models can be used to classify tissue samples as either benign or malignant and identify the specific cancer types. AI models help to enhance the accuracy of diagnosis and reduce the chances of errors during diagnosis. AI also provides accurate measurements for clinical decisions, besides classification, and quantitates histological features. For example, AI models can predict tumor cell density, assess tumour infiltrating lymphocytes, and others (Wang and Summers, 2012).

4.2 Automated Tumor Grading and Staging

Tumor grading and staging are integral components of cancer diagnosis, and provide information about the aggressiveness of the tumor and the extent of its spread. In the past, tumor grading and staging were done manually by oncologists. Artificial intelligence (AI) however, has shed new light on these evaluations, enabling an objective and consistent approach using data analysis. The technology allows imaging data to be used in conjunction with machine learning to classify the tumour by its grade, which is a measure of its degree of differentiation and aggressiveness. Such models can help to recognize patterns corresponding to various grades and classify tumors with high precision and stratify patients based on their risks. Likewise, AI can assist in staging using imaging data that will help identify the size of the tumor, the presence of lymph nodes and metastases. Notably, the implementation of AI in grading and staging not only increases accuracy and reliability of the process but also makes it much faster. Thus doctors get valuable information on time and their treatment decisions are made with more information (Villaruz and Socinski, 2013).

4.3 AI-Assisted Biopsy Interpretation

Biopsy evaluation of tissue samples is another important aspect to the diagnosis of lung cancer. AI helps to make evaluation of biopsies more efficient and accurate.

Through deep learning, artificial intelligence is able to analyze histopathology images and make a reliable assessment based on the results. Deep learning algorithms have proven themselves capable of recognizing cancerous cells in the biopsies with unprecedented precision and can recognize morphological changes indicating early stages of cancer development. Meanwhile, AI can be used to analyze the molecular components related to cancerous cells. The AI algorithms can also include information about genetic abnormalities in cells, which can be used to provide a comprehensive assessment of the tumor's pathology. Standardization is another benefit of the use of AI in the evaluation of biopsies. In the case of diagnosis, by assisting with artificial intelligence, the process can be more standardized and reduce the differences that specialists might have in the process of making the diagnosis (Wang et al., 2021).

4.4 Integration of Radiology and Pathology

Data obtained from both radiology and pathology would form an important milestone in the journey of a cancer patient with respect to the understanding of the nature of the malignant tumors. Historically, these two specialties were studied separately and therefore it was impossible to correlate the results that were achieved by different approaches (Wu and Hicks, 2021). In healthcare, AI helps to integrate these various data sources and create a more holistic diagnostic approach. The imaging data obtained by a CT scan can be used in an AI model with data obtained via the study of histological slides. Therefore, an AI system could allow doctors to study the relationships between imaging characteristics and histopathological characteristics of the cancerous growths. Moreover, the data of radiological and pathological findings can be leveraged for the development of predictive models in the future for tumor progression and the success of treatment plans (Xu et al., 2019).

5. RADIOMICS IN PULMONARY ONCOLOGY

The application of radiomics to the medical sphere implies a method of extracting high dimensional features from images and using the data collected from these processes. Thus, radiomics provides additional information about a tumor that cannot be seen with the naked eye. Radiomics is being actively implemented in the field of pulmonary oncology, providing the ability to diagnose, predict outcome and establish a therapy plan for patients. The technology consists in conversion of image data into radiomic features. AI technologies have proved their importance in radiomics due to the ability of machines to extract, choose and analyze the most important data regarding images. Machine learning technologies can help identify patterns in radiomic data that can predict a patient's condition. For example, the information in the data can be used to determine if the tumor is aggressive, and how it might affect a patient's health. Moreover, radiomics may provide a better insight into the reaction of the disease to different treatments. Radiomics may also be a powerful way of integrating various data types pertaining to cancer, including genomics and clinical data. Therefore, it is beneficial to gain a wider understanding of the tumor heterogeneity and provide personalized treatment to patients (Yip and Aerts, 2016).

6. AI IN PERSONALIZED THERAPY

The concept of personalized therapy, which is sometimes referred to as precision medicine, seeks to design treatment strategies that consider the unique attributes of patients and their cancers. Personalized therapy is especially crucial in treating lung cancer because of its heterogeneity and differential treatment responses. Artificial intelligence technology has been found to offer a platform for personalizing the management of lung cancers through data analysis. Artificial intelligence systems can incorporate information from various sources like genomics, images, and clinical records and analyze it to formulate the most appropriate treatment strategies (Yu et al., 2018). Machine learning algorithms have been used to determine how individual patients may react to certain therapies and thus help choose the best treatment options. Personalized therapy not only improves the success rate of treatments but also helps minimize the risk of complications. Artificial intelligence algorithms can also facilitate personalized therapy in lung cancers by optimizing treatment plans through data analysis. For instance, artificial intelligence can help in choosing the best therapeutic strategies that may involve chemotherapy, radiation, and immunotherapy among others (Zhang et al., 2021). Table 1 summarizes the diverse applications of Artificial Intelligence in personalized lung cancer therapy, including treatment selection, drug response prediction, radiotherapy planning, and monitoring of patient outcomes. It highlights how AI-driven approaches optimize treatment strategies by improving precision, reducing adverse effects, and supporting individualized patient care.

Table 1. Applications of artificial intelligence in personalized lung cancer therapy and treatment optimization

Applications	Techniques Used	Significance	References
Personalized lung cancer therapy	Machine learning, multimodal data integration	Improves individualized treatment outcomes	Zhao et al., 2018
Therapy selection and optimization	Treatment recommendation systems	Supports evidence-based therapy planning	Tizhoosh and Pantanowitz, 2018
Precision medicine and targeted therapy	Genomic sequencing, ML models	Advances precision oncology	Topol, 2019
Integrated patient assessment	Deep learning, diagnostic platforms	Enhances prediction accuracy	Subramanian and Simon, 2010
Treatment outcome prediction	Predictive modeling, decision support	Improves patient management	Silva et al., 2018
Combination therapy optimization	Clinical trial and real-world analytics	Optimizes therapy sequencing	Smeltzer et al., 2020
Adaptive treatment monitoring	Real-time analytics	Improves survival outcomes	Singh et al., 2020
Immunotherapy response prediction	Genomic and proteomic analysis	Enhances treatment effectiveness	Sollini et al., 2017
Detection of immunotherapy resistance	Response monitoring systems	Improves resistance management	Saba et al., 2019
Biomarker discovery	Multi-omics analysis, ML	Supports precision treatment	Sun et al., 2016
Treatment-response signature analysis	Integrated omics analysis	Improves immunotherapy prediction	Wang and Summers, 2012
PD-L1 assessment automation	Deep learning, pathology imaging	Enhances diagnostic consistency	Villaruz and Socinski, 2013
PD-L1 spatial pattern analysis	Image segmentation algorithms	Predicts immunotherapy response	Wang et al., 2021
TMB-based immunotherapy prediction	Genomic analytics, ML integration	Enhances immune-response prediction	Wu and Hicks, 2021
Integrated biomarker modeling	Multi-parameter predictive modeling	Supports personalized immunotherapy	Xu et al., 2019
AI-assisted radiation therapy	Deep learning, contouring systems	Improves radiation precision	Yip and Aerts, 2016
Automated tumor contouring	CNNs, image segmentation	Enhances treatment consistency	Yu et al., 2018
Radiation dose optimization	Predictive modeling, simulation	Reduces treatment complications	Zhang et al., 2021

6.1 Precision Medicine in Lung Cancer

Precision oncology of lung cancer is defined by using molecular and genetic knowledge to make informed decisions about the therapy of patients with this type of cancer. The latest advancements in genomic sequencing technologies allowed scientists to find multiple genetic mutations that could cause this disease, thus creating new options for targeted therapeutic approaches. It was AI that made it possible to analyze genomic data and find actionable mutations that could become the targets of certain medications. Machine learning systems could analyze vast genomic datasets to find connections between various mutations and therapeutic success. Predictive algorithms could also be designed using such connections to suggest the best therapy options and increase the odds of successful treatment. AI could be used to find out which patients had a higher likelihood of responding positively to specific treatment methods thanks to their genetic makeup. Moreover, AI helped integrate genetic data into comprehensive analyses along with clinical and imaging information (Zhao et al., 2018).

6.2 Treatment Selection and Optimization

The selection of treatment for patients with lung cancer is a very complicated procedure that requires consideration of many factors, such as properties of the tumor, the general condition of the patient, and other factors. The use of AI can facilitate the selection process through the analysis of huge amounts of information and making recommendations based on reliable scientific facts. For example, machine learning algorithms can assess different types of therapy and their effectiveness and recommend a certain option. AI can be used to optimize the treatment process since it can select the most effective combinations of different approaches. Moreover, AI technology allows predicting the effectiveness of various treatment regimens by using the data from clinical trials and observational studies. It increases the efficiency of the chosen treatment method and helps to avoid potential risks associated with side effects. Besides, adaptive therapy can be conducted based on the continuous assessment of patient's conditions (Tizhoosh and Pantanowitz, 2018).

6.3 AI in Immunotherapy

6.3.1 Biomarker Discovery

The biomarker discovery is a vital element of immunotherapy because it helps to determine patients who will be most responsive to certain immunotherapeutic drugs. AI plays a crucial role in accelerating the discovery of biomarkers through big data analytics based on information gained from genomics, proteomics, and clinical research (Topol, 2019). The traditional way of finding biomarkers tends to be rather slow and limited, while AI-based techniques have the potential to sift through extensive volumes of data to find unknown biomarkers linked with treatment effects. One of the advantages of using machine learning to analyze biomarker data is that it allows identifying multidimensional biomarker signatures (Subramanian and Simon, 2010). The machine learning algorithms could combine various data sources ranging from genomics and proteomics to imaging techniques to reveal the underlying connections between different biomarkers and treatment effects. Thus, using AI to detect biomarkers would help to create prediction models and select optimal immunotherapies for particular individuals. Besides, AI-driven biomarker discovery contributes to personalized medicine since it could make targeted therapy even more personalized due to identification of new biomarkers and their subsequent implementation in practices (Silva et al., 2018).

6.3.2 PD-L1 Expression

Another very popular biomarker, which has been studied widely as a predictor of the response to immunotherapy in patients with lung cancer, is programmed death-ligand 1 or PD-L1 expression. Interaction between PD-L1 and its receptor – the programmed death-1 on immune cells leads to inhibition of the immune response and allows cancer cells to avoid detection. Consequently, assessment of PD-L1 expression in tumors is an important step in assessing whether patients are candidates for receiving immune checkpoint inhibitors (Bray et al., 2018). Artificial intelligence has contributed significantly to making this process much more reliable and accurate through development of algorithms capable of analyzing digital pathology images obtained after immunohistochemical staining. Deep learning algorithms are capable of quantifying PD-L1 expression levels and identifying patterns associated with different levels of its expression. At the same time, artificial intelligence systems have the potential to be used to create more complex models based on integrating information from different biomarkers along with data about the patient's conditions (Smeltzer et al., 2020).

6.3.3 Tumor Mutational Burden (TMB)

Tumor mutational burden (TMB) is defined as the total quantity of mutations within a tumor genome and is gaining importance as a biomarker in predicting response to immunotherapy. A high level of TMB usually results in a higher neoantigen load, thus improving cancer immunity against tumors. However, the estimation of TMB in clinical applications poses difficulties, especially in determining the meaning of TMB in specific cases. In this regard, the use of artificial intelligence (AI) can be vital for analyzing TMB data, as AI processes information from large-scale genomic datasets to find patterns that determine treatment efficacy. The use of machine learning algorithms helps predict cancer patient outcomes and incorporate TMB data into the analysis process. The application of AI-based technologies allows researchers to detect optimal thresholds for high and low levels of TMB, thus enhancing patient stratification. Another benefit of AI application in this context is that it facilitates the combination of TMB data with other indicators, including the expression of PD-L1 and infiltration by immune cells. The use of multi-biomarker predictive models will significantly increase their efficiency in predicting treatment outcomes (Singh et al., 2020).

6.4 AI in Radiation Therapy

The use of radiotherapy is among the key ways to manage lung cancer, and AI technologies have advanced this type of treatment dramatically. For instance, an area where AI can help significantly improve the effectiveness of radiotherapy is contouring. This process is related to the identification of tumors that will be subjected to radiation. The importance of accurate contouring cannot be underestimated as it allows providing radiation treatment while avoiding healthy body parts. AI technology has proven to be efficient when it comes to contouring as deep learning models can accurately draw contours in relatively little time. Moreover, AI technology can assist in optimizing radiation dose through simulation of different possible scenarios. In addition, machine learning models can identify an optimal set of characteristics for patients, allowing for effective treatment plans and minimizing risks associated with radiation (Sollini et al., 2017).

7. AI FOR PROGNOSIS AND SURVIVAL PREDICTION

Lung cancer prognosis and survival predictions have significant clinical value in the management of lung cancer patients. Prognostication involves the use of various clinical and pathological parameters that are usually employed to predict survival and determine the most appropriate treatment strategy. Prognostic prediction models are commonly developed using conventional machine learning algorithms. However, there are certain limitations associated with such models as they are only based on clinical and pathological parameters that might fail to incorporate other vital parameters. With advances in technology, artificial intelligence (AI) has been identified as a promising approach that could improve the accuracy of lung cancer prognosis and survival prediction models. In addition, AI technologies are known to leverage several types of data such as imaging and genomics in order to generate a model that could accurately predict survival outcomes and disease progression. Through the analysis of large amounts of data, these models are able to extract vital features that could influence disease outcomes. In addition, AI-driven models are known to generate risk scores that would provide insight into potential patient outcomes (Saba et al., 2019).

8. AI IN TREATMENT MONITORING

Monitoring treatment is crucial when assessing the success of treatment and the presence of cancer recurrence or progression. With the development of AI, it became possible to analyze patients' information promptly, and conclusions about treatment efficacy can be drawn much earlier than before. It allows physicians to modify their methods of treating patients in time, and thus improve patients' conditions. AI can help track the dynamics of tumor growth and morphological changes through the analysis of images acquired during different periods of the treatment process (Bahado-Singh et al., 2022). The use of deep learning algorithms will allow identifying even the slightest changes that can be used to assess whether treatment is effective or not. At the same time, AI can take into account data obtained from multiple sources such as imaging results, biomarker levels, and clinical history, and thus make more accurate decisions. Besides, AI can provide personalized treatment based on how patients react to treatment Pastorino et al., 2019).

9. INTEGRATION OF MULTI-OMICS DATA WITH AI

Multi-omics data integration, such as genomics, proteomics, transcriptomics, and metabolomics, is an innovative method for the study of lung cancer. Multi-omics datasets offer profound knowledge about the molecular processes involved in the growth and development of cancers. Nevertheless, due to their high level of complexity and multidimensionality, multi-omics data necessitate sophisticated tools for their investigation, which makes the use of artificial intelligence crucial for analyzing them. AI techniques can process multi-omics data by discovering pathways, biomarkers, and drug targets. Machine learning can detect intricate connections between biological levels, giving a comprehensive picture of the biological processes occurring within tumors. The combination of multi-omics information with clinical and imaging data can help construct detailed profiles of patients. These profiles can be used for predicting treatment response, assessing disease progression, and discovering novel therapeutic targets (Wang and Summers, 2012).

10. ETHICAL, LEGAL, AND REGULATORY CONSIDERATIONS

One of the significant ethical, legal, and regulatory issues arising from AI integration in pulmonary oncology is data privacy. Data privacy becomes an issue when handling large amounts of data that may contain sensitive patient information. The protection of the confidentiality and integrity of the data is vital to protect the interests of the patients and maintain their trust. Furthermore, transparency and interpretability are also some of the challenges associated with the use of AI. Some of the AI algorithms, especially those based on deep learning, are not transparent, and their decision-making processes cannot be interpreted easily. In such cases, the clinicians and regulators may find it challenging to understand how AI works. Explainable AI models should be developed to ensure transparency in the decision-making process. Additionally, regulatory frameworks need to be developed to govern AI technology in healthcare settings. It is vital to ensure that the AI systems used in healthcare are safe and effective (Villaruz and Socinski, 2013 and (Wang et al., 2021).

11. FUTURE PERSPECTIVES AND EMERGING TRENDS

There is a bright future for AI in the field of pulmonary oncology, as AI applications are expected to undergo groundbreaking changes that will revolutionize how lung cancers are diagnosed and treated. With continued advancements in technology, artificial intelligence is likely to go beyond its current supportive role and become a key part of clinical decisions. High-quality datasets, advancements in AI algorithms, and incorporation of emerging innovations, such as cloud computing and high-performance computing technologies, have paved the way for these changes. They will make it possible for clinicians to benefit from increasingly accurate AI models capable of meeting the challenges posed by lung cancers (Wu and Hicks, 2021). One of the key areas of future development includes the emergence of end-to-end systems incorporating different types of data, including imaging and genomics data, in order to generate a holistic patient profile that enables clinicians to make better-informed decisions when it comes to lung cancer patients' care.

Moreover, the integration of real-time data obtained from wearable devices and remote monitoring technologies will ensure constant patient evaluation, enabling healthcare professionals to implement proactive and adaptive approaches to treating patients. The transition is characterized by a shift in paradigms from reactive to predictive and preventive cancer care (Xu et al., 2019). Moreover, innovations in AI are projected to facilitate cooperation between medical professionals and AI technologies, thus fostering evidence-based and efficient decision-making processes. Instead of displacing healthcare professionals, the implementation of AI will assist in enhancing their performance, delivering data-driven solutions and relieving cognitive load. To make it happen, current barriers such as data interoperability, ethical concerns, and compliance with regulations should be addressed. When done successfully, AI may play a pivotal role in shaping the future of precision oncology (Yip and Aerts, 2016).

11.1 Explainable AI (XAI)

The advent of explainable artificial intelligence (XAI) marks another important trend in AI studies since it focuses on explaining machine learning algorithms and enhancing their transparency and interpretability. XAI technology can be applied in the field of pulmonary oncology in order to make machine-learning algorithms understandable for doctors who use them in medical practice. The issue of interpretability of algorithms remains an obstacle to the implementation of AI in the area of pulmonary oncology. Machine learning methods, particularly deep learning algorithms, have been criticized due to the "black-box problem", referring to the difficulty of understanding how a particular solution has been reached. In this regard, explainable artificial intelligence serves as a tool for explaining how a certain decision is made. Methods like feature importance, saliency maps, and attention mechanism help to pinpoint areas or features of a model, which make an algorithm generate predictions. Explainable AI is especially significant in terms of complying with regulatory and ethical requirements for introducing AI algorithms in health care. Clinicians should be able to understand why a certain recommendation is suggested, which helps to establish accountability in case of errors (Yu et al., 2018).

11.2 Federated Learning in Healthcare

One of the revolutionary ways of training AI models is through federated learning which offers an interesting solution to issues surrounding data privacy and security. In conventional ML, data obtained from various institutions are consolidated into one place to train AI models, posing risks to patient data privacy and security. Through federated learning, models are trained from data kept in decentralized datasets without transmitting confidential data (Alowais et al., 2023). In pulmonary oncology, federated learning can facilitate collaboration between healthcare institutions to develop AI models while maintaining patient confidentiality. Federated learning involves local training of AI models using the data in each institution, and the parameters are only exchanged between collaborating institutions. Not only does federated learning enable organizations to develop AI models while ensuring data privacy, but also it increases the generalizability of AI models by utilizing more diverse datasets obtained from different parties. The application of federated learning can help increase collaborative efforts among institutions and regions, hence, accelerating the development of AI tools (Zhang et al., 2021).

11.3 AI-Powered Digital Twins for Cancer Patients

AI-driven digital twins are considered a remarkable innovation within the realm of personalized medicine and imply the development of a virtual representation of each particular patient. Within the framework of pulmonary oncology, the digital twins can assist in modeling the tumor growth and progression, as well as predicting the treatment outcomes using virtual tools. Digital twins are created on the basis of various types of information related to imaging, genomics, and clinical records of a patient (Zhao et al., 2018). Thanks to digital twins, clinicians will have the possibility to conduct multiple experiments concerning the potential impact of treatment options on patients' health and make predictions regarding their outcomes. Therefore, the application of digital twins will allow reducing the risks associated with incorrect and inappropriate treatment of a patient. For instance, digital twins might be used for testing the impact of chemotherapy, immunotherapy, and radiation therapy as the primary means of treating lung cancer and determining the most suitable strategy. Moreover, the introduction of digital twins implies continuous monitoring and modification of a treatment strategy by integrating the up-to-date information regarding the patient's health (Tizhoosh and Pantanowitz, 2018).

11.4 Integration with Robotics and IoT

AI with robotics and the Internet of Things (IoT) represents another interesting trend in the field of pulmonary oncology. Robotic technology is currently employed for carrying out surgical operations and performing minimally invasive interventions with very high precision. AI technology further augments the performance of robotic systems through real-time guidance and reduced risk of complications associated with surgery. Besides, there is an increasing role played by IoT in pulmonary medicine. Devices such as wearable sensors and other technological innovations connected to one another via IoT continuously monitor a variety of physiological parameters in patients. These may include breathing rate, pulse and even activity levels among other things. Through analysis of the information generated by sensors, AI identifies potential problems associated with disease progression or possible side effects of particular types of therapy. Overall, integration of AI, robotics and IoT technologies into pulmonary medicine creates a connected healthcare environment, which will contribute to better treatment results and outcomes achieved through personalized and proactive approaches to disease management (Topol, 2019).

11.5 Real-World Clinical Implementation

The implementation of AI into real-world clinical settings will be a crucial step in ensuring that its full potential in pulmonary oncology is harnessed. While many studies on AI have produced impressive findings, its implementation in actual clinical settings will entail overcoming various practical barriers. For instance, it may require ensuring the availability of reliable data, integration of AI technology with healthcare delivery systems, and training healthcare practitioners on how to use it. One of the crucial aspects of implementing AI in healthcare settings is the development of easy-to-use and seamless AI applications. The design of such systems should not interfere with other operations, and users should be able to make sense out of it (Subramanian and Simon, 2010). It may also call for collaboration among clinicians, data scientists, and engineers to develop effective AI technologies. In addition, the implementation of AI technology in health care may demand validation, regulation, and continuous monitoring. Silva et al. (2018) suggest that AI technology should be continuously evaluated to ensure that it meets clinical requirements. With time, the implementation process will help overcome current barriers and enable the incorporation of AI in routine medical practices (Smeltzer et al., 2020).

12. CONCLUSION

AI has become a game changer for pulmonary oncology and has brought significant changes in diagnosing, treating, predicting, and even managing lung cancers. Due to its ability to integrate modern imaging, biomarker analyses, machine learning, deep learning, radiomics, and multi-omics approaches, it has positively impacted clinical workflows and helped to develop personalized treatment programs. Moreover, due to innovative imaging techniques, biomarkers detection, risk stratification, and predictive models based on various types of big data, early diagnosis and timely treatment have improved patient outcomes and increased patients' survival chances. In addition, through applications in histopathology, immunotherapy, radiation therapy, and prognosis, AI has positively affected the field of pulmonary oncology. However, despite all promising developments, there are still many obstacles that prevent the use of artificial intelligence in clinics. The lack of high-quality data, issues with interpretability, ethical dilemmas, privacy, and regulatory policies are among them. Nevertheless, with emerging technologies such as explainable AI, federated learning, digital twin creation, robotics, IoT applications, AI will become even more important for the field of pulmonary oncology.

REFERENCES

Alowais, S. A., Alghamdi, S. S., Alsuhebany, N., Alqahtani, T., Alshaya, A. I., Almohareb, S. N., Aldairem, A., Alrashed, M., Bin Saleh, K., & Badredin, H. A. (2023). Revolutionizing healthcare: The role of artificial intelligence in clinical practice. *BMC Medical Education, 23*(1), 689. DOI: 10.1186/s12909-023-04698-z PMID: 37740191

Bahado-Singh, R., Vlachos, K. T., Aydas, B., Gordevicius, J., Radhakrishna, U., & Vishwesvaraiah, S. (2022). Precision oncology: Artificial intelligence and DNA methylation analysis of circulating cell-free DNA for lung cancer detection. *Frontiers in Oncology, 12*, 790645. DOI: 10.3389/fonc.2022.790645 PMID: 35600397

Bray, F., Ferlay, J., Soerjomataram, I., Siegel, R. L., Torre, L. A., & Jemal, A. (2018). Global cancer statistics 2018: GLOBOCAN estimates of incidence and mortality worldwide for 36 cancers in 185 countries. *CA: a Cancer Journal for Clinicians, 68*(6), 394–424. DOI: 10.3322/caac.21492 PMID: 30207593

Pastorino, U., Silva, M., Sestini, S., Sabia, F., Boeri, M., Cantarutti, A., Sverzellati, N., Sozzi, G., Corrao, G., & Marchiano, A. (2019). Prolonged lung cancer screening reduced 10-year mortality in the MILD trial: New confirmation of lung cancer screening efficacy. *Annals of Oncology : Official Journal of the European Society for Medical Oncology, 30*(7), 1162–1169. DOI: 10.1093/annonc/mdz117 PMID: 30937431

Saba, L., Biswas, M., Kuppili, V., Cuadrado Godia, E., Suri, H. S., Edla, D. R., & Suri, J. S. (2019). The present and future of deep learning in radiology. *European Journal of Radiology, 114*, 14–24. DOI: 10.1016/j.ejrad.2019.02.038 PMID: 31005165

Saul, E. E., Guerra, R. B., Saul, M. E., da Silva, L. L., Aleixo, G. F. P., Matuda, R. M. K., & Lopes, G. (2020). The challenges of implementing low-dose computed tomography for lung cancer screening in low- and middle-income countries. *Nature Cancer, 1*(12), 1140–1152. DOI: 10.1038/s43018-020-00142-z PMID: 35121933

Shafiq-Ul-Hassan, M., Latifi, K., Zhang, G., Ullah, G., Gillies, R., & Moros, E. (2018). Voxel size and gray level normalization of CT radiomic features in lung cancer. *Scientific Reports, 8*(1), 10545. DOI: 10.1038/s41598-018-28895-9 PMID: 30002441

Siegel, R. L., Miller, K. D., & Jemal, A. (2019). Cancer statistics, 2019. *CA: a Cancer Journal for Clinicians, 69*(1), 7–34. DOI: 10.3322/caac.21551 PMID: 30620402

Silva, M., Schaefer-Prokop, C. M., Jacobs, C., & Prokop, M. (2018). Detection of subsolid pulmonary nodules in lung cancer screening: Complementary sensitivity of visual reading and computer-aided diagnosis. *Investigative Radiology*, *53*(8), 441–449. DOI: 10.1097/RLI.0000000000000464 PMID: 29543693

Singh, A., Sengupta, S., & Lakshminarayanan, V. (2020). Explainable deep learning models in medical image analysis. *Journal of Imaging*, *6*(6), 52. DOI: 10.3390/jimaging6060052 PMID: 34460598

Smeltzer, M. P., Wynes, M. W., Lantuejoul, S., & Govindan, R. (2020). The International Association for the Study of Lung Cancer global survey on molecular testing in lung cancer. *Journal of Thoracic Oncology*, *15*(9), 1434–1448. DOI: 10.1016/j.jtho.2020.05.002 PMID: 32445813

Sollini, M., Cozzi, L., Chiti, A., & Kirienko, M. (2017). Texture analysis and machine learning to characterize suspected lung nodules and lung cancer: A narrative review. *European Journal of Radiology*, *90*, 1–9. PMID: 29362138

Subramanian, J., & Simon, R. (2010). Gene expression-based prognostic signatures in lung cancer: Ready for clinical use? *Journal of the National Cancer Institute*, *102*(7), 464–474. DOI: 10.1093/jnci/djq025 PMID: 20233996

Sun, W., Zheng, B., & Qian, W. (2016). Computer aided lung cancer diagnosis with deep learning algorithms. *Proceedings of SPIE Medical Imaging*, *9785*, 97850Z. DOI: 10.1117/12.2216307

Tizhoosh, H. R., & Pantanowitz, L. (2018). Artificial intelligence and digital pathology: Challenges and opportunities. *Journal of Pathology Informatics*, *9*(1), 38. DOI: 10.4103/jpi.jpi_53_18 PMID: 30607305

Topol, E. J. (2019). High-performance medicine: The convergence of human and artificial intelligence. *Nature Medicine*, *25*(1), 44–56. DOI: 10.1038/s41591-018-0300-7 PMID: 30617339

Tunali, I., Gillies, R. J., & Schabath, M. B. (2019). Application of radiomics and artificial intelligence for lung cancer precision medicine. *Cold Spring Harbor Molecular Case Studies*, *5*(6), a003111.

Vaid, A., Somani, S., Russak, A. J., Freitas, J. K., Chaudhry, F., Paranjpe, I., Johnson, K. W., Lee, S. J., & Miotto, R. (2021). Machine learning to predict mortality and critical events in COVID-19 positive New York City patients. *NPJ Digital Medicine*, *3*, 40.

Villaruz, L. C., & Socinski, M. A. (2013). The role of anti-angiogenesis in non-small-cell lung cancer: An update. *Current Oncology Reports, 15*, 346–355. PMID: 25947099

Wang, L., Alexander, C. A., Wu, H., & Wang, J. (2021). Integrating artificial intelligence in lung cancer care: Current applications and future directions. *Seminars in Cancer Biology, 72*, 216–230.

Wang, S., & Summers, R. M. (2012). Machine learning and radiology. *Medical Image Analysis, 16*(5), 933–951. DOI: 10.1016/j.media.2012.02.005 PMID: 22465077

Wu, J., & Hicks, C. (2021). Breast cancer type classification using machine learning. *Journal of Personalized Medicine, 11*(2), 61. DOI: 10.3390/jpm11020061 PMID: 33498339

Xu, Y., Hosny, A., Zeleznik, R., Parmar, C., Coroller, T., Franco, I., Mak, R. H., & Aerts, H. J. W. L. (2019). Deep learning predicts lung cancer treatment response from serial medical imaging. *Clinical Cancer Research, 25*(11), 3266–3275. DOI: 10.1158/1078-0432.CCR-18-2495 PMID: 31010833

Yip, S. S. F., & Aerts, H. J. W. L. (2016). Applications and limitations of radiomics. *Physics in Medicine and Biology, 61*(13), R150–R166. DOI: 10.1088/0031-9155/61/13/R150 PMID: 27269645

Yu, K. H., Beam, A. L., & Kohane, I. S. (2018). Artificial intelligence in healthcare. *Nature Biomedical Engineering, 2*(10), 719–731. DOI: 10.1038/s41551-018-0305-z PMID: 31015651

Zhang, B., He, X., Ouyang, F., Gu, D., Dong, Y., Zhang, L., Mo, X., Huang, W., Tian, J., & Zhang, S. (2021). Radiomic machine-learning classifiers for prognostic biomarkers of advanced nasopharyngeal carcinoma. *Cancer Letters, 403*, 21–27. DOI: 10.1016/j.canlet.2017.06.004 PMID: 28610955

Zhao, W., Yang, J., Sun, Y., Li, C., Wu, W., Jin, L., Wang, X., & Xu, Z. (2018). 3D deep learning from CT scans predicts tumor invasiveness of ground-glass nodules. *Nature Communications, 9*, 1–8.

Chapter 7

AI in Pulmonary Oncology–Driven Innovations in Early Lung Cancer Detection and Risk Stratification

Rahul Kumar
http://orcid.org/0009-0000-1323-2220
Department of Microbiology, Graphic Era (Deemed to be) University, India

Mohammad Aves
http://orcid.org/0009-0008-9927-4410
Department of Computer Science and Engineering, Graphic Era (Deemed to be) University, India

ABSTRACT

The field of pulmonary oncology receives its transformative power from artificial intelligence (AI) which uses its capabilities to enhance early lung cancer detection and improve diagnostic accuracy and create personalized lung cancer treatment solutions. AI operates through its advanced algorithms which combine deep learning with radiomics and multimodal fusion models to deliver precise results when examining imaging data along with histopathology and genomic information. The automated system of AI technology which detects nodules through low-dose CT screening programs extends its capabilities by enabling segmentation and malignancy risk assessment. The combination of whole-slide imaging and AI technology in pathology assists in tumor grading and biomarker measurement and subtype

DOI: 10.4018/979-8-3373-7759-9.ch007

identification. AI-powered predictive analytics assist in developing personalized treatment plans while they estimate treatment effectiveness and resistance patterns and patient survival rates.

INTRODUCTION

Lung cancer continues to represent one of the most pressing global health challenges of the 21st century. The disease remains the top cause of cancer deaths around the world despite major medical advancements which have developed better diagnostic and treatment methods (Chhikara and Parang 2023). The high rate of lung cancer cases together with the disease's pattern of advanced stage diagnosis creates an essential burden which restricts available treatment methods and results in bad outcomes for patients. The field of precision medicine has developed through the use of genomic information for treatment and biomarker-based treatment methods which have produced better clinical results yet patients still experience delays in obtaining early diagnosis tools and personalized treatment methods and efficient patient progress tracking tools. The medical field needs fresh solutions which will build better systems to find lung cancer cases and to make better predictions about disease results and to design better treatment methods and to create a new system for lung cancer treatment throughout the world. Artificial Intelligence (AI) has emerged as a powerful transformation technology which impacts various industries including healthcare and biomedical research and population disease monitoring systems (Hussain et al. 2022). AI systems which use machine learning (ML) and deep learning (DL) technologies enable researchers to process complex clinical data and imaging data and molecular data faster and more accurately than what humans could accomplish through conventional methods.

The intricate nature of lung cancer diagnosis and treatment establishes it as a prime candidate for artificial intelligence-based solutions. AI has shown exceptional capabilities to enhance both clinical diagnostic performance and treatment decision-making accuracy through its ability to analyze low-dose computed tomography (LDCT) scans and digital pathology slides and its capacity to forecast treatment results and detect minor indications of patient outcomes (Rajendran et al., 2025). AI has begun to permeate oncology workflows which enable pulmonary medicine to use data analysis tools for automated disease pattern detection to assist clinicians during their decision-making processes. The process of understanding how AI will change pulmonary oncology requires two steps which include establishing global lung cancer statistics and studying the ways that technological advancements are changing established medical procedures (Dasgupta, 2024). The chapter offers a comprehensive examination of lung cancer as a worldwide health problem while studying how AI technology works to improve early detection methods and diagnosis procedures and treatment customization and clinical process improvement.

Overview of Lung Cancer as a Global Health Burden

Lung cancer represents a substantial challenge that impacts global health systems and economic systems and social systems. The World Health Organization reports that lung cancer cases reached about 2.2 million and caused 1.8 million deaths in 2022, which makes it the most deadly cancer according to their data (Al-Musawi et al., 2025). The disease continues to spread in various territories that include nations which undergo fast industrial growth and experience rising air pollution levels and have widespread tobacco consumption. The historical pattern shows that tobacco consumption served as the main threat which caused almost 85 percent of lung cancer cases but medical experts now recognize non-smoking-related lung cancer as an increasing medical issue that particularly affects women and people who belong to younger age groups (Zhao et al., 2025). Disease development includes crucial environmental and occupational exposures to substances such as radon asbestos particulate matter and diesel exhaust. The primary obstacle to decreasing lung cancer death rates stems from the disease's tendency to remain either asymptomatic or present with minimal symptoms during its early development stages. Most patients arrive at medical facilities with either advanced cancer or metastatic cancer because they have passed the point when doctors can use curative treatment methods. Countries experience inconsistent implementation of LDCT screening because the method requires funding and needs adequate facilities and because medical staff worries about false positive results and overdiagnosis issues. Lung cancer displays histological diversity through two main types which are non–small cell lung cancer (NSCLC) that makes up 85% of cases and small cell lung cancer (SCLC) which represents a more aggressive cancer type (Rodak et al., 2021). The challenges of diagnosis and prognosis and treatment remain distinct for each subtype of the disease. The combination of molecular profiling advances and targeted therapies research has enabled better treatment results for patients with genetic variations like EGFR mutations and ALK rearrangements and PD-L1 expression. Advanced-stage cancer management has experienced a fundamental change because of immunotherapy and especially immune checkpoint inhibitors. The development of treatment resistance together with the unavailability of molecular testing and the inconsistent expression of biomarkers has created obstacles that hinder scientific advancement. The economic impact of lung cancer treatment costs creates a significant financial burden for both patients and healthcare systems (Yousefi et al., 2023). The expenses originate from diagnostic tests and extended medical care and hospitalization stays and post-treatment assessments. The total impact increases because of indirect expenses which include lost work capacity and the burden on caregivers and early deaths. To achieve better patient outcomes through increased cancer detection rates and better resource use and customized treatment options healthcare systems require new methods to reduce their existing patient load (Table 1).

Table 1. Role of artificial intelligence in transforming oncology and pulmonary medicine

Domain	AI Applications	Impact on Oncology & Pulmonary Medicine
Early Detection & Screening	Automated nodule detection in CT/LDCT, Risk prediction algorithms, AI-assisted chest X-ray interpretation	Earlier diagnosis of lung cancer, Reduced false positives & false negatives, Improved population-level screening programs
Imaging Analysis (Radiology)	CNN-based CT & PET-CT image analysis, Segmentation & volumetric assessment, Radiomics feature extraction	More accurate tumor characterization, Quantification of tumor heterogeneity, Enhanced monitoring of disease progression
Digital Pathology	Whole-slide image (WSI) analysis, Histological subtype classification, Tumor grading & biomarker quantification	Faster and more accurate pathological diagnoses, Objective, reproducible measurements, Identification of subtle diagnostic features
Precision Oncology	Integration of genomics, proteomics, & clinical data, Prediction of mutation status (EGFR, ALK, KRAS), Treatment response prediction models	Personalized therapy selection, Early detection of drug resistance, Improved patient stratification
Clinical Decision Support	AI-assisted treatment planning, Predictive analytics for prognosis, Recommendation engines integrated with EHRs	Data-driven clinical decisions, Reduced clinician workload, Enhanced adherence to guidelines
Workflow Automation	Automated report generation, Prioritizing urgent radiology cases, Monitoring patient outcomes through AI-enabled EHRs	Streamlined clinical workflows, Reduced diagnostic delays, Improved resource allocation
Interdisciplinary Collaboration	AI-powered insights for tumor boards, Synthesis of multimodal data, Visualization tools for case discussions	Better integration of radiology, pathology, and oncology, More accurate and comprehensive decision-making
Population Health & Epidemiology	Predictive models for disease trends, AI-supported screening outreach, Identification of high-risk populations	More effective public health strategies, Enhanced early detection in underserved regions
Ethics & Safety	Bias detection systems, Explainable AI (XAI), Data privacy safeguards	Increased clinician trust, Reduced inequities in care, Safe and responsible AI adoption

AI FOUNDATIONS IN PULMONARY ONCOLOGY

Conceptual of AI, Machine Learning, and Deep Learning

AI functions as an extensive discipline within computer science which seeks to develop systems that can execute tasks which only human intelligence can perform through learning and reasoning and pattern recognition and decision making. The field of artificial intelligence includes machine learning as its main subfield that studies how to create algorithms which enable computers to acquire knowledge through data and enhance their performance without needing specific programming instructions (Islam et al., 2024). ML systems identify patterns and relationships within structured or unstructured datasets and use these learned patterns to make predictions, classifications, or recommendations. The three main ML approaches consist of supervised learning which works with labeled data, unsupervised learning which helps find hidden patterns, and reinforcement learning which supports decision-making in changing situations. Deep learning functions as an advanced ML category which uses artificial neural networks that contain multiple interconnected layers to create deep neural networks which model intricate non-linear correlations in high-dimensional datasets. Deep learning techniques demonstrate their capacity to extract multiple levels of features from medical images entire slide pathology scans genomic data and clinical records which contain natural language text. The biomedical field employs convolutional neural networks and recurrent neural networks and transformer architectures as the primary deep learning frameworks which researchers use in pulmonary oncology studies. The system architecture relies on artificial intelligence as its foundation machine learning supplies the scientific methods needed for data-driven educational programs while deep learning provides its sophisticated automated feature extraction capabilities. The three technologies create the fundamental computational system which powers current precision medicine practices to achieve better diagnostic results and predictive accuracy and customized treatment recommendations for lung cancer patients.

Data Modalities in Pulmonary Oncology

Researchers in pulmonary oncology study lung cancer through various data types which medical professionals use to develop complete patient profiles for better treatment assessment and testing methods. The complete anatomical and functional information from low-dose computed tomography (LDCT) and diagnostic CT and PET-CT and MRI systems serves as essential tools for screening and detecting pulmonary nodules and staging tumors and assessing treatment efficacy (Owens et al., 2023). Histopathology and cytopathology research investigates tissue biopsies together with whole-slide images (WSI) which allow scientists to study cellular structure and tumor development and environmental attributes that reveal histological subtype and tumor grade and biomarker expression. Digital pathology technology enables researchers to study high-resolution images together with AI tools which automatically identify vital features in the images. Omics research uses genomics data together with transcriptomics data and proteomics data and metabolomics data to construct lung cancer molecular structures which help scientists find actionable mutations and PD-L1 immune markers and pathways that determine patient outcomes and drug response and treatment resistance (Ashrafi et al., 2022). Scientists use high-dimensional datasets to develop precise cancer treatment techniques for their research work. The electronic health record system collects clinical data which contains information about demographics and smoking habits and existing medical conditions and laboratory test results and patient performance and treatment results over time. The actual data from the real world establishes background information which enables better assessment of risks and improves the precision of future predictions. The different data sources create a complete three-dimensional disease representation which helps doctors to improve their diagnostic work and create personalized treatment strategies and better handle patient cases in pulmonary oncology (Hao et al., 2025).

Integration of Multimodal Data for Comprehensive Decision Support to Oncology

The integration of multimodal data in pulmonary oncology has become essential for achieving comprehensive and precise clinical decision support, as no single data source can fully capture the biological complexity and clinical variability of lung cancer. The combination of imaging with histopathology and omics together with clinical data enables a complete evaluation which improves diagnostic accuracy and prognostic prediction and treatment planning for individual patients (Takamatsu, 2025). The development of artificial intelligence technologies has enabled researchers to create systems which use complex designs for processing diverse types of data that contain extensive information. Medical professionals commonly use convolutional neural networks (CNNs) to analyze various medical images which include CT and PET-CT and whole-slide pathology. These networks extract hierarchical spatial features which help identify nodules and segment tumors and classify different tumor subtypes (Hussain et al. 2024). The use of recurrent neural networks (RNNs) with long short-term memory (LSTM) models provides optimal results for studying sequential data and longitudinal data, which scientists can use to assess patients' medical history and laboratory test results and their response to treatment over time. In current research, transformer architectures function as advanced oncological tools because their attention system allows the analysis of intricate data sets that contain multiple types of information. The implementation of transformers across different data types enables decision-making processes through their ability to track relationships between medical imaging data and genomic information and clinical assessment results (Zhao et al., 2025). The architectural design enables organizations to perform predictive analytics while establishing risk categories and selecting treatments and identifying treatment resistance at an early stage. Multimodal AI-powered systems create patient-specific insights from multiple data sources through their advanced information processing capabilities, which represent a new achievement in precision pulmonary oncology that can transform clinical workflows to enhance patient results.

AI IN EARLY DETECTION AND SCREENING

AI in Low Dose CT (LDCT) Lung Cancer Screening Programs

The implementation of artificial intelligence (AI) has improved the operational capacity of low-dose CT (LDCT) lung cancer screening programs by solving essential problems which existed in early detection, diagnostic precision and operational workflow. The gold standard for population-based screening in high-risk groups requires LDCT implementation yet challenges arise because of excessive imaging data and difficulty observing nodules and diverse interpretation abilities which radiologists display. AI-powered algorithms which use deep learning techniques through convolutional neural network (CNN) models achieve better results in detecting and analyzing pulmonary nodules through their ability to study CT images with pixel-level detail (Aishwarya and Asuntha, 2025). The systems use automated processes to identify nodules and measure their dimensions and shapes while they identify suspicious lesions, which helps to decrease the chances of missing early-stage cancers through false negative results. The system uses AI to decrease false positive results by identifying which features are non-cancerous through their classification as scars or calcifications, which results in fewer unnecessary follow-up examinations and less patient anxiety. AI acts as an effective second opinion tool for radiologists in large screening programs by helping them identify critical cases, which improves diagnostic accuracy and speeds up their examination process. The artificial intelligence (AI) systems which operate on LDCT platforms produce real-world operational data that researchers use to improve their algorithms and develop algorithms which work across various demographic groups (Navarro-Garcia et al., 2025). The implementation of artificial intelligence in LDCT screening programs will improve lung cancer detection through two main advantages which include improved clinician performance and the ability to make decisions based on data.

Algorithms for Nodule Detection, Segmentation, and Classification

The implementation of algorithms for nodule detection and segmentation and classification serves as the foundational element of AI systems which assess lung cancer through their capacity to analyze low-dose CT scans and boost their ability to detect the disease in its initial stages. Nodule detection algorithms Progress through three stages which start with automatic candidate generation and use different methods to detect abnormal areas in three-dimensional medical scans. The primary method for studying lung nodules has shifted towards using convolutional neural networks because their 3D CNN variants permit direct learning of spatial and contextual features which include ground-glass opacities and small solid nodules that doctors frequently miss (Marinakis et al., 2024). The process of segmentation algorithms requires detection nodules which need to be precisely identified so that their boundaries become visible for calculating volume measurements and tracking tumor development and constructing treatment strategies. Advanced architectural designs such as U-Net and V-Net together with attention-based segmentation networks achieve pixel- and voxel-level precision by employing multi-scale features while maintaining detailed body structure information (Xu et al., 2024). The process of segmentation enables subsequent radiomics research by using its ability to gather numerical data about shape and texture and intensity patterns. The classification algorithms for lung nodules use handcrafted radiomic features together with deep learning-based representations to determine the likelihood of cancer in each detected nodule. The combination of hybrid CNN-radiomics models and ensemble learning together with transformer-based classifiers achieves accurate differentiation between benign and malignant nodules by combining multiple feature sets (Huang et al., 2025). Many modern systems use temporal data to measure interval growth through recurrent and sequential modeling methods. The combined algorithms create a complete system which improves diagnostic accuracy while decreasing observer differences and enabling faster clinical operations that lead to earlier lung cancer diagnosis and better patient results (Table 2).

Table 2. AI approaches for automated differentiation between benign and malignant pulmonary lesions

Aspect	Benign Lesions	Malignant Lesions	AI Methods Used	Reference
Imaging Characteristics	Smooth margins, well-defined edges, slow or no growth	Irregular/spiculated margins, heterogeneous density, rapid growth	CNNs, 3D-CNNs, Vision Transformers (ViT)	(Mannumadam Venugopal, 2024)
Radiomic Features	Low texture complexity, stable morphology	High heterogeneity, increased entropy, irregular shape descriptors	Radiomics + ML classifiers (SVM, Random Forest, XGBoost)	(Raptis et al., 2024)
Growth Dynamics	Minimal or no change over time	Significant volumetric increase on follow-up scans	Sequential models (RNNs, LSTMs), growth-rate prediction networks	(Tao et al., 2022)
Functional Imaging (PET-CT)	Lower SUV uptake	High SUV indicating hypermetabolic activity	Multimodal AI fusion (CNN + dense networks)	(Nakajo et al., 2025)
Histopathology Indicators	Organized cell patterns, low mitotic activity	Nuclear atypia, high mitotic index	Whole-slide image DL models (ResNet, EfficientNet)	(Ibrahim et al., 2022)
Omics Profile	Stable gene expression, non-oncogenic mutation patterns	Driver mutations, oncogenic pathways activated	Multi-omics integration models (transformers, GNNs)	(Yassine et al., 2026)
Risk Probability Output	Low malignancy probability scores	High malignancy risk scores with explainability maps	Explainable AI (Grad-CAM, SHAP)	(Akgündoğdu and Çelikbaş, 2025)
Clinical Integration	Often leads to surveillance or no intervention	Guides biopsy, staging, and active treatment decisions	Clinical decision-support AI systems	(Magrabi et al., 2019)

AI-Assisted Early Diagnosis From Chest X-Rays and Sputum Cytology

AI-assisted early diagnosis from chest X-rays and sputum cytology has emerged as a transformative approach in the early detection of lung cancer, especially in resource-limited settings where advanced imaging technologies like CT and PET-CT are unavailable. Deep learning systems work as artificial intelligence models that effectively analyze chest X-rays by detecting radiographic abnormalities which include small nodules and consolidations and atypical opacities that may be missed during standard clinical evaluations. Convolutional neural networks (CNNs) trained on large annotated datasets can detect early-stage lesions, quantify their characteristics, and provide malignancy probability scores which enable earlier referral for confirmatory imaging or specialist evaluation (Ogut, 2025).AI applications in sputum cytology together with radiographic assessment have enhanced the diagnostic accuracy of this economical testing method. The traditional method of sputum cytology testing shows two major problems because different observers test results through two separate processes which lead to unreliable results when they try to discover early signs of cancer. AI-powered image analysis of cytological smears enhances the identification of atypical cells through automated detection of nuclear irregularities, chromatin patterns, and cell morphology features. Machine learning classifiers can distinguish between three types of cellular changes which include benign and pre-malignant and malignant alterations with high precision to assist cytopathologists in making quick and accurate assessments. The combination of chest X-ray analytics with sputum cytology testing improves diagnostic accuracy because it provides a dual approach which helps to identify high-risk patients who smoke and those with chronic respiratory disease (Georgakopoulou et al., 2025). The combination of AI-enabled chest radiography and cytology analysis delivers an affordable and expandable solution which hospitals can use to improve their early lung cancer detection capabilities while reducing the time it takes to diagnose patients across different medical settings.

Real-World Evidence and Performance Validation in Population Screening

The AI systems that operate in lung cancer screening programs need both real-world evidence and performance validation to demonstrate their clinical effectiveness and operational reliability and safety features. AI algorithms achieve their best results in experimental research settings but actual environments bring about major shifts in medical imaging standards and patient population characteristics and disease distribution patterns and healthcare provider operations. The generalizability and strength of an AI model need assessment through validation tests that utilize data from multiple screening populations. Researchers conduct real-world studies in population-based low-dose CT (LDCT) programs to investigate essential outcomes which include early-stage lung cancer sensitivity metrics and false positive reduction specificity and nodule detection performance and its effects on patient follow-up procedures (Oudkerk et al., 2021).The algorithm performance research demonstrates its effectiveness in analyzing different CT scanner types and various acquisition protocols and different clinical settings. The national screening programs that national screening programs conduct in the United States, United Kingdom, and Asian countries have demonstrated that AI technology helps decrease the workload of radiologists while increasing their ability to detect medical conditions. The actual testing process evaluates how well AI systems function within clinical settings by measuring their impact on reporting times and team-based decision processes and subsequent diagnostic activities. The population-based data enables organizations to monitor algorithm performance changes and bias detection and safety hazard identification which assists in maintaining model accuracy across various population segments throughout time. The approval process for AI screening tools now requires companies to provide this evidence to regulatory agencies before they obtain certification.

AI IN HISTOPATHOLOGY AND CYTOPATHOLOGY

Digital Pathology and Whole-Slide Imaging Platforms

Digital pathology and whole-slide imaging (WSI) platforms have introduced revolutionary changes to traditional histopathological processes by providing researchers with the ability to digitize, store, analyze, and distribute tissue samples at unprecedented high-resolution levels. WSI technology enables users to transform entire tissue specimens into digital images which they can access from any location to conduct remote diagnostic work through telepathology and collaborative consultations (Evans et al., 2021). Pathologists can use gigapixel images to examine tissues from their complete structure down to the smallest cellular details while maintaining perfect clarity at every zoom level. WSI platforms deliver consistent imaging standards through their established protocols which include color calibration and contrast and spatial resolution measurements. Digital pathology workflows help oncology centers achieve faster results while improving record-keeping and decreasing differences between what different observers perceive. WSI establishes the core framework for AI-powered histopathology because deep learning systems require extensive digital databases with detailed annotations to acquire knowledge about complex cancer-related structural patterns. WSI enables lung cancer diagnosis through its support of automated tumor detection and segmentation and mitotic count assessment and PD-L1 biomarker quantification (Davri et al. 2023). The WSI system enables better workflow management through its integration with laboratory information systems which enhances quality control and enables research across multiple institutions. Digital slide repositories established through WSI technology help advance educational efforts while creating standardized processes and establishing worldwide reference materials. The implementation of digital pathology systems and WSI technology has transformed histopathological diagnostics through its enhanced diagnostic accuracy and AI-based analytical capabilities and the development of interconnected systems which support contemporary pulmonary oncology practices.

AI-Based Tissue Segmentation, Tumour Grading, and Biomarker Quantification

AI technologies for tissue segmentation and tumor grading and biomarker quantification function as effective instruments which improve the accuracy and speed and consistency of histopathological examinations used in lung cancer research. Digital pathology uses tissue segmentation as its basic work to separate different tissue types which include tumor areas and stroma and necrotic tissue and blood vessels and areas of inflammation. Deep learning models especially convolutional neural networks demonstrate their best performance when they identify these structures within complex tumor environments that include multiple tumor types (Khosravi et al., 2018). The process of automated segmentation benefits pathologists because it accelerates their work while reducing observer variability and delivering accurate measurements of tumor dimensions and environmental elements to researchers. AI systems evaluate tumor morphology through the analysis of nuclear atypia and mitotic figures and architectural patterns and tissue organization which enables them to classify tumors into distinct grades that predict patient outcomes and treatment success. The method provides essential advantages to lung adenocarcinoma and squamous cell carcinoma because even minor histological changes can determine which treatments doctors will prescribe. The introduction of AI-based systems for biomarker measurement represents a major advancement because it resolves past difficulties related to the manual scoring method used in immunohistochemistry tests. The algorithms enable accurate detection of PD-L1 and Ki-67 and ALK and EGFR biomarker expressions which yields objective results that medical professionals use to identify patients suitable for targeted therapy and immunotherapy (Restrepo et al., 2023). AI technology creates novel ways for healthcare workers to gain complete understanding of tissue samples by merging tissue structure details with molecular marker expression information. The automated systems enable researchers to conduct extensive testing while they improve diagnostic accuracy and support customized cancer treatment methods. The combination of AI-based systems for tissue segmentation and tumor grading and biomarker measurement has transformed pathology work because it produces data-driven measurements which hospitals need for contemporary lung cancer care (Table 3).

Table 3. Deep learning models for histological subtype classification in lung cancer

Subtype Classification Task	Deep Learning Model Used	Features Analyzed	Performance/Advantages	Applications in Pulmonary Oncology	References
Adenocarcinoma vs. Squamous Cell Carcinoma	Convolutional Neural Networks (CNNs)	Glandular patterns, keratinization, nuclear morphology	High accuracy (>90% in many studies); reduces inter-observer variability	Automated subtype diagnosis; supports treatment planning	(Nayak et al., 2026)
Small Cell Lung Carcinoma (SCLC) Identification	Deep Residual Networks (ResNet)	Cell size, chromatin texture, necrosis patterns	Effective for rare/complex subtypes; enhances early recognition	Guides therapy selection (e.g., chemo-sensitive tumors)	(Zhang et al., 2025)
Mixed/Variant Histology Classification	Inception Networks	Multi-scale features, heterogeneous tumor regions	Good performance on complex, mixed subtypes	Helps detect tumors with mixed differentiation	(Dong et al., 2022)
Subtype Prediction from Whole-Slide Images (WSI)	Slide-Level Multiple Instance Learning (MIL) Models	Patch-based tissue structures, contextual cues	Handles gigapixel WSI without pixel-level labels	Fully automated WSI analysis in digital pathology labs	(Fu et al., 2025)
Molecularly Informed Subtype Prediction	CNN + Transformer Hybrid Models	Morphology + spatial attention patterns	Predicts molecular correlates (e.g., EGFR/ ALK patterns) indirectly	Supports precision oncology and biomarker-guided therapy	(Parra-Medina et al., 2025)
Rare Subtype Detection (e.g., Large Cell Carcinoma)	DenseNet Models	Low-frequency morphological features	Improves detection of rare entities with limited training data	Enhances diagnostic completeness in complex cases	(Cooper et al., 2023)

Integration of Histopathological Features With Genomic Data for Precision Oncology

The combination of histopathological features with genomic data represents a significant development for precision oncology which provides deeper biological insights into lung cancer research. The fields of histopathology and genomics functioned as independent diagnostic methods which allowed histopathologists to study morphological patterns and genomics experts to investigate molecular changes. Artificial intelligence now establishes a connection between these two fields by using whole-slide images to extract high-dimensional features and connect them to genomic signatures that include EGFR ALK KRAS BRAF MET and TP53 mutations (Cheng and Shi, 2025). Deep learning models can identify subtle morphological changes that occur due to genetic mutations because they can process complex information which humans cannot understand. The AI system successfully predicts EGFR mutation status and PD-L1 expression from histopathology slides with high accuracy. The combination of genomic data and histological features produces multimodal models which improve predictions about treatment response and disease aggressiveness and survival outcomes. The models combine cellular morphology with tumor microenvironment features and immune infiltration patterns and molecular mutations to create integrated predictive systems. The multimodal approach becomes essential for therapy personalization because it guides treatment selection and determines immunotherapy eligibility and predicts patient outcomes. The combined histopathology genomic models enable researchers to discover biomarkers through their ability to extract molecular profiles from standard pathology slides without needing expensive genomic testing or tissue samples. The AI-powered systems enable multiple oncology disciplines to make better decisions while providing solutions that can function in areas which lack access to molecular testing facilities. The combination of histopathological and genomic data represents a major advancement which enables personalized treatment for lung cancer patients through a comprehensive data analysis of their specific tumor biology (Table 4).

Table 4. Case studies of AI in predictive pathology for lung cancer prognosis

Case Study	AI Model Used	Data Source	Predictive Outcome	Findings	References
Prediction of overall survival from WSIs	Convolutional Neural Networks (CNNs)	Whole-slide histopathology images	Overall survival (OS) risk stratification	AI identified morphological risk patterns, outperforming traditional grading systems.	(Lee, 2023)
AI-based tumor microenvironment analysis	Deep Learning + Spatial Analysis Models	Digitized H&E slides	Immune infiltration and stromal composition	Model predicted prognosis by quantifying tumor–immune interactions with high accuracy.	(Xie et al., 2024)
Morphology-driven EGFR mutation prediction	ResNet Models	Pathology WSIs + genomic data	EGFR mutation likelihood and associated prognosis	Enabled earlier prediction of EGFR-driven tumor behavior and treatment sensitivity.	(Haixian et al., 2025)

continued on following page

Table 4. Continued

Case Study	AI Model Used	Data Source	Predictive Outcome	Findings	References
Prognostic radiology–pathology fusion models	Multimodal CNN–MLP Hybrid Models	CT scans + pathology slides	Recurrence risk and progression-free survival	Fusion model improved prognosis prediction compared to single-modality models.	(Yang et al., 2025)
PD-L1 expression and immunotherapy response prediction	Transformer-based Pathology Models	IHC-stained pathology slides	Likelihood of immunotherapy response	Provided objective PD-L1 quantification and predicted treatment benefit more consistently than manual scoring.	(Cheng et al., 2025)
Risk prediction in early-stage lung adenocarcinoma	Multi-instance Learning (MIL) Models	WSI patches	Risk of postoperative recurrence	AI stratified patients into high-/low-risk groups, aiding decisions on adjuvant therapy.	(Tiwari et al., 2025)
Prognostic modeling using tumor grading automation	Automated Grading Models (CNN)	Histology images	Disease aggressiveness	Improved reproducibility of grading and correlated with long-term survival outcomes.	(Jaroensri et al., 2022)

RADIOMICS AND IMAGING BIOMARKERS

Concept and Workflow of Radiomics: Feature Extraction, Selection, and Modelling

Radiomics represents a developing field within medical imaging which transforms standard radiological scans into extensive quantitative data for tumor phenotype analysis and precision oncology treatment. The radiomics process starts with image acquisition and standardization which establishes uniform imaging standards through consistent imaging quality and slice thickness and contrast settings and scanner parameters that apply to both patients and medical facilities. The process continues with tumor segmentation which designates the specific area for analysis by using three methods which include manual and semi-automatic and AI-driven automated systems. The region of interest in the study exists through the process of radiomics which enables scientists to identify particular details that researchers will examine. The research includes first-order features which show how pixel intensities distribute through image processing and shape-based features which represent tumor geometry and margins and texture features which show how tumors contain multiple types of tissues through GLCM and GLRLM and wavelet-based transformation matrices (Elsayed et al., 2023). The workflow needs feature selection because radiomics generates thousands of features which contain unnecessary duplicate components and unproductive elements. The stable yet clinically relevant predictors can be identified through the application of LASSO regression and recursive feature elimination and principal component analysis and correlation-based filtering methods. The final stage involves modelling, where selected features are used to build predictive or prognostic models through machine learning algorithms, including random forests, support vector machines, gradient boosting, and increasingly, deep learning frameworks. The models undergo internal and external validation processes which test their ability to maintain performance standards across various population groups. Radiomics thus provides a non-invasive, reproducible method to infer tumor biology, forecast treatment response, and enhance clinical decision-making in lung cancer management (Martell et al., 2025).

Quantitative Imaging Biomarkers for Tumour Heterogeneity, Invasiveness, and Treatment Response

Quantitative imaging biomarkers function as essential tools for studying tumor heterogeneity and invasiveness and treatment response in lung cancer through their ability to provide information which exceeds what standard radiological assessments can show. The characteristic of aggressive cancers shows itself through tumor heterogeneity which manifests as varying degrees of cellular density and necrosis and vascularity and genetic diversity. Radiomic biomarkers obtained from CT and PET-CT and MRI studies can measure tumor heterogeneity through their ability to analyze texture features which include entropy and uniformity and gray-level co-occurrence metrics thereby detecting tumors with increased malignancy potential (Flaiban et al., 2025). The use of shape-based features which encompass irregularity and spiculation and volume changes functions as a non-invasive method to assess tumor invasiveness. PET metabolic biomarkers which include standardized uptake value (SUV) and metabolic tumor volume (MTV) enable structural imaging to evaluate biological aggressiveness and proliferative activity. Quantitative biomarkers enable treatment response assessment by providing early indicators of therapeutic effectiveness through their ability to detect initial tumor morphological and functional changes which precede traditional imaging detection. Dynamic contrast-enhanced

MRI, diffusion-weighted imaging, and changes in PET-based metabolic parameters enable monitoring of perfusion, cellularity, and metabolic shifts during chemotherapy, immunotherapy, or targeted therapy (Paudyal et al., 2021). Radiomic response signatures enable differentiation between actual progression and false progression in patients who received immunotherapy treatment. The use of these biomarkers in predictive models enhances patient classification accuracy while helping to determine the best treatment approaches and enabling flexible treatment methods. The quantitative imaging biomarkers create an effective non-invasive method that researchers can use to study tumor biology and monitor disease progression and develop customized treatment approaches for lung cancer patients.

Machine Learning in CT, PET-CT, and MRI for Phenotype Prediction

Machine learning (ML) has developed into a vital technology for lung cancer phenotype detection through its application in CT, PET-CT, and MRI. The technology enables researchers to analyze tumor biological characteristics that exceed visual observation limits. TheML models in CT imaging use nodule shape and texture and margin characteristics and density patterns to identify tumor aggressive behavior and metastatic potential and histological subtype and gene mutation status (Cheng et al., 2024). The algorithms random forests and support vector machines and deep learning methods extract radiomic features to learn from hundreds of features which show different patterns of heterogeneity and growth that match molecular activity. The machine learning models in PET-CT use metabolic information which PET-CT provides through SUV and total lesion glycolysis (TLG) and metabolic tumor volume (MTV) metrics to identify tumor metabolic characteristics and proliferation capacity and immune microenvironment behavior. The metabolic biomarkers help to detect tumors which display aggressive behavior and respond poorly to treatment. The process of MRI-based phenotype prediction uses functional sequences which include diffusion-weighted imaging (DWI) and dynamic contrast-enhanced MRI (DCE-MRI) and perfusion imaging to assess tumor cellularity and perfusion patterns and angiogenesis (Li et al., 2025). The development of ML models that use MRI features enables accurate predictions of tumor grade and hypoxia status and treatment sensitivity for patients with locally advanced lung cancer. The application of cross-modality machine learning models which combine CT structural data with PET metabolic markers and MRI functional parameters enables better phenotype prediction through the collection of complementary biological information. Integrated models enable precision oncology applications by predicting treatment response and recurrence risk and survival probabilities which empowers clinicians to customize treatments according to specific tumor characteristics of individual patients. The current field of ML-based phenotype prediction from multiple imaging modalities operates as the leading method for non-invasive tumor assessment in contemporary pulmonary oncology (Table 5).

Table 5. Role of deep radiomics and hybrid AI-imaging models in lung cancer

Category	Description	Advantages	Applications in Pulmonary Oncology	References
Deep Radiomics	Uses deep learning to automatically extract high-level imaging features from CT, PET-CT, or MRI without manual feature engineering.	Captures complex patterns, reduces human bias, and handles large imaging datasets.	Predicting tumor heterogeneity, mutation status (EGFR, KRAS), and treatment response.	(Avanzo et al., 2020)
Hybrid Radiomics (Handcrafted + Deep Features)	Combines traditional radiomic features with deep learning derived features for improved prediction accuracy.	Maximizes complementary strengths of both feature types; enhances robustness.	Risk stratification, recurrence prediction, and multi-parameter tumor characterization.	(Salmanpour et al., 2026)
AI-Imaging Genomic Models	Integrate imaging features with molecular/genomic data to infer tumor biology.	Enables non-invasive prediction of gene mutations and tumor microenvironment traits.	Predicting EGFR/ ALK status, immunotherapy biomarkers (PD-L1), and survival outcomes.	(Guo et al., 2025)
Multimodal Hybrid Models (Imaging + Clinical Data)	Merge imaging features with clinical variables such as age, smoking history, and performance status.	Improves generalizability and clinical applicability.	Personalized treatment planning and prognostic modelling.	(Kamrul et al., 2025)
Deep Learning Segmentation + Radiomics Models	Use automated tumor segmentation from deep networks as input for radiomic analysis.	Provides consistent tumor boundaries and improves feature reliability.	Automated nodule analysis, radiotherapy planning, and monitoring therapy response.	(Jyothi and Singh, 2023)
Time-Series Hybrid Models	Combine sequential imaging data with ML models to analyze tumor evolution.	Predicts early treatment response and captures changes over time.	Monitoring immunotherapy or targeted therapy outcomes.	(Hao et al., 2025)

Regulatory and Clinical Validation Aspects of Radiomic Models

Radiomic models require both regulatory approval and clinical validation studies to establish their safe operation and dependable performance and their suitability for use in lung cancer diagnosis and prognosis and treatment response evaluation. Radiomic models must undergo rigorous evaluation to meet standards set by regulatory bodies such as the U.S. FDA, EMA, and national health authorities. The evaluations assess system performance through testing which includes checking whether results stay consistent across different imaging devices and testing how the system performs under different scanning methods and evaluating the system's ability to maintain analysis results and understand the system's workings. Clinical validation typically proceeds through multi-phase studies, including retrospective testing, external validation across multiple institutions, and prospective clinical trials. The requirement is demonstrating that radiomic features remain consistent across different CT or PET-CT machines, ensuring that the model's predictions are not device dependent (Mo et al., 2025). A representative case report highlights the importance of such validation. The radiomic model which predicts treatment response after stereotactic body radiotherapy (SBRT) underwent clinical testing in a multicenter pilot study that included 68 patients who had early stage non–small cell lung cancer (NSCLC). The researchers collected imaging data from three CT scanner types and used these images to extract radiomic features which predicted local control at 12 months (Wang et al., 2019). The model achieved an AUC of 0.82 in internal validation and 0.79 in external cohorts, demonstrating its generalizability (Shung et al., 2020). A 65-year-old male patient with stage IB adenocarcinoma showed post-treatment CT texture changes which the model predicted would indicate recurrence three months before radiologists identified it (Goel et al., 2017). The model successfully predicted progressive disease according to follow-up results. Regulatory decisions need case-based evidence which demonstrates the clinical importance of radiomics as a non-invasive biomarker that can be used in regular lung cancer treatment.

AI IN PERSONALIZED LUNG CANCER THERAPY

Precision Oncology and the Paradigm of AI-Guided Treatment Decisions

Precision oncology together with AI-based treatment decision systems establishes a new framework for diagnosing and characterizing and treating lung cancer through its ability to deliver tailored treatment solutions. Standard medical approaches depend on wide-ranging patient data while using restricted genetic data, which fails to represent the complete tumor complexity and patient-specific treatment outcomes. The complete predictive models developed by AI research combine extensive genomic profiles together with diverse radiomic signatures and histopathologic features and clinical records and immune biomarkers and actual patient results (Takamatsu, 2025). The models can reveal hidden patterns which human thought processes find difficult to understand, thereby helping doctors choose therapies based on the specific genetic and structural and environmental attributes of tumors. AI uses machine learning algorithms for predicting how patients will respond to targeted therapies and chemotherapy and immunotherapy by examining biomarkers which include EGFR mutations and ALK rearrangements and KRAS variants and PD-L1 expression levels (Lococo et al., 2024). The artificial intelligence system provides dynamic treatment optimization because it learns from patient information and detects new resistance patterns while recommending treatment alternatives through its machine learning capabilities. The AI-driven decision-support systems simulate potential treatment outcomes which help multidisciplinary tumor board meetings develop patient-specific treatment plans that deliver optimal evidence-based medical care. The artificial intelligence system assists in creating patient risk groups which lets healthcare professionals treat patients who face the highest risks while stopping unnecessary procedures for patients with less severe conditions. Artificial intelligence functions as an advanced cognitive assistant for medical professionals because it helps them reach precise decisions based on reliable data throughout their work (Kothinti, 2024). The field of precision oncology will experience a fundamental transformation because artificial intelligence systems will provide targeted lung cancer treatment that creates individualized patient care solutions.

AI in Predicting Therapeutic Response and Resistance to Chemotherapy, Targeted Therapy, and Immunotherapy

The application of AI technology enables researchers to create predictive models which assess how lung cancer patients will respond to various chemotherapy and targeted therapy and immunotherapy treatments. Doctors use clinical characteristics and a small number of biomarkers to make treatment choices, but this method fails to recognize the complete tumor diversity and the evolving molecular features of tumors. AI-based systems use radiomics, genomics, transcriptomics, histopathology, and clinical data to build predictive models which show how specific treatments will affect different tumors. AI evaluates tumor structure and tumor growth and genetic changes to determine which platinum-based chemotherapy treatments will work for patients while avoiding treatments that would not help them and would cause harmful effects. Machine learning models examine genomic patterns through the analysis of specific mutations which include EGFR and ALK and KRAS and ROS1 and BRAF together with imaging data to predict treatment outcomes and identify early signs of molecular resistance which involve secondary mutations and pathway reactivation (Manik et al., 2022). AI boosts immunotherapy response prediction through its assessment of PD-L1 expression and tumor mutational burden (TMB) and immune infiltration patterns and radiomic biomarkers which indicate tumor microenvironment characteristics. Deep learning techniques can differentiate true progression from pseudoprogression and identify early non-responders which enables timely treatment strategy adjustments. AI-based dynamic response monitoring uses serial imaging together with circulating biomarkers to enable early identification of treatment failures. The predictive information enables doctors to create customized treatment plans which decrease the need for trial-and-error methods while increasing patient survival rates. AI enables precision oncology through its ability to deliver data-driven solutions which predict treatment response and resistance patterns thus improving lung cancer treatment (Table 6).

Table 6. Integration of AI with key molecular profiles in lung cancer

Molecular Marker	AI Methods Used	Data Inputs	AI-Enhanced Capabilities	Clinical Applications	References
EGFR Mutations	CNNs, radiomics + ML models, WSI-based DL	CT scans, histopathology slides, genomic sequencing	Predict EGFR mutation probability; detect subtle morphological correlates	Non-invasive mutation prediction, candidate selection for EGFR-TKI therapy	(Moscalu et al., 2023)
ALK Rearrangements	Deep learning classifiers, multimodal fusion models	PET-CT, MRI, WSI, molecular testing	Identify imaging patterns linked to ALK; integrate structural + genomic features	Early detection, therapy matching for ALK inhibitors	(Marouf et al., 2025)
KRAS Mutations	Radiogenomic models, ResNet variants	CT texture features, pathology WSIs	Predict KRAS mutation likelihood; identify radiomic heterogeneity signatures	Risk stratification, prognosis estimation, targeted therapy planning	(Ortuño-Miquel et al., 2025)
PD-L1 Expression	Transformer models, AI-driven IHC quantification	Digital pathology slides, IHC staining images	Automated PD-L1 scoring; predict immune microenvironment activity	Immunotherapy eligibility, prediction of response to checkpoint inhibitors	(Wasinger et al., 2025)
Multigene Integrated Profiling	Hybrid AI models (imaging + genomics), graph neural networks	WSI, CT, multi-omics datasets	Capture interactions between genetic pathways and imaging phenotypes	Comprehensive precision oncology, multi-marker treatment recommendations	(Albaradei, 2025)

Predictive Analytics for Patient Stratification and Outcome Forecasting

Predictive analytics has become a cornerstone of modern lung cancer treatment because it allows doctors to categorize patients better while they can predict patient outcomes with exceptional accuracy. AI-based predictive systems use machine learning (ML) models which combine clinical data with radiological information and molecular data and demographic details to discover hidden risk patterns that standard approaches cannot detect. The models predict overall survival and progression-free survival and relapse risk while they use tumour biology and treatment history and response likelihood to create distinct prognostic groups for patients. The research team used supervised ML algorithms such as random forests and Cox-survival models and gradient boosting machines to study extensive datasets and develop customized risk assessment tools (Wang et al., 2022). Tumour imaging analytics use radiomics-derived signatures to create multiple predictive capabilities which measure tumour typicality and display how tumours spread their aggressive characteristics. The models achieve their highest level of accuracy through genomic marker testing which includes EGFR and ALK and KRAS and MET and PD-L1 expression. The AI-powered forecasting tools enable active monitoring because they update their predictions based on new data which includes follow-up scans and circulating tumour DNA (ctDNA) profiles. The systems from Rouvinov et al. (2026) provide instant risk updates through their ability to track changing patient conditions. The predictive algorithms enable healthcare providers to identify patients who will develop treatment resistance or extreme toxicity. The analytics in clinical operations enhance decision-making capabilities while they help choose appropriate clinical trials and establish value-based care procedures. Predictive analytics enable lung cancer treatment to shift from a reactive approach to a proactive method which delivers personalized treatment that boosts patient results and improves resource allocation (Dasgupta, 2024).

Case Studies: AI-Driven Clinical Decision Support Systems for Individualized Therapy

AI-based Clinical Decision Support Systems (CDSS) have started to change personalized lung cancer treatment procedures because their systems use various types of medical data which include radiology and genomics and pathology and clinical records to help clinicians make decisions based on established research. The case study presents a 62-year-old male patient who has stage IIIA non-small cell lung cancer (NSCLC) and received CT imaging and PET-CT staging along with tumour genomic sequencing (Forde et al., 2018). The institution implemented an AI-based

CDSS system which used radiomic tumour signatures together with circulating tumour DNA (ctDNA) dynamics and EGFR/KRAS mutation status to develop a customized treatment plan for the patient (Cherukuri et al., 2025). The system evaluated more than two thousand measurement points which covered tumor shape variability and patterns of metabolic activity and the past results from matching patients. The study showed a standard chemoradiation treatment would result in a high probability of poor response which reached 78 percent while the study showed targeted therapy with immunotherapy would provide a positive response probability of 64 percent (Pilard et al., 2021). The oncology board chose to administer osimertinib together with pembrolizumab based on CDSS recommendations instead of using traditional cisplatin-based treatment methods. The same CDSS system conducted serial monitoring which detected early biomarker response through decreased ctDNA levels and unchanged radiomic feature development that demonstrated successful disease management. An AI-based clinical decision support system used MRI radiomics and PD-L1 expression data to assist immunotherapy selection for a 55-year-old woman diagnosed with metastatic adenocarcinoma according to Zhang et al. 2025. The system identified high potential for immunotherapy advantages while showing risk for immune-related side effects which led to development of monitoring procedures and dose management techniques. The AI-powered CDSS system demonstrates important advantages because it helps doctors make precise treatment choices while minimizing the need for treatments that need to be tested during multiple therapeutic sessions. The CDSS improves its accuracy through data acquisition which enables safer and more effective lung cancer management solutions.

DISCUSSION

The application of artificial intelligence (AI) throughout the complete process of pulmonary oncology which includes screening diagnosis and treatment planning until longitudinal patient tracking represents a major breakthrough for contemporary cancer treatment. The integration of AI systems into clinical pathways and electronic health record (EHR) systems delivers decision support capabilities that operate in real time while enabling automatic image evaluation and patient risk assessment and choice of treatment. AI-powered multidisciplinary tumour boards (MDTs) develop better shared decision-making capabilities through their ability to combine imaging results and histopathology and genomic information and clinical findings into precise treatment recommendations. This system enables oncologists and radiologists and pathologists to perform their duties with higher accuracy while retaining human control during difficult situations that require complex decision-making. The success of clinical implementation depends on how humans and artificial intelligence systems work together. Through its analytical capabilities which include detecting minute imaging irregularities and measuring biomarkers and forecasting treatment outcomes and verifying reporting accuracy AI assists clinicians in their work. The advantages associated with this situation create difficulties that need to be resolved. The process of implementing ethical standards requires organizations to deal with four key issues which include bias detection and algorithmic transparency and safeguarding personal data and determining responsibility for actions. The major obstacle to trust in AI systems for clinical use exists because clinicians require both AI output results and the system's prediction methods to be understandable. The combination of different data quality levels and the absence of established standards and the limited capability to test outside boundaries and the presence of regulatory barriers create difficulties for organizations that want to implement their solutions on a large scale. AI systems demonstrate considerable proficiency in three areas which include developing personalized lung cancer treatments and creating effective screening systems and enhancing their ability to forecast outcomes. The research work in deep radiomics and multimodal fusion models and federated learning and real-world validation will create more advanced clinical AI applications which will demonstrate enhanced safety features.

CONCLUSION

The field of pulmonary oncology is undergoing rapid transformation because AI technology enables medical professionals to identify diseases at earlier stages while achieving better diagnostic results and creating treatment plans that fit each individual patient. The implementation of AI in clinical settings becomes effective when the system uses validated testing methods together with clear algorithm specifications and built-in ethical protections. Although current AI systems still face issues with reliability and bias and interoperability and trust problems, ongoing technological development will lead to systems that enhance human judgment instead of replacing it. The future of lung cancer treatment will benefit from improved data standardization methods and advanced imaging-genomic predictive systems and machine learning-based clinical decision support tools. The responsible use of AI technology will create better patient results while creating a new personalized cancer treatment standard.

REFERENCES

Aishwarya, K. V., & Asuntha, A. (2025). A survey on comparative study of lung nodules applying machine learning and deep learning techniques. *Multimedia Tools and Applications*, *84*(5), 2127–2181. DOI: 10.1007/s11042-024-20009-0

Akgündoğdu, A., & Çelikbaş, Ş. (2025). Explainable deep learning framework for brain tumor detection: Integrating LIME, Grad-CAM, and SHAP for enhanced accuracy. *Medical Engineering & Physics*, *144*(1), 104405. DOI: 10.1016/j.medengphy.2025.104405 PMID: 40925692

Al-Musawi, J. M., Al-Shadeedi, F., Shakir, N. A., & Ibrahim, S. Q. (2025). Epidemiological Characteristics of Lung Cancer Patients in the Middle Euphrates Region of Iraq: Retrospective Analysis from the Middle Euphrates Cancer Center (2018-2023). *Al-Rafidain Journal of Medical Sciences (ISSN 2789-3219)*, *8*(2), 63-70.

Albaradei, S. (2025). AI-Driven Approaches to Utilization of Multi-Omics Data for Personalized Diagnosis and Treatment of Cancer: A Comprehensive Review. *Computer Modeling in Engineering & Sciences*, *145*(3), 2937–2970. DOI: 10.32604/cmes.2025.072584

Ashrafi, A., Akter, Z., Modareszadeh, P., Modareszadeh, P., Berisha, E., Alemi, P. S., Chacon Castro, M. C., Deese, A. R., & Zhang, L. (2022). Current landscape of therapeutic resistance in lung cancer and promising strategies to overcome resistance. *Cancers (Basel)*, *14*(19), 4562. DOI: 10.3390/cancers14194562 PMID: 36230484

Avanzo, M., Wei, L., Stancanello, J., Vallieres, M., Rao, A., Morin, O., Mattonen, S. A., & El Naqa, I. (2020). Machine and deep learning methods for radiomics. *Medical Physics*, *47*(5), e185–e202. DOI: 10.1002/mp.13678 PMID: 32418336

Cheng, C. H., & Shi, S. S. (2025). Artificial intelligence in cancer: Applications, challenges, and future perspectives. *Molecular Cancer*, *24*(1), 274. DOI: 10.1186/s12943-025-02450-3 PMID: 41168799

Cheng, D. O., Khaw, C. R., Mccabe, J., Pennycuick, A., Nair, A., Moore, D. A., Janes, S. M., & Jacob, J. (2024). Predicting histopathological features of aggressiveness in lung cancer using CT radiomics: A systematic review. *Clinical Radiology*, *79*(9), 681–689. DOI: 10.1016/j.crad.2024.04.022 PMID: 38853080

Cheng, Y., Lama, N., Chen, M., Amidi, E., Ramzanpour, M., Rahman, M. A., Xiu, J., Helmstetter, A., Dickman, L., Ribeiro, J. R., Ghani, H., Oberley, M., Spetzler, D., & Sledge, G. W. (2025). Synergistic H&E and IHC image analysis by AI predicts cancer biomarkers and survival outcomes in colorectal and breast cancer. *Communications Medicine*, *5*(1), 328. DOI: 10.1038/s43856-025-01045-9 PMID: 40750675

Cherukuri, S. P., Kaur, A., Goyal, B., Kukunoor, H. R., Sahito, A. F., Sachdeva, P., Yerrapragada, G., Elangovan, P., Shariff, M. N., Natarajan, T., Janarthanan, J., Richard, S., Pallikaranai Venkatesaprasath, S., Karuppiah, S. S., Iyer, V. N., Helgeson, S. A., & Arunachalam, S. P. (2025). Artificial Intelligence-Enhanced Liquid Biopsy and Radiomics in Early-Stage Lung Cancer Detection: A Precision Oncology Paradigm. *Cancers (Basel)*, *17*(19), 3165. DOI: 10.3390/cancers17193165 PMID: 41097693

Chhikara, B. S., & Parang, K. (2023). Global Cancer Statistics 2022: the trends projection analysis. *Chemical biology letters, 10*(1), 451-451.

Cooper, M., Ji, Z., & Krishnan, R. G. (2023). Machine learning in computational histopathology: Challenges and opportunities. *Genes, Chromosomes & Cancer*, *62*(9), 540–556. DOI: 10.1002/gcc.23177 PMID: 37314068

Dasgupta, S. (2024). Next-generation cancer phenomics: A transformative approach to unraveling lung cancer complexity and advancing precision medicine. *OMICS: A Journal of Integrative Biology*, *28*(12), 585–595. DOI: 10.1089/omi.2024.0175 PMID: 39435580

Dasgupta, S. (2024). Next-generation cancer phenomics: A transformative approach to unraveling lung cancer complexity and advancing precision medicine. *OMICS: A Journal of Integrative Biology*, *28*(12), 585–595. DOI: 10.1089/omi.2024.0175 PMID: 39435580

Davri, A., Birbas, E., Kanavos, T., Ntritsos, G., Giannakeas, N., Tzallas, A. T., & Batistatou, A. (2023). Deep learning for lung cancer diagnosis, prognosis and prediction using histological and cytological images: A systematic review. *Cancers (Basel)*, *15*(15), 3981. DOI: 10.3390/cancers15153981 PMID: 37568797

Dong, X., Li, M., Zhou, P., Deng, X., Li, S., Zhao, X., Wu, Y., Qin, J., & Guo, W. (2022). Fusing pre-trained convolutional neural networks features for multi-differentiated subtypes of liver cancer on histopathological images. *BMC Medical Informatics and Decision Making*, *22*(1), 122. DOI: 10.1186/s12911-022-01798-6 PMID: 35509058

Elsayed, B., Alksas, A., Shehata, M., Mahmoud, A., Zaky, M., Alghandour, R., Abdelwahab, K., Abdelkhalek, M., Ghazal, M., Contractor, S., El-Din Moustafa, H., & El-Baz, A. (2023). Exploring neoadjuvant chemotherapy, predictive models, radiomic, and pathological markers in breast cancer: A comprehensive review. *Cancers (Basel)*, *15*(21), 5288. DOI: 10.3390/cancers15215288 PMID: 37958461

Evans, A. J., Vajpeyi, R., Henry, M., & Chetty, R. (2021). Establishment of a remote diagnostic histopathology service using whole slide imaging (digital pathology). *Journal of Clinical Pathology*, *74*(7), 421–424. DOI: 10.1136/jclinpath-2020-206762 PMID: 32611763

Flaiban, E., Orhan, K., Gonçalves, B. C., Lopes, S. L. P. D. C., & Costa, A. L. F. (2025). Radiomics in Action: Multimodal Synergies for Imaging Biomarkers. *Bioengineering (Basel, Switzerland)*, *12*(11), 1139. DOI: 10.3390/bioengineering12111139 PMID: 41301095

Forde, P. M., Chaft, J. E., Smith, K. N., Anagnostou, V., Cottrell, T. R., Hellmann, M. D., Zahurak, M., Yang, S. C., Jones, D. R., Broderick, S., Battafarano, R. J., Velez, M. J., Rekhtman, N., Olah, Z., Naidoo, J., Marrone, K. A., Verde, F., Guo, H., Zhang, J., & Pardoll, D. M. (2018). Neoadjuvant PD-1 blockade in resectable lung cancer. *The New England Journal of Medicine*, *378*(21), 1976–1986. DOI: 10.1056/NEJMoa1716078 PMID: 29658848

Fu, F., Zhang, X., Wang, Z., Xie, L., Fu, M., Peng, J., Wu, J., Wang, Z., Guan, T., He, Y., Lin, J.-S., Zhu, L., & Dai, W. (2025). A pathology-attention multi-instance learning framework for multimodal classification of colorectal lesions. *Frontiers in Pharmacology*, *16*, 1592950. DOI: 10.3389/fphar.2025.1592950 PMID: 40548052

Georgakopoulou, V. E., Spandidos, D. A., & Corlateanu, A. (2025). Diagnostic tools in respiratory medicine. *Biomedical Reports*, *23*(1), 112. DOI: 10.3892/br.2025.1990 PMID: 40420977

Goel, R., Moore, W., Sumer, B., Khan, S., Sher, D., & Subramaniam, R. M. (2017). Clinical practice in PET/CT for the management of head and neck squamous cell cancer. *AJR. American Journal of Roentgenology*, *209*(2), 289–303. DOI: 10.2214/AJR.17.18301 PMID: 28731808

Guo, Y., Li, T., Gong, B., Hu, Y., Wang, S., Yang, L., & Zheng, C. (2025). From Images to Genes: Radiogenomics Based on Artificial Intelligence to Achieve Non-Invasive Precision Medicine in Cancer Patients. *Advancement of Science*, *12*(2), 2408069. DOI: 10.1002/advs.202408069 PMID: 39535476

Haixian, L., Shu, P., Zhao, L., Chunfeng, L., & Lun, L. (2025). Machine learning approaches for EGFR mutation status prediction in NSCLC: An updated systematic review. *Frontiers in Oncology*, *15*, 1576461. DOI: 10.3389/fonc.2025.1576461 PMID: 40708937

Hao, L., Wang, C., Che, J., Sun, M., & Wang, Y. (2025). Deep learning-based time series prediction in multispectral and hyperspectral imaging for cancer detection. *Frontiers in Medicine*, *12*, 1605865. DOI: 10.3389/fmed.2025.1605865 PMID: 40823576

Huang, Y., Li, Q., Chen, H., Zhou, X., Han, Q., Lu, H., Cui, N., & Cao, Q. (2025). A novel approach to integrating Vision Transformers and machine learning for robust lung nodule classification using CT imaging. *Journal of Radiation Research and Applied Sciences*, *18*(3), 101672. DOI: 10.1016/j.jrras.2025.101672

Hussain, D., Al-Masni, M. A., Aslam, M., Sadeghi-Niaraki, A., Hussain, J., Gu, Y. H., & Naqvi, R. A. (2024). Revolutionizing tumor detection and classification in multimodality imaging based on deep learning approaches: Methods, applications and limitations. *Journal of X-Ray Science and Technology*, *32*(4), 857–911. DOI: 10.3233/XST-230429 PMID: 38701131

Hussain, H. K., Tariq, A., Gill, A. Y., & Ahmad, A. (2022). Transforming healthcare: The rapid rise of artificial intelligence revolutionizing healthcare applications. *BULLET: Jurnal Multidisiplin Ilmu*, *1*(02), 592216.

Ibrahim, A., Lashen, A., Toss, M., Mihai, R., & Rakha, E. (2022). Assessment of mitotic activity in breast cancer: Revisited in the digital pathology era. *Journal of Clinical Pathology*, *75*(6), 365–372. DOI: 10.1136/jclinpath-2021-207742 PMID: 34556501

Islam, M. T., Al Mamun, M. A., Khan, O. U., Akeem, A. B., Mohammad, H., Hamdache, A., & Elmouki, I. (2024). Emerging Trends In Artificial Intelligence Learning Methods: Deep Learning And Machine Learning Innovation In Computer Science. *Nanotechnology Perceptions*, *20*(13), 1150–1173. DOI: 10.62441/nano-ntp.vi.2598

Jaroensri, R., Wulczyn, E., Hegde, N., Brown, T., Flament-Auvigne, I., Tan, F., Cai, Y., Nagpal, K., Rakha, E. A., Dabbs, D. J., Olson, N., Wren, J. H., Thompson, E. E., Seetao, E., Robinson, C., Miao, M., Beckers, F., Corrado, G. S., Peng, L. H., & Chen, P. H. C. (2022). Deep learning models for histologic grading of breast cancer and association with disease prognosis. *NPJ Breast Cancer*, *8*(1), 113. DOI: 10.1038/s41523-022-00478-y PMID: 36192400

Jyothi, P., & Singh, A. R. (2023). Deep learning models and traditional automated techniques for brain tumor segmentation in MRI: A review. *Artificial Intelligence Review*, *56*(4), 2923–2969. DOI: 10.1007/s10462-022-10245-x

Kamrul, S. M., Jobair, H. F. M., Bofan, H., Cheng, J. Q., & Huanying, G. (2025). Multimodal Models in Healthcare: Methods, Challenges, and Future Directions for Enhanced Clinical Decision Support. *Information (Basel), 16*(11), 971. DOI: 10.3390/info16110971

Khosravi, P., Kazemi, E., Imielinski, M., Elemento, O., & Hajirasouliha, I. (2018). Deep convolutional neural networks enable discrimination of heterogeneous digital pathology images. *EBioMedicine, 27*, 317–328. DOI: 10.1016/j.ebiom.2017.12.026 PMID: 29292031

Kothinti, R. R.Rishi Reddy Kothinti. (2024). Deep learning in healthcare: Transforming disease diagnosis, personalized treatment, and clinical decision-making through AI-driven innovations. *World J Adv Res Rev, 24*(2), 2841–2856. DOI: 10.30574/wjarr.2024.24.2.3435

Lee, M. (2023). Recent advancements in deep learning using whole slide imaging for cancer prognosis. *Bioengineering (Basel, Switzerland), 10*(8), 897. DOI: 10.3390/bioengineering10080897 PMID: 37627783

Li, X. M., Nguyen, T., Sparks, H. D., Sung, K., & Chiang, J. (2025). Quantitative Dynamic Contrast-Enhanced Magnetic Resonance Imaging (DCE-MRI) in Hepatocellular Carcinoma: A Review of Emerging Applications for Locoregional Therapy. *Bioengineering (Basel, Switzerland), 12*(8), 870. DOI: 10.3390/bioengineering12080870 PMID: 40868383

Lococo, F., Ghaly, G., Flamini, S., Campanella, A., Chiappetta, M., Bria, E., Vita, E., Tortora, G., Evangelista, J., Sassorossi, C., Congedo, M. T., Valentini, V., Sala, E., Cesario, A., Margaritora, S., Boldrini, L., & Mohammed, A. (2024). Artificial intelligence applications in personalizing lung cancer management: State of the art and future perspectives. *Journal of Thoracic Disease, 16*(10), 7096–7110. DOI: 10.21037/jtd-24-244 PMID: 39552872

Magrabi, F., Ammenwerth, E., McNair, J. B., De Keizer, N. F., Hyppönen, H., Nykänen, P., Rigby, M., Scott, P. J., Vehko, T., Wong, Z. S.-Y., & Georgiou, A. (2019). Artificial intelligence in clinical decision support: Challenges for evaluating AI and practical implications. *Yearbook of Medical Informatics, 28*(01), 128–134. DOI: 10.1055/s-0039-1677903 PMID: 31022752

Manik, M. M. T. G., Hossain, S., Ahmed, M. K., Rozario, E., Miah, M. A., Moniruzzaman, M., & Saimon, A. S. M.Mia Md Tofayel Gonee Manik. (2022). Integrating genomic data and machine learning to advance precision oncology and targeted cancer therapies. *Nanotechnology Perceptions, 18*(2), 219–243. DOI: 10.62441/nano-ntp.v18i2.5443

Mannumadam Venugopal, S. (2024). Can Vision Transformers Be the Next State-of-the-Art Model for Oncology Medical Image Analysis? *AI in Precision Oncology*, *1*(6), 286–305. DOI: 10.1089/aipo.2024.0023

Marinakis, I., Karampidis, K., & Papadourakis, G. (2024). Pulmonary nodule detection, segmentation and classification using deep learning: A comprehensive literature review. *BioMedInformatics*, *4*(3), 2043–2106. DOI: 10.3390/biomedinformatics4030111

Marouf, A. A., Rokne, J. G., & Alhajj, R. (2025). Integrating Multi-Omics and Medical Imaging in Artificial Intelligence-Based Cancer Research: An Umbrella Review of Fusion Strategies and Applications. *Cancers (Basel)*, *17*(22), 3638. DOI: 10.3390/cancers17223638 PMID: 41301005

Martell, M. B., Linton-Reid, K., Chen, M., & Aboagye, E. O. (2025). Radiomics for lung cancer diagnosis, management, and future prospects. *Clinical Radiology*, *86*, 106926. DOI: 10.1016/j.crad.2025.106926 PMID: 40344812

Mo, Q., Cui, J., Jia, S., Zhang, Y., Xiao, Y., Liu, C., . . . Zhao, M. (2025). Stacking Ensemble Learning-based Models Enabling Accurate Diagnosis of Cardiac Amyloidosis using SPECT/CT: an International and Multicentre Study. medRxiv, 2025-06.

Moscalu, M., Moscalu, R., Dascălu, C. G., arcă, V., Cojocaru, E., Costin, I. M., arcă, E., & erban, I. L. (2023). Histopathological images analysis and predictive modeling implemented in digital pathology—Current affairs and perspectives. *Diagnostics (Basel)*, *13*(14), 2379. DOI: 10.3390/diagnostics13142379 PMID: 37510122

Nakajo, M., Hirahara, D., Hirahara, M., Eizuru, Y., Tani, A., Kanzaki, F., & Yoshiura, T. (2025). Artificial intelligence in oncological positron emission tomography: Advancing image analysis and interpretation. *Clinical Radiology*, •••, 107187. PMID: 41401681

Navarro-Garcia, D., Marcos, A., Beets-Tan, R., Blomqvist, L., Bodalal, Z., Deandreis, D., Crispin-Ortuzar, M., Gallagher, F., Giandini, T., Graves, M. J., Lassau, N., Maier-Hein, K., Prelaj, A., Schader, P., Schlemmer, H.-P., Sedlaczek, O., Vaiani, M., & Perez-Lopez, R. (2025). Real-world radiology data for artificial intelligence-driven cancer support systems and biomarker development. *ESMO Real World Data and Digital Oncology*, *8*, 100120. DOI: 10.1016/j.esmorw.2025.100120 PMID: 41647703

Nayak, K., Kadavigere, R., Pendem, S., Mane, P. R., Sampathila, N., Pattath Sankaran, P., & Siddeshappa, N. (2026). Diagnostic Accuracy of Artificial Intelligence Models for Differentiation of Squamous Cell Carcinoma and Adenocarcinoma of Lung—A Systematic Review. *Diagnostics (Basel)*, *16*(3), 500. DOI: 10.3390/diagnostics16030500 PMID: 41681818

Ogut, E. (2025). Artificial intelligence in clinical medicine: Challenges across diagnostic imaging, clinical decision support, surgery, pathology, and drug discovery. *Clinics and Practice*, *15*(9), 169. DOI: 10.3390/clinpract15090169 PMID: 41002784

Ortuño-Miquel, S., Roca, R., Alenda, C., Aranda, F., Martínez-Banaclocha, N., Amador, S., & Gil, D. (2025). Deep Learning Model-Based Architectures for Lung Tumor Mutation Profiling: A Systematic Review. *Cancers (Basel)*, *17*(22), 3619. DOI: 10.3390/cancers17223619 PMID: 41300986

Oudkerk, M., Liu, S., Heuvelmans, M. A., Walter, J. E., & Field, J. K. (2021). Lung cancer LDCT screening and mortality reduction—Evidence, pitfalls and future perspectives. *Nature Reviews. Clinical Oncology*, *18*(3), 135–151. DOI: 10.1038/s41571-020-00432-6 PMID: 33046839

Owens, C. A. R. A., Hindocha, S. U. M. E. E. T., Lee, R. I. C. H. A. R. D., Millard, T. H. O. M. A. S., & Sharma, B. H. U. P. I. N. D. E. R. (2023). The lung cancers: staging and response, CT, 18F-FDG PET/CT, MRI, DWI: review and new perspectives. *The British Journal of Radiology*, *96*(1148), 20220339. DOI: 10.1259/bjr.20220339 PMID: 37097296

Parra-Medina, R., Guerron-Gomez, G., Mendivelso-González, D., Gil-Gómez, J. H., Alzate, J. P., Gomez-Suarez, M., Polo, J. F., Sprockel, J. J., & Mosquera-Zamudio, A. (2025). Deep learning in histopathology images for prediction of oncogenic driver molecular alterations in lung cancer: A systematic review and meta-analysis. *Translational Lung Cancer Research*, *14*(5), 1756–1769. DOI: 10.21037/tlcr-2024-1196 PMID: 40535093

Paudyal, R., Grkovski, M., Oh, J. H., Schöder, H., Nunez, D. A., Hatzoglou, V., Deasy, J. O., Humm, J. L., Lee, N. Y., & Shukla-Dave, A. (2021). Application of community detection algorithm to investigate the correlation between imaging biomarkers of tumor metabolism, hypoxia, cellularity, and perfusion for precision radiotherapy in head and neck squamous cell carcinomas. *Cancers (Basel)*, *13*(15), 3908. DOI: 10.3390/cancers13153908 PMID: 34359810

Pilard, C., Ancion, M., Delvenne, P., Jerusalem, G., Hubert, P., & Herfs, M. (2021). Cancer immunotherapy: It's time to better predict patients' response. *British Journal of Cancer*, *125*(7), 927–938. DOI: 10.1038/s41416-021-01413-x PMID: 34112949

Rajendran, A., Angelin Rajan, R., Balasubramaniyam, S., & Elumalai, K. (2025). AI-Enhanced Predictive Imaging in Precision Medicine: Advancing Diagnostic Accuracy and Personalized Treatment. *iRadiology*, *3*(4), 261–278. DOI: 10.1002/ird3.70027

Raptis, S., Ilioudis, C., & Theodorou, K. (2024). Uncovering the diagnostic power of radiomic feature significance in automated lung cancer detection: An integrative analysis of texture, shape, and intensity contributions. *BioMedInformatics*, *4*(4), 2400–2425. DOI: 10.3390/biomedinformatics4040129

Restrepo, J. C., Dueñas, D., Corredor, Z., & Liscano, Y. (2023). Advances in genomic data and biomarkers: Revolutionizing NSCLC diagnosis and treatment. *Cancers (Basel)*, *15*(13), 3474. DOI: 10.3390/cancers15133474 PMID: 37444584

Rodak, O., Peris-Diaz, M. D., Olbromski, M., Podhorska-Okołów, M., & Dzięgiel, P. (2021). Current landscape of non-small cell lung cancer: Epidemiology, histological classification, targeted therapies, and immunotherapy. *Cancers (Basel)*, *13*(18), 4705. DOI: 10.3390/cancers13184705 PMID: 34572931

Rouvinov, K., Naamneh, R., Yakobson, A., Najjar, W., Abu Amna, M., Soklakova, A., Abu Zeid, E. E. D., Brenner, R., Asla, M., Ghalion, F. A., Abu Juma'a, A., Meirovitz, A., & Shalata, W. (2026). The Transformative Potential of Liquid Biopsies and Circulating Tumor DNA (ctDNA) in Modern Oncology. *Diagnostics (Basel)*, *16*(4), 523. DOI: 10.3390/diagnostics16040523 PMID: 41750672

Salmanpour, M. R., Mehrnia, S. S., Jabarzadeh Ghandilu, S., Safahi, Z., Falahati, S., Taeb, S., Mousavi, G., Maghsudi, M., Shariftabrizi, A., Hacihaliloglu, I., & Rahmim, A. (2026). Handcrafted vs. Deep Radiomics vs. Fusion vs. Deep Learning: A Comprehensive Review of Machine Learning-Based Cancer Outcome Prediction in PET and SPECT Imaging. *Journal of Imaging Informatics in Medicine*, •••, 1–50. DOI: 10.1007/s10278-025-01804-z PMID: 41612111

Shung, D. L., Au, B., Taylor, R. A., Tay, J. K., Laursen, S. B., Stanley, A. J., Dalton, H. R., Ngu, J., Schultz, M., & Laine, L. (2020). Validation of a machine learning model that outperforms clinical risk scoring systems for upper gastrointestinal bleeding. *Gastroenterology*, *158*(1), 160–167. DOI: 10.1053/j.gastro.2019.09.009 PMID: 31562847

Takamatsu, M. (2025). Transforming histologic assessment: artificial intelligence in cancer diagnosis and personalized treatment: Molecular Diagnostics. *British Journal of Cancer*, *133*(12), 1765–1775. DOI: 10.1038/s41416-025-03206-y PMID: 40993310

Takamatsu, M. (2025). Transforming histologic assessment: artificial intelligence in cancer diagnosis and personalized treatment: Molecular Diagnostics. *British Journal of Cancer*, *133*(12), 1765–1775. DOI: 10.1038/s41416-025-03206-y PMID: 40993310

Tao, G., Zhu, L., Chen, Q., Yin, L., Li, Y., Yang, J., Ni, B., Zhang, Z., Koo, C. W., Patil, P. D., Chen, Y., Yu, H., Xu, Y., & Ye, X. (2022). Prediction of future imagery of lung nodule as growth modeling with follow-up computed tomography scans using deep learning: A retrospective cohort study. *Translational Lung Cancer Research, 11*(2), 250–262. DOI: 10.21037/tlcr-22-59 PMID: 35280310

Tiwari, A., Ghose, A., Hasanova, M., Faria, S. S., Mohapatra, S., Adeleke, S., & Boussios, S. (2025). The current landscape of artificial intelligence in computational histopathology for cancer diagnosis. *Discover. Oncology, 16*(1), 438. DOI: 10.1007/s12672-025-02212-z PMID: 40167870

Wang, J., Shen, L., Zhong, H., Zhou, Z., Hu, P., Gan, J., Luo, R., Hu, W., & Zhang, Z. (2019). Radiomics features on radiotherapy treatment planning CT can predict patient survival in locally advanced rectal cancer patients. *Scientific Reports, 9*(1), 15346. DOI: 10.1038/s41598-019-51629-4 PMID: 31653909

Wang, M., Greenberg, M., Forkert, N. D., Chekouo, T., Afriyie, G., Ismail, Z., Smith, E. E., & Sajobi, T. T. (2022). Dementia risk prediction in individuals with mild cognitive impairment: A comparison of Cox regression and machine learning models. *BMC Medical Research Methodology, 22*(1), 284. DOI: 10.1186/s12874-022-01754-y PMID: 36324086

Wasinger, G., Koeller, M. C., & Compérat, E. (2025). Pathology in the artificial intelligence era: Practical insights for immunohistochemistry and molecular pathology. *Diagnostic Histopathology, 31*(7), 416–423. DOI: 10.1016/j.mpdhp.2025.04.003

Xie, T., Huang, A., Yan, H., Ju, X., Xiang, L., & Yuan, J. (2024). Artificial intelligence: Illuminating the depths of the tumor microenvironment. *Journal of Translational Medicine, 22*(1), 799. DOI: 10.1186/s12967-024-05609-6 PMID: 39210368

Xu, Y., Quan, R., Xu, W., Huang, Y., Chen, X., & Liu, F. (2024). Advances in medical image segmentation: A comprehensive review of traditional, deep learning and hybrid approaches. *Bioengineering (Basel, Switzerland), 11*(10), 1034. DOI: 10.3390/bioengineering11101034 PMID: 39451409

Yang, H., Yang, M., Chen, J., Yao, G., Zou, Q., & Jia, L. (2025). Multimodal deep learning approaches for precision oncology: A comprehensive review. *Briefings in Bioinformatics, 26*(1), bbae699. DOI: 10.1093/bib/bbae699 PMID: 39757116

Yassine, E. L., Wang, S. L., & Ali, T. A. A. (2026). Hybrid GNN-Transformer model for multi-omic cancer classification with interpretable pathway-driven feature selection. *PeerJ. Computer Science, 12*, e3415. DOI: 10.7717/peerj-cs.3415

Yousefi, M., Jalilian, H., Heydari, S., Seyednejad, F., & Mir, N. (2023). Cost of lung cancer: A systematic review. *Value in Health Regional Issues*, *33*, 17–26. DOI: 10.1016/j.vhri.2022.07.007 PMID: 36201970

Zhang, R., Peng, W., Wang, Y., Jiang, Y., Wang, J., Zhang, S., Li, Z., Shi, Y., Chen, F., Feng, Z., & Xiao, W. (2025). MRI radiomics model for predicting tumor immune microenvironment types and efficacy of anti-PD-1/PD-L1 therapy in hepatocellular carcinoma. *BMC Medical Imaging*, *25*(1), 211. DOI: 10.1186/s12880-025-01751-9 PMID: 40597775

Zhang, X., Liu, J., Zhou, W., Lu, J., Wu, L., Li, Y., Wang, Y., Wang, Z., & Cai, J. (2025). Deep learning enhances precision diagnosis and treatment of non-small cell lung cancer: Future prospects. *Translational Lung Cancer Research*, *14*(8), 3196–3215. DOI: 10.21037/tlcr-2025-187 PMID: 40948833

Zhao, J., Li, M., Niu, L., Zhao, Y., & Song, X. (2025). Lung cancer in non-smoking women (LCINSW): From risk factors to precision therapy. *Cancer and Metastasis Reviews*, *44*(4), 74. DOI: 10.1007/s10555-025-10289-9 PMID: 41028595

Chapter 8
Artificial Intelligence in Pulmonary Imaging

Norhene Gargouri
http://orcid.org/0000-0003-1613-2115
Digital Research Center of Sfax, Tunisia

Nesrine Charfi
Independent Researcher, Tunisia

Malek Laadhar
http://orcid.org/0009-0006-3501-5423
Independent Researcher, Tunisia

Wiem Feki
Faculté de Médecine de Sfax, Tunisia

ABSTRACT

Interstitial lung diseases represent a clinically challenging group of pulmonary disorders, for which early detection and accurate diagnosis are essential. High-resolution computed tomography provides detailed visualization of lung structures; however, manual interpretation is time-consuming and requires substantial specialized expertise. This chapter examines the integration of advanced artificial intelligence techniques with pulmonary imaging to automate the recognition of patterns in interstitial lung diseases. Three Vision Transformer architectures are systematically evaluated on high resolution chest imaging datasets to classify six primary pulmonary patterns. Attention maps, gradient-weighted class activation mapping visualizations, and performance metrics are employed to enhance interpretability and support clinical trust. The results demonstrate that the Swin Transformer pro-

DOI: 10.4018/979-8-3373-7759-9.ch008

vides superior accuracy and explainability. Furthermore, quantitative biomarkers facilitate objective monitoring of disease progression and support personalized treatment strategies.

INTRODUCTION

The human lung, a complex network of branching airways and delicate alveoli, represents one of the most challenging targets for precise medical imaging. Minor textural changes, such as subtle variations in tissue density, faint reticular patterns, or small nodules, can signal the onset of serious pulmonary conditions. Detecting these subtle features typically requires highly trained radiologists with extensive clinical experience.

The prevalence of respiratory diseases, particularly the heterogeneous group of interstitial lung diseases, is increasing worldwide. Interstitial lung diseases encompass more than two hundred chronic lung disorders, including idiopathic pulmonary fibrosis, hypersensitivity pneumonitis, and connective tissue disease-related forms. Depending on the population studied and the diagnostic methods employed, prevalence ranges from thirty to eighty cases per one hundred thousand individuals. Beyond statistics, patients often undergo repeated imaging, experience delayed treatment, and suffer progressive loss of lung function. These factors collectively increase healthcare costs and reduce quality of life. Early and accurate diagnosis is therefore essential, yet conventional methods often require twelve to twenty-four months, during which irreversible lung damage may occur. These challenges highlight the urgent need for reliable, consistent imaging tools to support clinical decision-making.

High-resolution computed tomography scans, the cornerstone of interstitial lung disease diagnosis, generate hundreds of slices per patient, all of which require meticulous evaluation. Radiologists in busy medical centers face heavy workloads, which can lead to fatigue and variability in interpretation. Studies indicate that up to twenty percent of expert assessments disagree when identifying subtle signs of interstitial lung diseases, underscoring the limitations of human-only visual assessment. Consequently, automated tools capable of providing precise, consistent, and rapid analysis are increasingly necessary.

Recent advances in artificial intelligence have transformed the analysis of medical imaging. Early computer-assisted diagnosis systems relied on handcrafted features, including texture, shape, and intensity. However, these approaches were limited by rules defined by experts and failed to capture complex interactions within lung tissue. Deep learning techniques, particularly convolutional neural networks, address this limitation by learning hierarchical features directly from imaging data. While convolutional neural networks excel at detecting local patterns, they often struggle to capture global contextual information, which is essential for diffuse and heterogeneous diseases such as interstitial lung diseases.

Vision Transformers and related architectures offer a promising solution. By dividing images into patches and modeling interactions across the entire image, these models capture both local details and long-range dependencies. Self-attention mechanisms highlight key regions within the images, improving interpretability and facilitating clinical trust in artificial intelligence-assisted decision-making.

This chapter explores the intersection of advanced imaging and artificial intelligence-based analysis for the diagnosis of interstitial lung diseases. It evaluates three leading transformer models the Vision Transformer, the Data-Efficient Image Transformer, and the Swin Transformer comparing their performance, strengths, and limitations for automated recognition of interstitial lung disease patterns. In addition to classification accuracy, the chapter emphasizes explainable artificial intelligence methods, including attention maps and gradient-weighted class activation mapping visualizations, to ensure outputs are interpretable by clinicians. Quantitative biomarkers derived from radiomics-style analysis are also extracted to objectively quantify disease progression and support personalized treatment planning.

By integrating artificial intelligence, quantitative analysis, and clinical validation, this chapter provides a comprehensive roadmap for automated, reliable, and interpretable pulmonary image analysis.

Objectives of the Chapter

1. To evaluate and compare the performance of three Vision Transformer architectures the Vision Transformer, the Data-Efficient Image Transformer, and the Swin Transformer for classifying six pulmonary patterns in high-resolution chest imaging: fibrosis, ground-glass opacity, consolidation, emphysema, micronodules, and healthy tissue.
2. To incorporate explainable artificial intelligence techniques, including attention maps and gradient-weighted class activation mapping visualizations, to enable clinicians to understand and trust model predictions.
3. To extract quantitative biomarkers related to fibrosis, emphysema, and airway remodeling to support disease monitoring and personalized patient care.
4. To propose an integrated artificial intelligence-assisted workflow that reduces radiologist workload, enhances diagnostic consistency, and supports precision medicine in the management of interstitial lung diseases.

BACKGROUND

Early automated approaches for pattern classification in interstitial lung diseases relied on handcrafted features and conventional machine learning techniques. With the emergence of deep learning, convolutional neural networks became the dominant paradigm for pulmonary image analysis. Pioneering work by Anthimopoulos et al. (2016) demonstrated the effectiveness of convolutional neural network-based architectures for interstitial lung disease pattern classification in high-resolution computed tomography images, establishing a strong baseline for data-driven analysis of lung texture.

Despite their success, convolutional neural networks are inherently limited by local receptive fields, which restrict their ability to model long-range spatial dependencies. This limitation is particularly significant for accurately characterizing diffuse and heterogeneous patterns in interstitial lung diseases. To address these challenges, Vision Transformers have emerged as a promising alternative for medical image analysis. By decomposing images into patches and leveraging self-attention mechanisms, Transformer-based models explicitly capture global contextual relationships across the entire image from the earliest layers. Several Transformer variants have been proposed to tackle issues related to data efficiency, scalability, and computational complexity, making them increasingly suitable for pulmonary imaging applications.

Recent studies have highlighted the potential of Vision Transformers for medical image analysis, particularly in pulmonary imaging:

- In 2025, Borno et al. (2025) integrated the Data-Efficient Image Transformer within a federated learning framework to classify medical images, demonstrating efficient learning on distributed datasets while preserving privacy. Gradient-weighted class activation mapping visualizations provided interpretable model decisions.
- In 2024, the Vision Transformer for interstitial lung disease, a pure Vision Transformer model, was trained to detect disease patterns directly from computed tomography images. It established a baseline for Vision Transformer applications in interstitial lung disease classification and showed promising performance compared to traditional convolutional neural network approaches (Saha et al., 2024).
- In 2023, a hierarchical Swin Transformer with shifted-window attention was proposed for interstitial lung disease classification. This architecture effectively captured both local and global contextual information, outperforming convolutional neural networks and standard Vision Transformer models while

providing interpretable visualizations to support clinical validation (Masood et al., 2023).

While these studies demonstrate the promise of Transformer-based architectures, most focus on individual models and lack systematic comparisons across multiple Transformer variants evaluated on standardized datasets encompassing diverse interstitial lung disease patterns.

Our Contributions in this Chapter Include

1. Developing a unified pipeline for preprocessing, training, and evaluating Transformer-based models on a real-world interstitial lung disease dataset.
2. Systematically comparing the performance of the three models across all six pulmonary pattern classes using standard metrics, including accuracy, F1-score, precision, and recall.
3. Incorporating explainable artificial intelligence techniques and interactive visualization tools to enhance clinical interpretability and trust in automated predictions.

By situating our work within this historical and methodological context (Greenspan et al., 2016; Palani et al., 2024; Rangel et al., 2024), this chapter provides a clear rationale for applying and comparing Transformer-based models in pulmonary image analysis and demonstrates their potential to overcome the limitations of traditional convolutional neural networks and handcrafted feature methods.

MAIN FOCUS OF THE CHAPTER

Pulmonary Imaging Modalities

Pulmonary imaging has undergone remarkable evolution, progressing from basic X-ray examinations to advanced three-dimensional volumetric techniques. Each imaging modality provides a distinct perspective on lung structure and function, highlighting different aspects of respiratory health. A thorough understanding of these tools is essential to appreciate how artificial intelligence-driven analysis is transforming modern radiology.

Chest radiography remains the most widely used and accessible imaging technique. It is rapid, cost-effective, and associated with low radiation exposure, making it well suited for routine screening and initial clinical assessment. However, as a two-dimensional projection, chest radiography compresses the complex three-dimensional lung anatomy into overlapping planes, which can obscure early or subtle pathological changes. This inherent limitation reduces its reliability for the accurate diagnosis of diffuse interstitial lung diseases.

Computed tomography, particularly high-resolution computed tomography, is the central imaging technique for the diagnosis of interstitial lung diseases. High-resolution computed tomography provides highly detailed visualization of lung parenchyma, enabling the identification of key indicators such as micronodules, reticulations, honeycombing, and ground-glass opacities. Thin-slice acquisition and advanced reconstruction algorithms reveal subtle structural changes, but this level of detail also requires radiologists to review hundreds of images per scan, an increasingly demanding task in busy clinical environments.

Positron emission tomography adds a functional dimension by visualizing metabolic activity within lung tissue. Although it is not routinely employed in standard evaluation of interstitial lung diseases, positron emission tomography can help differentiate active inflammation from established fibrosis in complex or ambiguous cases, providing valuable complementary information.

Magnetic resonance imaging, historically limited by low pulmonary signal and rapid signal decay, is gaining relevance due to innovations such as ultrashort echo time sequences. While still not a mainstream tool for lung assessment, magnetic resonance imaging offers radiation-free functional insights and shows promise for longitudinal follow-up, perfusion analysis, and pediatric imaging.

Together, these imaging modalities form a comprehensive foundation for diagnosing and characterizing pulmonary disease. Among them, computed tomography remains the cornerstone for the detection and classification of interstitial lung diseases and represents the most suitable basis for artificial intelligence and transformer-based diagnostic approaches. As artificial intelligence continues to advance, integrating its capabilities with these diverse imaging techniques is expected to enhance diagnostic accuracy, accelerate clinical decision-making, and reveal subtle disease patterns that are currently beyond human perception.

Computed Tomography (CT): Interstitial Lung Disease

Interpreting high-resolution computed tomography images requires a high degree of radiological expertise, built upon years of training and clinical experience. Radiologists must carefully evaluate subtle textural and structural abnormalities within the lung parenchyma such as ground-glass opacities or fibrotic reticulations and integrate these findings with clinical and functional data. Despite its critical role, this diagnostic process remains time-consuming, cognitively demanding, and inherently subjective. Moreover, it is affected by inter-observer variability, even among experienced specialists, which can lead to diagnostic inconsistencies and suboptimal therapeutic decisions. These challenges are particularly pronounced in interstitial lung diseases, where early and accurate identification of disease patterns is essential for guiding treatment strategies and improving patient outcomes.

In recent years, the emergence of artificial intelligence and deep learning has opened new perspectives in medical imaging. AI-based systems have the potential to assist radiologists by automating the detection, segmentation, and classification of pulmonary abnormalities in high-resolution Chest radiography scans. Unlike traditional computer-aided diagnosis systems that rely on handcrafted features, modern deep learning approaches especially convolutional neural networks and, more recently, transformer-based architectures learn complex hierarchical representations directly from imaging data, achieving state-of-the-art results in image recognition and classification.

Integrating such artificial intelligence systems into clinical workflows offers several advantages:

- Reducing the diagnostic burden on radiologists through fast and reproducible analyses;
- Minimizing inter-observer variability by providing objective and standardized results;
- Enabling quantitative assessment of disease extent and progression over time;
- Supporting personalized medicine through patient stratification based on imaging phenotypes.

In this context, the exploration of advanced artificial intelligence models such as Vision Transformer, Data-efficient Image Transformer, and Swin Transformer represents a significant step toward robust, automated classification of clinically relevant pulmonary patterns in high-resolution chest computed tomography images. By leveraging their ability to model long-range dependencies and capture both local and global contextual information, these architectures have the potential to surpass conventional convolutional neural network-based methods and provide radiologists with powerful, interpretable decision-support tools. While Vision Transformers have shown strong performance in general computer vision tasks, their comparative evaluation in the specific context of pulmonary pattern classification, particularly on real-world high-resolution chest computed tomography datasets, remains limited. This gap underscores the need for systematic studies assessing their applicability, efficiency, and interpretability in medical imaging.

This chapter therefore aims to evaluate and compare three state-of-the-art Vision Transformer architectures; Vision Transformer, Data-efficient Image Transformer, and Swin Transformer for the automated classification of six clinically significant pulmonary patterns observed in high-resolution chest computed tomography scans.

- **Fibrosis:** Scarring and thickening of lung tissue, leading to loss of elasticity and impaired gas exchange, visible as reticular opacities or honeycombing.
- **Ground-glass opacity:** A hazy increase in lung attenuation that does not obscure pulmonary vessels, often associated with early-stage inflammation or fibrosis.
- **Consolidation:** Dense, opaque lung regions caused by fluid replacing air, typically due to infection or alveolar damage.
- **Emphysema:** Destruction of alveolar walls and enlargement of air spaces, appearing as low-attenuation areas with reduced vascular markings.
- **Micronodules:** Small (<3 mm) round opacities that may indicate infection, sarcoidosis, or early fibrosis.
- **Healthy:** Normal lung tissue with no structural abnormalities.

The objective of this work is to develop a robust classification system capable of distinguishing among these six classes using Vision Transformer models trained on high-resolution Chest radiography images. Ultimately, the system seeks to support clinical decision-making by providing accurate, explainable, and reproducible pattern recognition for interstitial lung diseases.

Quantification of Emphysema and Fibrosis

The classification of lung patterns in medical imaging has traditionally relied on handcrafted techniques, including radiomics, texture analysis, and gradient-based descriptors. While these methods can capture certain structural and intensity details, they depend heavily on expert knowledge and often produce inconsistent results when applied to datasets from different institutions. This variability limits their clinical utility, particularly for interstitial lung diseases, which are characterized by highly heterogeneous and diffuse imaging patterns.

With the advent of deep learning, particularly convolutional neural networks, the landscape of lung pattern classification has changed significantly. Architectures such as Visual Geometry Group Network, Residual Network, and Densely Connected Convolutional Network have demonstrated success in identifying lung abnormalities, including pneumonia, cancer, and fibrosis, from chest radiographs and high-resolution computed tomography scans. However, convolutional neural networks primarily focus on local features within limited receptive fields, which makes capturing long-range dependencies or global context challenging. This limitation is critical when analyzing interstitial lung diseases, where pathological changes often extend across large and complex regions of the lung. Furthermore, convolutional neural networks generally require large annotated datasets to achieve optimal performance and are prone to overfitting when trained on smaller medical datasets, a common constraint in clinical research.

To address these challenges, researchers have explored more versatile architectures capable of modeling both local details and global context. Vision Transformers have emerged as a promising alternative. Adapted from Transformer models originally developed for natural language processing, Vision Transformers analyze images by dividing them into patches and processing these patches through a Transformer encoder. This approach enables Vision Transformers to capture long-range spatial relationships from the earliest layers, mitigating the local bias observed in convolutional neural networks. Instead of relying solely on translation invariance, Vision Transformers effectively model broader spatial interactions, which is particularly valuable for medical images where abnormalities are distributed across large areas.

Despite their potential, Vision Transformers have limitations. They generally require extensive pretraining on very large datasets and demand substantial computational resources, making direct application to medical imaging with limited labeled data challenging. To overcome this, researchers introduced the Data-Efficient Image Transformer, which achieves strong performance with smaller pretraining datasets. When combined with distributed learning frameworks, the Data-Efficient Image Transformer enables training on decentralized medical datasets while preserving patient privacy and maintaining model interpretability through gradient-weighted class activation mapping visualizations. Building on these advances, Saha and colleagues developed a Vision Transformer specifically designed for classifying interstitial lung disease patterns in computed tomography scans, demonstrating notable improvements in accuracy compared to traditional convolutional neural network methods.

More recently, the Swin Transformer introduced a hierarchical, shifted-window mechanism that enhances vision model architectures. Unlike standard Vision Transformers that process fixed-size patches, the Swin Transformer generates multi-scale features, combining the local hierarchical feature extraction strengths of convolutional neural networks with the global context modeling of Transformers. This architecture has quickly become a versatile and powerful approach for a wide range of computer vision tasks, including applications in medical imaging.

This chapter addresses a gap in the literature by systematically comparing three Vision Transformer variants the Vision Transformer, the Data-Efficient Image Transformer, and the Swin Transformer for classifying six lung tissue patterns in high-resolution computed tomography scans: fibrosis, ground-glass opacity, consolidation, emphysema, micronodules, and normal tissue. The main contributions of this study include:

- Developing a unified workflow for preprocessing and training Transformer models on a real-world interstitial lung disease dataset.
- Thoroughly evaluating the performance of the three architectures across all lung patterns using standard quantitative metrics.
- Incorporating explainable artificial intelligence techniques and interactive visualization tools to enhance model transparency and support clinical decision-making.

Beyond classification, Transformer models also facilitate the extraction of quantitative imaging biomarkers essential for monitoring diseases such as emphysema, fibrosis, and airway remodeling. By combining attention maps with segmentation masks, the models can quantify:

- Fibrotic burden: the volume or percentage of lung tissue affected by fibrosis.
- Emphysema extent: regions of low attenuation corresponding to damaged alveoli.
- Airway remodeling: measurements of airway wall thickness, lumen area, and structural changes.

These artificial intelligence-derived biomarkers provide automated, reproducible, and sensitive tools for tracking disease progression, improving prognostic accuracy, and supporting personalized treatment strategies. Coupling these quantitative features with explainable artificial intelligence techniques, such as gradient-weighted class activation mapping visualizations, ensures that results remain interpretable and clinically meaningful.

By integrating accurate pattern classification with quantitative biomarker extraction, this study demonstrates how Transformer-based models can enhance automated assessment of interstitial lung diseases and pave the way for more reliable, transparent, and actionable analysis of pulmonary disorders in medical imaging.

Radiomics and Predictive Modeling in Lung Diseases

Radiomics is an emerging field in medical imaging that focuses on extracting quantitative features from radiological images, including texture, shape, intensity, and spatial patterns, to reveal information that may not be apparent to the human eye. Unlike conventional visual assessment, radiomics provides a numerical representation of lung tissue characteristics, enabling reproducible and objective analyses.

In the context of interstitial lung diseases, radiomic features can capture subtle variations in fibrosis, emphysema, ground-glass opacities, and micronodules. These quantitative features form the foundation for predictive modeling, facilitating disease classification, monitoring of disease progression, and assessment of treatment response. By converting complex imaging data into measurable and analyzable parameters, radiomics supports more precise and personalized clinical decision-making in pulmonary medicine.

Dataset Preparation

The dataset used in this study originates from the MedGIFT-HUG database (Depeursinge et al., 2012), developed in collaboration with Geneva University Hospitals for interstitial lung disease research. It consists of high-resolution computed tomography images annotated by expert radiologists according to dominant pulmonary patterns. After preprocessing, a total of 2,307 images were retained across six classes: fibrosis, ground-glass opacity, micronodule, consolidation, emphysema, and healthy tissue.

Class imbalance was present, with fibrosis accounting for more than thirty-two percent of the dataset. To address this imbalance and improve model generalization, several data augmentation strategies were applied:

- Rotation: Images were rotated within a range of plus or minus fifteen degrees to simulate variations in patient positioning.
- Translation: Images were shifted along horizontal and vertical axes to introduce spatial variability.
- Horizontal flipping: Images were flipped horizontally, which is clinically valid for axial lung slices.

All images were resized to 224 by 224 pixels and intensity-normalized to facilitate model convergence. Since high-resolution computed tomography images were in grayscale, they were duplicated across three channels to match the input format expected by pretrained neural networks.

Transformer-Based Modeling for Predictive Analysis

Modern medical imaging presents a complex array of challenges, and interstitial lung disease exemplifies this complexity. Radiological images of interstitial lung diseases are characterized by heterogeneous textures, diffuse opacities, and intricate spatial patterns that are often subtle yet clinically significant. Traditional convolutional neural networks have demonstrated effectiveness in extracting local features; however, they are inherently limited in capturing long-range dependencies and relationships between regions. This limitation is particularly important in interstitial lung diseases, where the distinction between subtypes may depend on nuanced spatial interactions.

Transformer architectures, originally developed for natural language processing, have emerged as powerful alternatives for medical image analysis. Their ability to model global context, facilitated by attention mechanisms, allows them to analyze high-dimensional computed tomography images with unprecedented sensitivity to structural and textural variations.

Among the most prominent transformer-based models in medical imaging are the Vision Transformer, the Data-Efficient Image Transformer, and the Swin Transformer. Each model offers unique advantages:

- The Vision Transformer provides comprehensive extraction of global features across the entire image.
- The Data-Efficient Image Transformer is particularly effective in scenarios with limited annotated data, reducing the need for extensive pretraining.
- The Swin Transformer combines fine-grained local attention with hierarchical global context, capturing both local details and large-scale spatial relationships.

Together, these models are transforming predictive analysis in interstitial lung diseases, converting high-dimensional computed tomography data into rich, interpretable representations that enhance clinical decision-making and support more precise and personalized patient care.

Vision Transformer (ViT)

The Vision Transformer represents a significant departure from convolution-centric approaches (Vaswani et al., 2017). Rather than sliding kernels over images, the Vision Transformer divides an image into patches, effectively treating pixels as words in a visual sentence. Each patch is flattened, embedded into a high-dimensional space, and then processed through a transformer encoder. Positional embeddings are incorporated to preserve spatial relationships, a step of critical importance in medical imaging, where anatomical orientation carries diagnostic significance.

What distinguishes the Vision Transformer is its self-attention mechanism. Every patch interacts with every other patch, allowing the model to capture long-range dependencies without relying on local receptive fields or hierarchical pooling. This capability enables the identification of patterns such as ground-glass opacities or fibrotic networks that extend across large regions of the lung. Multi-head attention layers further diversify the model's focus: one head might capture small-scale reticulations, while another interprets the global lung architecture. The result is a rich mosaic of features that integrates both micro-level and macro-level information into a cohesive representation.

The strength of the Vision Transformer lies in its expressive power. With sufficient data, it can capture subtle variations in tissue texture, inter-patient heterogeneity, and complex radiomic patterns. In interstitial lung diseases, these distinctions are often critical, as minor textural changes can indicate different disease subtypes. Moreover, the patch-based approach aligns with radiomics principles: each embedding functions as a local descriptor, while attention maps reveal which regions drive model predictions. This combination provides clinicians with both accuracy and interpretability, a rare and valuable characteristic in artificial intelligence systems.

However, the Vision Transformer has a notable limitation. Unlike convolutional neural networks, it does not possess inductive biases such as locality and translation invariance. As a result, it requires large datasets for optimal performance, which poses a challenge in medical imaging, where annotated data are often limited. Transfer learning and pretraining on large image collections can mitigate this challenge, but data scarcity remains a significant hurdle.

In summary, the Vision Transformer advances interstitial lung disease classification by bridging local and global features through self-attention, offering a framework that learns long-range dependencies while maintaining fine-grained patch-level information.

Data-Efficient Image Transformer

While the Vision Transformer performs exceptionally well with large datasets, real-world medical imaging often operates under significant constraints (Touvron et al., 2021). Annotated computed tomography scans are expensive and time-consuming to acquire. The Data-Efficient Image Transformer addresses this challenge by reconciling high transformer capacity with limited data availability. It achieves this balance through a teacher-student knowledge distillation framework. A pretrained convolutional neural network serves as the teacher, guiding the transformer, the student, by transferring inductive biases such as recognition of local textures and translation invariance. The result is a model capable of learning robust features from fewer annotated samples.

The architecture of the Data-Efficient Image Transformer mirrors that of the Vision Transformer in terms of patch embedding and attention processing, but it introduces distillation tokens. These tokens capture complementary information from the teacher network, enhancing feature generalization and enabling the model to focus on diagnostically relevant patterns, such as reticulations, honeycombing, or subtle ground-glass opacities. The combination of global attention from the transformer and local insights derived from the convolutional neural network allows the model to learn efficiently, reducing overfitting while improving predictive reliability.

From a practical perspective, the Data-Efficient Image Transformer offers computational efficiency. By optimizing attention mechanisms and leveraging knowledge distillation, it achieves performance comparable to the Vision Transformer without requiring massive datasets or prohibitive training time. For interstitial lung disease classification, this translates to models that train faster, can be deployed in clinical environments, and remain capable of interpreting complex radiological patterns.

Interpretability is a central feature. Visualization of attention maps highlights which regions of the image influence predictions, fostering clinician trust and facilitating model validation. The Data-Efficient Image Transformer thus bridges the gap between high-capacity transformer models and the practical realities of limited medical data, making it a valuable tool in artificial intelligence-driven radiology.

Swin Transformer

The Swin Transformer introduces a structured and hierarchical approach to transformer-based vision models (Liu et al., 2021). While earlier transformer architectures are highly effective at capturing global relationships, they become computationally demanding when applied to high-resolution medical images and are less efficient at modeling localized details. The Swin Transformer overcomes these challenges by adopting a window-based attention strategy. Instead of computing attention across the entire image, the image is partitioned into non-overlapping regions, and attention is calculated within each region. This design substantially reduces computational complexity while maintaining sensitivity to fine-scale textures, which are essential for distinguishing subtle pathological variations in interstitial lung diseases.

A defining feature of the Swin Transformer is its shifted-window attention mechanism. In successive layers, the attention windows are deliberately shifted, allowing information to flow between neighboring regions. This progressive interaction enables the model to construct a hierarchical representation of the image. Such a structure supports multi-scale feature extraction, resembling the layered organization of convolutional neural networks. Through this process, the model captures both localized textural patterns and broader anatomical configurations that are critical for accurate characterization of interstitial lung diseases. As spatial resolution gradually decreases and feature depth increases across layers, complex lung structures are abstracted while preserving diagnostically important local details.

The balance between localized precision and global contextual understanding makes the Swin Transformer particularly well suited for high-resolution volumetric lung imaging. Its window-based attention mechanism accommodates images of varying sizes, ensuring computational efficiency and adaptability across heterogeneous clinical datasets. In the context of interstitial lung disease classification, the Swin Transformer demonstrates strong performance by accurately identifying diffuse ground-glass patterns, localized fibrotic regions, and abnormalities across multiple spatial scales. The resulting attention maps further enhance interpretability by clearly indicating which anatomical regions contribute most to the model's predictions, thereby supporting clinical validation and decision-making.

Overall, the Swin Transformer integrates the hierarchical feature learning strengths of convolutional neural networks with the global contextual modeling capabilities of transformer architectures. This hybrid design enables simultaneous detailed local analysis and comprehensive lung assessment, offering a practical and powerful framework for predictive modeling in advanced pulmonary medical imaging.

RESULTS

All models were trained on a GPU-enabled server using PyTorch, with the following configuration: a batch size of 32, 10 training epochs, and an input image resolution of 224 × 224 pixels. Optimization was performed using the Adam optimizer with a learning rate of 1×10^{-4}, which was empirically selected to ensure stable convergence across all architectures. Stratified splitting ensured that 80% of images were used for training and 20% for validation, preserving class distribution. Performance was evaluated using accuracy, macro F1-score, precision, recall, and confusion matrices.

All experiments were conducted in a controlled software environment designed to support efficient processing of high-resolution medical images. The computational system operated on the Ubuntu Server operating system based on Linux, selected for its stability, flexibility, and compatibility with deep learning workflows. The PyTorch framework served as the primary platform for model development, training, and evaluation. Additional core libraries included the PyTorch vision module for image processing and data augmentation, the scientific learning library for data preprocessing and performance evaluation, the plotting library for result visualization, and the numerical computing library for efficient mathematical operations. Supplementary utility packages were employed to ensure reliable data loading, structured analysis, and full experiment reproducibility.

To guarantee a fair and unbiased comparison, the three transformer-based architectures the Vision Transformer, the Data-Efficient Image Transformer, and the Swin Transformer were trained under identical experimental conditions. Each model was trained for ten epochs using a batch size of thirty-two images. All input images were resized to a resolution of two hundred twenty-four by two hundred twenty-four pixels to comply with architectural input requirements. Learning rate values and optimization strategies were kept consistent across all models so that performance differences could be attributed solely to architectural design rather than training configuration.

Model performance on the six-class interstitial lung disease classification task was assessed using multiple complementary evaluation metrics. Overall accuracy quantified the proportion of correctly classified images across the entire dataset, providing a general indicator of performance. However, because the dataset exhibited class imbalance, additional metrics were required for a balanced evaluation. The macro-averaged F1-score was therefore calculated by computing the F1-score independently for each class and then averaging the results, ensuring equal importance for both frequent and rare patterns. Precision and recall were also computed for each class. Precision measured the proportion of correctly identified samples among all predictions assigned to a given class, reflecting susceptibility to false positive errors. Recall measured the proportion of correctly identified samples among all true instances of a class, highlighting the risk of false negatives. Finally, confusion matrices were generated to visually compare predicted labels with ground truth annotations, enabling identification of systematic misclassifications and evaluation of model reliability across all pulmonary patterns.

The Vision Transformer model demonstrated strong baseline performance, achieving an overall classification accuracy of ninety-five percent and a macro-averaged F1-score of ninety-four percent. The results presented in Table 1 confirm the model's capacity to capture global contextual relationships within high-resolution computed tomography slices of the lung.

Table 1. Performance of the vision transformer

Class	Precision	Recall	F1-score	Support
Consolidation	0.96	0.96	0.96	141
Emphysema	0.79	0.86	0.82	125
Fibrosis	0.97	0.91	0.94	604
Ground-glass opacity	0.93	0.99	0.96	435
Micronodules	0.98	0.97	0.98	393
Normal tissue	0.98	0.99	0.98	147

The Vision Transformer achieved high F1-scores across most pulmonary patterns, with values exceeding ninety-four percent in all categories except emphysema. Emphysema remained the most challenging class due to its heterogeneous appearance and overlap with normal low-attenuation lung regions, which resulted in reduced precision. Despite this limitation, the model showed strong reliability for high-support classes such as fibrosis, ground-glass opacity, and micronodules, demonstrating its effectiveness in learning dominant interstitial lung disease features.

The Data-Efficient Image Transformer achieved improved performance compared to the Vision Transformer, reaching an overall accuracy of ninety-six percent and a macro-averaged F1-score of ninety-five percent as presented in table 2. This improvement highlights the effectiveness of knowledge distillation strategies when working with limited medical imaging datasets.

Table 2. Performance of the data-efficient image transformer

Class	Precision	Recall	F1-score	Support
Consolidation	0.93	0.99	0.96	141
Emphysema	0.84	0.87	0.86	109
Fibrosis	0.98	0.94	0.96	601
Ground-glass opacity	0.99	0.98	0.98	446
Micronodules	0.95	0.99	0.97	392
Normal tissue	0.99	0.97	0.98	157

This model delivered balanced performance across all pulmonary patterns, with noticeable gains in minority classes. The improvement was particularly evident in emphysema detection, where both precision and recall increased compared to the Vision Transformer. High recall values across most classes indicate reduced risk of missed pathological cases, an essential requirement in clinical imaging applications.

The Swin Transformer achieved the strongest results among all evaluated models as presented in Table 3, reaching an overall accuracy of ninety-eight percent and a macro-averaged F1-score of ninety-eight percent.

Table 3. Performance of the Swin transformer

Class	Precision	Recall	F1-score	Support
Consolidation	0.99	1.00	1.00	127
Emphysema	0.84	0.95	0.89	99
Fibrosis	0.99	0.97	0.98	610
Ground-glass opacity	1.00	0.99	1.00	445
Micronodules	1.00	1.00	1.00	408
Normal tissue	1.00	1.00	1.00	157

The Swin Transformer delivered exceptional performance across nearly all pulmonary patterns. Perfect classification was achieved for micronodules and normal tissue, while ground-glass opacity and consolidation also reached flawless F1-scores. Fibrosis classification remained highly accurate, reflecting the model's ability to distinguish fibrotic structures reliably as presented in Table 4. Even emphysema, the most challenging category, achieved a strong F1-score, demonstrating the model's sensitivity to subtle and diffuse low-attenuation patterns.

Table 4. Global comparison of model performances

Model	Accuracy (%)	Macro F1-score (%)
Vision Transformer	95	94
Data-Efficient Image Transformer	96	95
Swin Transformer	98	98

The comparative analysis reveals a clear progression in performance across the three architectures. The Vision Transformer establishes a strong baseline but shows limitations in handling subtle and heterogeneous patterns. The Data-Efficient Image Transformer improves robustness through knowledge distillation, reducing overfitting in limited-data scenarios. The Swin Transformer consistently outperforms both alternatives by integrating hierarchical representations with localized attention mechanisms, resulting in superior accuracy, balanced classification, and enhanced clinical reliability.

DISCUSSION

The experimental findings provide valuable insight into the relationship between architectural design choices and training methodologies in transformer-based medical image classification systems. The Vision Transformer demonstrates strong performance when applied to radiological patterns that are clearly defined and well represented in the training dataset. However, its effectiveness decreases when confronted with subtle imaging variations and imbalanced class distributions. Unlike convolutional neural networks, the Vision Transformer does not incorporate built-in spatial inductive biases, making it highly dependent on large volumes of annotated data to learn robust representations. This dependency poses a significant limitation in clinical research settings, where curated medical datasets are often scarce.

This limitation is particularly pronounced in the context of interstitial lung diseases. High-resolution computed tomography images of these conditions are not only limited in availability but also exhibit substantial variability due to differences in imaging protocols, scanner configurations, patient positioning, and disease evolution. As a result, a standard Vision Transformer may struggle to generalize effectively unless supported by extensive data augmentation strategies or strong regularization techniques. These requirements can restrict its practical deployment in real-world clinical environments, where data diversity and annotation resources are constrained.

The Data-Efficient Image Transformer addresses several of these challenges through the incorporation of knowledge distillation, a training paradigm in which a larger, pretrained teacher model guides the learning process of a smaller student model. This mechanism enhances feature learning from limited annotated data, accelerates convergence, and mitigates overfitting. A notable advantage of this approach is its improved handling of class imbalance, which is critical when dealing with rare interstitial lung disease subtypes such as usual interstitial pneumonia and non-specific interstitial pneumonia. By stabilizing optimization and refining feature representations under data scarcity, the Data-Efficient Image Transformer demonstrates that carefully designed training strategies can compensate for some of the inherent constraints of medical imaging datasets. Its improved generalization across heterogeneous cases reinforces its potential suitability for clinical deployment.

The Swin Transformer represents a further evolution by combining the global modeling capabilities of transformers with locality principles inspired by convolutional neural networks. Its hierarchical architecture, based on windowed self-attention, enables simultaneous analysis of fine-grained structures such as micronodules and subtle reticular patterns, as well as broader manifestations including diffuse fibrosis and honeycombing. This multi-scale representation is particularly well suited to interstitial lung disease pattern recognition, where diagnostic interpretation often depends on both local texture details and global spatial context. The shifted window mechanism further enhances the model's capacity to capture long-range dependencies while maintaining computational efficiency, avoiding the prohibitive costs associated with full self-attention across high-resolution images.

The consistent performance of the Swin Transformer across a wide spectrum of interstitial lung disease subtypes, including rare and visually subtle manifestations, highlights its robustness and adaptability to high-resolution chest imaging datasets. These results demonstrate the practical advantages of integrating hierarchical feature aggregation with localized attention mechanisms in complex radiological classification tasks.

Taken together, the findings emphasize that architectural innovation plays a decisive role in addressing the spatial and textural complexity inherent in interstitial lung disease imaging. Models that incorporate hierarchical representations and refined attention strategies are better equipped to capture diagnostically relevant patterns. Among the evaluated approaches, the Swin Transformer emerges as the most clinically viable solution, offering a compelling balance between accuracy, robustness, and scalability.

Beyond quantitative performance metrics, clinical relevance was ensured through close collaboration with an experienced radiologist, who systematically reviewed and validated model predictions. This human-in-the-loop evaluation strengthens the reliability of the results and bridges the gap between algorithmic output and expert clinical judgment, a critical requirement for real-world implementation.

Given the rarity and heterogeneity of interstitial lung diseases, artificial intelligence–driven diagnostic systems hold substantial promise for accelerating and standardizing radiological assessment. Automated identification of key imaging patterns can significantly reduce the burden of manual interpretation, enabling clinicians to make faster and more consistent decisions, potentially leading to earlier diagnosis and improved patient outcomes. Moreover, such systems enhance reproducibility across multi-center studies and support longitudinal patient follow-up.

Future research directions may include the integration of multimodal data sources, such as clinical information and pulmonary function measurements, with transformer-based imaging analysis to further improve diagnostic accuracy. Additionally, exploring semi-supervised or self-supervised learning strategies in combination with the Swin Transformer could alleviate the dependence on large labeled datasets, thereby extending applicability to even rarer disease subtypes. Overall, this study highlights the transformative potential of advanced transformer architectures in medical imaging and lays the groundwork for their effective integration into clinical workflows for improved management of patients with interstitial lung diseases.

INTEGRATION INTO RADIOLOGY WORKFLOWS

Explainable Artificial Intelligence plays a key role in integrating deep learning systems into real-world radiology workflows. In clinical practice especially for the diagnosis of Interstitial Lung Diseases radiologists must understand not only what a model predicts but also *why* it arrives at a particular decision. Models that visually highlight the regions influencing their predictions allow clinicians to verify diagnostic relevance, improve trust in automated systems, and potentially detect subtle pathological patterns that may otherwise remain unnoticed.

Gradient-weighted Class Activation Mapping (Selvaraju et al., 2017) is one of the most widely used explainable artificial intelligence techniques for visualizing decision-making in deep neural networks. Initially designed for convolutional neural networks, Gradient-weighted Class Activation has since been successfully adapted for transformer-based models, including ViT, DeiT, and Swin Transformer. Its goal is to generate a class-specific heatmap that highlights the spatial regions of an input image contributing most strongly to a given prediction.

Let:

- I denote the input image,
- y^c the predicted score for class c,
- $A^k \in \mathbb{R}^{u*v}$ the kth feature map from a convolutional or attention layer.

Gradient-weighted Class Activation is computed as follows:

(a) Forward Pass: The input image I is passed through the model to obtain the class score:

$$y^c = f(I)$$

(b) Gradient Computation: Compute the gradient of the target class score y^c with respect to the feature maps A^k:

$$\frac{\partial y^c}{\partial A^k} \in \mathbb{R}^{u*v}$$

(c) Importance Weights: For each feature map, compute the importance weight α_k^c by averaging the gradients over the spatial dimensions:

$$\alpha_k^c = \frac{1}{u.v} \sum_{i=1}^{u} \sum_{j=1}^{v} \frac{\partial y^c}{\partial A_{ij}^k}$$

(d) Class Activation Map Generation: Combine the feature maps with their importance weights and apply ReLU to focus on positive contributions:

$$L_{Grad-CAM}^c = RELU\left(\sum_k \alpha_k^c A^k\right)$$

(e) Visualization: Resize $L_{Grad-CAM}^c$ to match the input image size and overlay it to highlight regions that most influenced the model's prediction.

Gradient-weighted Class Activation Mapping offers several important advantages for medical image interpretation. It is a model-agnostic technique, making it applicable to both convolutional neural networks -based architectures and more recent Vision Transformers. It provides intuitive visualizations that can be easily interpreted by clinicians, helping them understand the regions that influence the model's decision. Additionally, Gradient-weighted Class

Activation Mapping is fully compatible with multi-class prediction, allowing the generation of separate heatmaps for each predicted class.
Gradient-weighted Class Activation Mapping plays a crucial role in interpreting interstitial lung diseases detection models by highlighting discriminative regions in high-resolution Chest radiography scans corresponding to patterns such as fibrosis, ground-glass opacity, consolidation, emphysema, and micronodules. It enhances clinical interpretation by helping radiologists verify the model's reasoning, thereby increasing confidence in automated predictions. Gradient-weighted Class Activation is also capable of revealing subtle textural and morphological features that may be difficult to detect visually, supporting earlier diagnosis. Furthermore, it can be integrated with transformer-based architectures, where Gradient-weighted Class Activation Mapping visualizations complement ViT attention maps to provide insights at both the patch level and the global contextual level. Finally, Gradient-weighted Class Activation supports multi-class explanations, generating distinct heatmaps for several coexisting interstitial lung diseases patterns, which is particularly valuable for understanding overlapping pulmonary pathologies.

Figure 1. Example of application of Grad-CAM to CT image

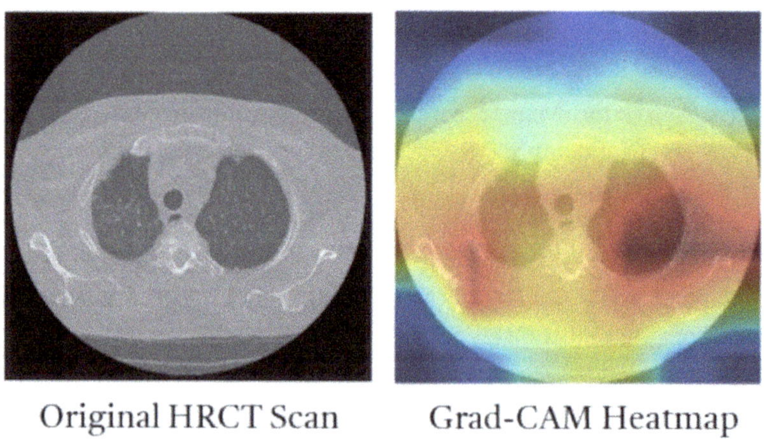

The explainable artificial intelligence analysis further reinforces the credibility and trustworthiness of the proposed diagnostic system by clearly identifying the image regions and visual characteristics that contribute to each classification outcome. By making the decision process transparent, the system allows radiologists to directly compare algorithmic predictions with their own clinical interpretation, thereby fostering confidence and enabling constructive human–machine collaboration. These visual explanations not only clarify how the model reaches its conclusions but also serve as valuable educational tools, assisting clinicians in recognizing subtle radiological patterns associated with different pulmonary conditions in computed tomography images. Feedback from the collaborating radiologist indicated a high level of satisfaction, particularly highlighting the system's usefulness and practicality within routine clinical workflows.

SUMMARY

This chapter examined the transformative role of artificial intelligence in lung image analysis, with particular emphasis on the automated interpretation of high-resolution computed tomography scans for interstitial lung diseases. These disorders represent a heterogeneous and relatively rare group of pulmonary conditions that present significant diagnostic challenges. Early identification requires the recognition of subtle, diffuse, and often overlapping radiological patterns, which places a heavy burden on manual assessment. Traditional diagnostic workflows rely extensively on the expertise of radiologists, a process that is both time-intensive and subject to inter-observer variability. These limitations underscore the urgent need for automated systems capable of delivering consistent, accurate, and timely diagnostic support.

A comprehensive comparative analysis was conducted involving three state-of-the-art transformer-based architectures: the Vision Transformer, the Data-efficient Image Transformer, and the Swin Transformer. All models demonstrated strong capability in identifying complex pulmonary patterns, including fibrosis, ground-glass opacities, consolidations, emphysema, micronodules, and normal lung tissue. Among them, the Swin Transformer consistently achieved superior accuracy and robustness. Its hierarchical design and shifted window attention mechanism enabled an effective balance between global contextual understanding and fine-grained texture analysis, making it particularly well suited for the intricate spatial characteristics of computed tomography lung images. These results highlight the importance of architectural innovation in addressing the unique demands of pulmonary imaging.

A notable strength of this work was the continuous collaboration with an experienced clinical radiologist, who systematically reviewed model predictions, classification outputs, and visual explanations. His feedback informed multiple stages of the study, including error interpretation, image preprocessing refinements, and the selection of clinically meaningful imaging biomarkers. This close interaction ensured that the system's outputs were aligned with real-world diagnostic expectations. The radiologist expressed strong confidence in the model's classification accuracy and emphasized the practical value of the explainability mechanisms for daily clinical use.

Explainable artificial intelligence methods, such as gradient-weighted class activation mapping and attention-based visual representations, played a pivotal role in clinical validation rather than merely serving as trust-enhancing tools. By explicitly identifying the anatomical lung regions that influenced each prediction, these techniques allowed clinicians to verify whether the highlighted areas corresponded to established radiological signatures of interstitial lung diseases. This concordance between model-driven attention and expert knowledge strengthens the integration of automated analysis with human expertise, while also revealing subtle pathological patterns that may be overlooked during routine visual inspection.

In addition to classification, the proposed framework enabled the extraction of quantitative imaging biomarkers related to fibrotic burden, emphysema distribution, and airway structural alterations. These objective measures support consistent monitoring of disease progression, evaluation of treatment response, and personalized therapeutic decision-making. In the context of interstitial lung diseases, where annotated data are scarce and variability is high, such automated biomarkers provide critical decision-support value. Overall, the combination of advanced deep learning architectures, rigorous evaluation procedures, and sustained clinician involvement resulted in a system that reduces analysis time while maintaining high diagnostic reliability. The radiologist's endorsement further underscores the potential of this approach for integration into routine clinical workflows.

SOLUTIONS AND RECOMMENDATIONS

This chapter's results endorse using hierarchical Transformer architectures as an effective approach for automated analysis of interstitial lung diseases. These models excel by blending localized attention with global context awareness, making them well-suited to handle the varied and widespread patterns of lung abnormalities. To boost transparency and build clinician confidence, we urge embedding explainable AI tools right into the diagnostic process. This allows for easy verification of predictions and fosters greater trust in automated systems. Looking ahead, AI tools should evolve past simple classification to routinely pull out key quantitative biomarkers from images such as levels of fibrosis, emphysema severity, and airway alterations. These metrics would support precise, objective evaluations and track disease progression over time. Robustness demands standardized image preprocessing steps and fair evaluation metrics, particularly to counter class imbalances and promote reliable results across diverse clinical data.

Above all, ongoing partnerships with radiologists are crucial during development and testing. This keeps model outputs practical, trustworthy, and fully integrated into everyday radiology practice.

FUTURE RESEARCH DIRECTIONS

Future work should focus on expanding hierarchical Transformer models to larger multi-center datasets while incorporating advanced self-supervised pre-training on diverse computed tomography scans to improve performance across different scanner types and patient groups; developing hybrid architectures that combine Vision Transformers with diffusion models or graph neural networks to capture detailed spatial relationships in interstitial lung diseases and enhance segmentation of subtle fibrotic patterns; exploring dynamic localization-guided loss functions with adaptive weighting based on real-time attention maps to optimize multi-task learning for classification, segmentation, and biomarker extraction simultaneously; integrating federated learning approaches to enable privacy-preserving training on distributed clinical data and speed up deployment in practical settings; and conducting prospective clinical trials to validate explainable artificial intelligence outputs against radiologist consensus, measuring gains in diagnostic efficiency, agreement between observers, and patient outcomes.

CONCLUSION

This chapter has shown how artificial intelligence can meaningfully support clinicians in understanding and managing interstitial lung diseases through the analysis of high-resolution computed tomography images. These diseases are complex, rare, and often difficult to recognize at an early stage because their radiological signs are subtle, diffuse, and highly variable. Relying solely on visual assessment places a heavy burden on radiologists and can lead to variability in interpretation, especially in demanding clinical environments.

By carefully examining three transformer-based models, namely the Vision Transformer, the Data-efficient Image Transformer, and the Swin Transformer, this work demonstrated that advanced attention-based architectures are well suited to capturing both fine textural details and broader spatial patterns in lung images. Among them, the Swin Transformer proved particularly effective due to its hierarchical structure and localized attention strategy, which align naturally with the anatomical and pathological characteristics of lung tissue. The strong and consistent performance observed across multiple pulmonary patterns highlights the robustness of this approach in real clinical scenarios.

A central strength of this study lies in its close collaboration with a practicing radiologist. Continuous expert review ensured that model predictions, visual explanations, and quantitative outputs were not only technically sound but also clinically meaningful. Explainable artificial intelligence techniques played a crucial role in this process by clearly highlighting the lung regions that influenced each decision, allowing the radiologist to verify results, understand model behavior, and gain confidence in the system's outputs.

Beyond classification, the extraction of quantitative imaging biomarkers provided an objective and reproducible way to describe disease extent and progression. Such measurements offer valuable support for follow-up, treatment planning, and personalized patient care, particularly in conditions where consistent monitoring is essential.

Overall, this chapter underscores the value of combining advanced artificial intelligence methods with clinical expertise. When thoughtfully designed and rigorously validated, these systems do not replace the radiologist but instead act as reliable partners, reducing workload, enhancing consistency, and ultimately contributing to more timely and informed care for patients affected by interstitial lung diseases.

REFERENCES

Anthimopoulos, M., Christodoulidis, S., Ebner, L., Christe, A., & Mougiakakou, S. (2016). Lung pattern classification for interstitial lung diseases using a deep convolutional neural network. *IEEE Transactions on Medical Imaging*, *35*(5), 1207–1216. DOI: 10.1109/TMI.2016.2535865 PMID: 26955021

Borno, M. N. A., Shovon, M. S. H., Sikder, M. D., Rimi, I. F., Alahmadi, T. J., & Moni, M. A. (2025). Federated Learning with LoRA Optimized DeiT and Multiscale Patch Embedding for Secure Eye Disease Recognition. arXiv preprint arXiv:2505.06982.

Depeursinge, A., Vargas, A., Platon, A., Geissbuhler, A., Poletti, P. A., & Müller, H. (2012). BuInterstitial Lung Diseases in a reference multimedia database for interstitial lung diseases. *Computerized Medical Imaging and Graphics*, *36*(3), 227–238. DOI: 10.1016/j.compmedimag.2011.07.003 PMID: 21803548

Greenspan, H., Van Ginneken, B., & Summers, R. M. (2016). Guest editorial deep learning in medical imaging: Overview and future promise of an exciting new technique. *IEEE Transactions on Medical Imaging*, *35*(5), 1153–1159. DOI: 10.1109/TMI.2016.2553401

Liu, Z., Lin, Y., Cao, Y., Hu, H., Wei, Y., Zhang, Z., . . . Guo, B. (2021). Swin transformer: Hierarchical vision transformer using shifted windows. In Proceedings of the IEEE/CVF international conference on computer vision (pp. 10012-10022).

Masood, A., Naseem, U., & Razzak, I. (2023, April). Multi-scale swin transformer enabled automatic detection and segmentation of lung metastases using CT images. In 2023 IEEE 20th international symposium on biomedical imaging (ISBI) (pp. 1-5). IEEE. DOI: 10.1109/ISBI53787.2023.10230663

Palani, M., Rajagopal, S., & Chintanpalli, A. K. (2024). A systematic review on feature extraction methods and deep learning models for detection of cancerous lung nodules at an early stage–the recent trends and challenges. *Biomedical Physics & Engineering Express*, *11*(1), 012001. DOI: 10.1088/2057-1976/ad9154 PMID: 39530659

Rangel, G., Cuevas-Tello, J. C., Nunez-Varela, J., Puente, C., & Silva-Trujillo, A. G. (2024). A survey on convolutional neural networks and their performance limitations in image recognition tasks. *Journal of Sensors*, *2024*(1), 2797320. DOI: 10.1155/2024/2797320

Saha, S., Kumar, A., & Nandi, D. (2024). ViT-ILD: A vision transformer-based neural network for detection of interstitial lung disease from CT images. *Procedia Computer Science*, *235*, 779–788. DOI: 10.1016/j.procs.2024.04.074

Selvaraju, R. R., Cogswell, M., Das, A., Vedantam, R., Parikh, D., & Batra, D. (2017). Grad-cam: Visual explanations from deep networks via gradient-based localization. In *Proceedings of the IEEE international conference on computer vision* (pp. 618-626). DOI: 10.1109/ICCV.2017.74

Touvron, H., Cord, M., Douze, M., Massa, F., Sablayrolles, A., & Jégou, H. (2021, July). Training data-efficient image transformers & distillation through attention. In *International conference on machine learning* (pp. 10347-10357). PMLR.

Vaswani, A., Shazeer, N., Parmar, N., Uszkoreit, J., Jones, L., Gomez, A. N., & Polosukhin, I. (2017). Attention is all you need. *Advances in Neural Information Processing Systems*, •••, 30.

KEY TERMS AND DEFINITIONS

Artificial Intelligence: Systems built on computers that mimic human-like intelligence for tasks such as analyzing data to learn patterns, spotting features, and reaching decisions—especially useful in fields like medical image processing.

Attention Mechanism: A technique in models that helps zero in on the key parts of an image during prediction, boosting both performance and the ability to understand what the model "sees."

Computed Tomography: An imaging method that creates clear, slice-by-slice views of the body's interior by combining X-rays captured from various angles.

Explainable Artificial Intelligence: Approaches that reveal how AI models arrive at their outputs, making them clearer for people—crucial in medicine and other high-stakes areas where trust matters.

Interstitial Lung Diseases: A range of ongoing lung conditions involving swelling and scarring in the tissue around the air sacs, which gradually worsens breathing over time.

Radiomics: A way to pull out dozens of quantitative traits from medical scans, offering reliable, objective descriptions of tissues for deeper analysis.

Self-Attention: In transformers, a process that weighs connections across every element of an image input, helping capture distant spatial links effectively.

Transformer Architecture: A neural network design relying on attention instead of convolutions, excelling at grasping broad context and intricate patterns across images.

Vision Transformer: A transformer model tailored for vision tasks, treating images as patch sequences to learn global features and richer visual relationships.

Chapter 9
AI in Pulmonary Imaging: Advances in Detection, Quantification, and Clinical Integration

Muskan Muskan Tamboli
http://orcid.org/0009-0000-0289-9468
Symbiosis Institute of Health Sciences, India

Vaishnavi Deshmukh
Symbiosis Institute of Health Sciences, India

Milind Chunkhare
http://orcid.org/0000-0001-9299-2075
Symbiosis International University, India

Sammita Jadhav
Symbiosis Institute of Health Sciences, India

ABSTRACT

Artificial intelligence (AI) is changing the way we look at pulmonary imaging by enhanced diagnosis and accurate findings for various lung disorders. The chapter deals with integration of AI in different modalities of medical imaging right from chest x-ray to computed tomography. In chest x-ray imaging, the AI algorithms can detect abnormalities, pneumonia, tuberculosis and nodules, often exceeding expectations of a radiologists. In computed tomography, AI integration facilitates lung cancer screening, achieving up to 99% accuracy in detecting the malignancies. It can also predict the malignancy accurately. Other than this it can quantify diseases like emphysema, fibrosis, airway modelling, COPD & ILD biomarkers. Combining

DOI: 10.4018/979-8-3373-7759-9.ch009

the radionomics with clinical findings can estimate predictive models to provide personalised treatment plans. The chapter addresses AI tools utilized in existing workflow to assist effective aids in clinical judgements.

1. INTRODUCTION

Artificial intelligence (AI) has evolved from an academic computational framework into a medical imaging technology that provides substantial clinical benefits which now drives current medical imaging practices. Imaging tests function as essential diagnostic methods in pulmonary medicine because they enable medical professionals to track patient progress from initial diagnosis to assessment of their response to treatment. Global health statistics show that respiratory diseases which include pneumonia tuberculosis chronic obstructive pulmonary disease interstitial lung diseases pulmonary embolism and lung cancer rank among the most frequent causes of death and illness. Physicians depend on chest radiography and computed tomography (CT) as essential diagnostic tools for these medical conditions, but their ability to interpret results has become more limited because of human factors and systemic issues and technological constraints (Pesapane et al., 2018).

The worldwide volume of radiological imaging studies has experienced dramatic growth during the last twenty years because of three main factors which include population aging and increased screening initiatives and technological progress in imaging. The number of radiologists who have received training does not match the current requirements for radiological services. The existing workforce imbalance leads to higher reporting demands, extended time needed for results, and increased potential for diagnostic mistakes. The pulmonary imaging field faces persistent challenges which include detection problems for lung nodules and interstitial changes and early infectious infiltrates and small pulmonary emboli. Inter-observer variability makes it harder to interpret results, especially for diseases that show diverse imaging patterns which include ILD and early-stage lung cancer.

The artificial intelligence system creates an approach which enables scientists to analyze images in a scalable manner that produces consistent results through its ability to analyze images with high efficiency according to (Litjens et al., 2017) and (Hosny et al., 2018). The artificial intelligence systems which use machine learning and deep learning methods can detect intricate relationships in extensive imaging databases. The combination of convolutional neural networks and vision transformers with hybrid multimodal architectures enables scientists to achieve expert-level results across multiple pulmonary imaging tasks which involve detecting abnormalities and classifying diseases and performing quantitative assessments. Modern AI systems have developed advanced capabilities which let them learn from unprocessed pixel information because they need this information to detect small spatial and texture characteristics which humans find difficult to see. The clinical environment needs to use artificial intelligence as a technology which enhances the capabilities of radiologists and pulmonologists instead of seeing it as a tool that replaces these medical professionals. The implementation of artificial intelligence systems in medical environments needs to follow human–AI collaboration as its central concept. The AI system acts as a decision-support system which helps doctors diagnose medical conditions through improved diagnostic accuracy while decreasing their mental effort and creating standardized medical reports and enabling personalized medicine delivery although the doctors remain in control of patient assessment and treatment. The pulmonary imaging field needs this cooperative model because accurate diagnosis depends on clinical information together with physiological measurements and long-term evaluation of patients.

The implementation of AI has introduced a fundamental change that permits medical professionals to assess radiological images through numeric measurements instead of their previous method of visual assessments. The traditional process of radiological interpretation depends on radiologists who assess images through their personal visual interpretation. AI uses its technology to create an exact measurement system which evaluates imaging characteristics including emphysema severity and fibrotic progression and airway structural changes and blood vessel irregularities. The imaging biomarkers show consistent measurement results which medical professionals can use to monitor patient progress while also predicting their lung capacity and developing prognostic assessment tools. The new field of radiomics expands upon existing scientific methods by using high-dimensional imaging data to create predictive models which include both clinical data and molecular data.

The chapter provides medical students and early-career clinicians with a complete technical framework that explains AI applications in pulmonary imaging. The chapter examines chest radiographs and CT imaging to study three areas which include automated detection of pulmonary abnormalities and quantitative imaging and radiomics and practical integration of AI into radiology workflows. The authors aim to equip readers with skills to assess AI technologies in respiratory medicine through their focus on clinical relevance and methodological principles and future development paths.

Figure 1. Adapted from prior frameworks in medical image analysis and radiomics (Hosny et al., 2018; Lambin et al., 2012; Litjens et al., 2017)

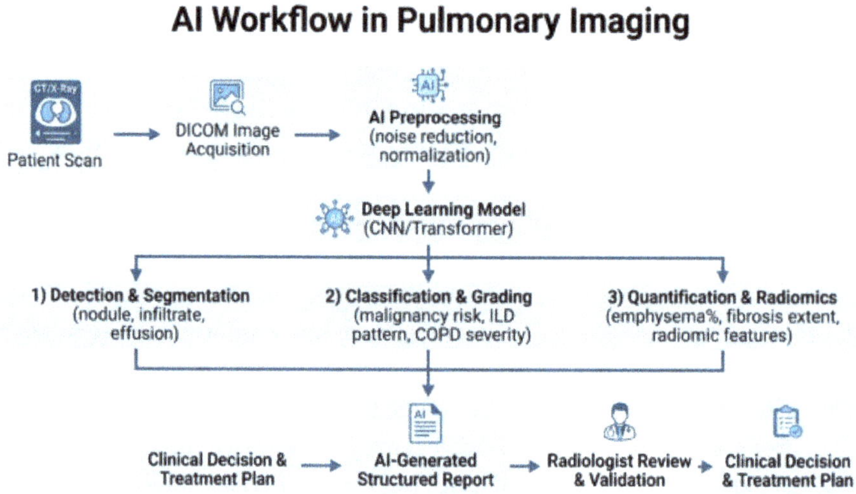

2. CHEST RADIOGRAPHS: AUTOMATED DETECTION OF NODULES, INFILTRATES, AND EFFUSIONS

Artificial intelligence algorithms can look at chest x-rays to find things like nodules, pneumonia, tuberculosis and effusions. This helps doctors decide what to do. Some studies put together show that artificial intelligence is very good at diagnosing things: it can find pneumonia 88% of the time and it is correct about 90% of the time when it says someone does not have pneumonia(Adam Essa, 2025).

Artificial intelligence is almost as good as doctors who look at x-rays for a living. When artificial intelligence looks at x-rays to find lung nodules, which can be cancer it finds them 72% of the time and it is correct about 95% of the time when it says someone does not have a nodule(Adam Essa, 2025).

Using intelligence to look at x-rays again after a doctor has already looked at them helps doctors find more things that they missed the first time. This makes doctors about 9 to 10 percent better at finding things. It does not make them much worse, at avoiding false alarms. When we actually use Artificial Intelligence it usually has trouble finding small or complicated growths but it can find about 90 percent of the bigger growths. One study that looked at how Artificial Intelligence can find growths on chest x-rays found that Artificial Intelligence systems can correctly identify growths about 56 to 95 percent of the time and are very good at finding solid or hardened growths(Adam Essa, 2025). When Artificial Intelligence and a radiologist work together to look at the x-rays they can find more growths, which is especially helpful for radiologists who are not as experienced. Artificial Intelligence is really good, at finding growths on chest x-rays, the bigger ones(Megat Ramli et al., 2025).

Pneumonia is a problem. Doctors use something called Deep CNN ensembles to look at pictures of lungs which are called CXRs to see if people have pneumonia. These computer programs are really good at finding pneumonia in kids and adults(-Togunwa et al., 2025). They are right about 94 to 97 percent of the time. Found that they are very good at finding pneumonia in kids and they are right about 96 percent of the time. These computer programs are only as good as the information they are given to learn from(Togunwa et al., 2025).

In some places there are not doctors to look at all the pictures of lungs. That is where computers can help. For example in Nigeria a computer program was able to find pneumonia in kids 95 percent of the time(Togunwa et al., 2025). This is really helpful because there are not doctors, in some of these places so the computer can give a second opinion. Pneumonia detection is very important. These computer programs can be very helpful. Pneumonia is a disease and finding it early is very important(Togunwa et al., 2025).

Tuberculosis is a problem. AI-based computer aided detection systems are really good at finding Tuberculosis cases in clinics where people first go to see a doctor. For example in a study in China they used computers with AI to look at pictures before a doctor saw them. This helped find people with Tuberculosis who were showing symptoms(Jiang et al., 2025). It also meant that doctors who look at pictures called radiologists had work to do because they only had to look at the pictures that the computer thought might be a problem. The computer was especially good at finding Tuberculosis in clinics that are far away from big cities. This is news, for places that do not have a lot of money or resources because it means they can use computers to help with screening for Tuberculosis(Jiang et al., 2025).

Modern chest x ray tools that use intelligence also find problems like fluid in the lungs and other issues. In a study that was approved by the FDA artificial intelligence helped doctors who look at x rays to find a lot of problems with the chest like fluid in the lungs and tumors(Anderson et al., 2024). The artificial intelligence was very good at finding problems and doctors who're not specialists in reading x rays were able to find problems just as well as specialists when they used the artificial intelligence. When doctors use these systems they can see if there might be fluid in the lungs or air, in the chest cavity and that helps them decide if they need to look at the x ray away(Anderson et al., 2024).

Triage and limited resources: AI can look at chest X-rays fast and find the urgent cases. For instance an AI that the FDA says is okay to use can send out warnings about problems within minutes(*Deep Learning-Based Algorithm for Automatic*

Detection of Incidental Pulmonary Embolism on Contrast-Enhanced CT: A Multicenter Multivendor Study | Radiology Advances | Oxford Academic, n.d.). This warning can show that someone has a case of pneumonia or fluid in their lungs. In places where there are not doctors who can look at X-rays AI can help sort out who needs attention first. Some studies have shown that using AI to look at X-rays and then having a doctor check them can help find more cases of pneumonia or tuberculosis in clinics that do not have a lot of resources. AI can look at chest X-rays. Find problems and then doctors can review them. This way doctors can focus on the cases that AI says are urgent, like pneumonia or tuberculosis(Jiang et al., 2025) (Togunwa et al., 2025).

Artificial intelligence on chest radiographs is really good at finding nodules and infiltrates like pneumonia and tuberculosis quickly and correctly. Artificial intelligence works well with common problems and big lesions(Togunwa et al., 2025) (Adam Essa, 2025). The best use of intelligence may be to help decide which cases need to be looked at right away or to double check the work of the first doctor to catch anything that was missed. Artificial intelligence on chest radiographs can be a help, in this way(Adam Essa, 2025)(Anderson et al., 2024).

3. COMPUTED TOMOGRAPHY (CT): LUNG CANCER SCREENING, ILD, PULMONARY EMBOLISM

Computer Tomography imaging is really helpful for doctors. Artificial Intelligence is used for finding lung cancer, interstitial lung disease and pulmonary embolism. Artificial Intelligence is also used for things. Deep learning makes Computer Tomography imaging better and more accurate for lung cancer and interstitial lung disease and pulmonary embolism. This is a help, for doctors who use Computer Tomography imaging.

Lung Cancer Screening is very important for finding out if someone has cancer. This is done by looking at pictures of the lungs, which are taken with a machine called a chest CT scanner. The pictures can be taken with a dose of radiation which is safer for people. Artificial Intelligence or AI for short is really good at helping computers look at these pictures. Find any problems(Arshad et al., 2025). Lung Cancer Screening uses something called CNNs which're like special tools that can find tiny spots on the lungs called nodules. These nodules can be cancer. It is very important to find them. The CNNs are very good at finding these nodules. Can even tell if they are cancer or not(Arshad et al., 2025).

Some people have written reviews about how these CNNs work. They say that the CNNs can find and mark the nodules with a degree of accuracy. They can even look at the shape and texture of the nodules to figure out if they are cancer. This is called radiomics. The radiomics models are very good at telling if a nodule is cancer or not and they can do this with a degree of accuracy around 99 percent(Arshad et al., 2025). This is very helpful for doctors who are trying to diagnose Lung Cancer. Lung Cancer Screening and Nodule Detection are very important, for saving lives. Ai is making it easier to do this. Artificial intelligence based risk models, such as the Sybil deep learning model can tell us if someone is likely to get lung cancer in the future from one low dose computed tomography scan. This is better than the methods we use(Arshad et al., 2025).

When we look at pictures of the lungs artificial intelligence can help doctors by checking the pictures and reducing the number of wrong diagnoses. It also helps doctors focus on the parts of the lung that're more likely to have cancer. If we combine the information from the lung pictures with information about the patient, such, as how old they're if they smoke we can get a better idea of how bad the cancer is and what might happen to the patient(Arshad et al., 2025).

Interstitial Lung Disease is a condition. High-resolution CT scans are really important for diagnosing Interstitial Lung Disease and keeping an eye on it. Artificial Intelligence helps with both of these things(Mei et al., 2023). Deep learning classifiers are able to tell the types of Interstitial Lung Disease apart on a CT scan. For example they can tell the difference between pulmonary fibrosis and other types by looking at the tiny patterns in the scan(Mei et al., 2023).

One example of this is a kind of Artificial Intelligence called a transformer-based AI. This Artificial Intelligence uses CT scans and other clinical data to categorize Interstitial Lung Disease into five groups. It can even predict the risk of survival, over a three-year period(Mei et al., 2023). Deep learning can measure how much fibrosis is in the lungs and it can give us some signs of how bad the disease is. It can see things like ground-glass and honeycombing in the lungs. The amount of fibrosis that deep learning finds is related to how the lungs are working. If deep learning finds a lot of fibrosis it means the lungs are not working well(Hoffmann et al., 2025). This is helpful because deep learning can help doctors find lung problems like lung disease early on. Deep learning can also help doctors see how the disease is progressing and what might happen to the patient. Deep learning is really good at looking at the lungs and finding problems, like fibrosis(Hoffmann et al., 2025) (Mei et al., 2023).

Pulmonary Embolism is a deal. Doctors really like to use something called CT angiography to check for Pulmonary Embolism. This is the way to find out if someone has Pulmonary Embolism. Some people made computer programs that can look at pictures from CT scans to find problems with Pulmonary Embolism(*Deep Learning-Based Algorithm for Automatic Detection of Incidental Pulmonary Embolism on Contrast-Enhanced CT: A Multicenter Multivendor Study | Radiology Advances | Oxford Academic*, n.d.). These programs can even find problems when the doctor did not order the CT scan to look for Pulmonary Embolism. For example some researchers tried out a computer program called CINA-iPE. They used this program to look at lots of CT scans that were done for reasons(*Deep Learning-Based Algorithm for Automatic Detection of Incidental Pulmonary Embolism on Contrast-Enhanced CT: A Multicenter Multivendor Study | Radiology Advances | Oxford Academic*, n.d.). The program was able to find Pulmonary Embolism in these scans 87.8 percent of the time. It was also correct 92.0 percent of the time when it said someone did not have Pulmonary Embolism(*Deep Learning-Based Algorithm for Automatic Detection of Incidental Pulmonary Embolism on Contrast-Enhanced CT: A Multicenter Multivendor Study | Radiology Advances | Oxford Academic*, n.d.).

The computer program was really fast. It could look at the pictures. Give the doctor an answer in about one and a half minutes. This is great because doctors can get the information they need quickly to help people, with Pulmonary Embolism. This Artificial Intelligence can point out CT studies that need to be looked at right away so doctors can diagnose Pulmonary Embolism faster. On CTPA studies these Deep Learning models have given very similar results in the first reports(Arshad et al., 2025).

So the thing about CT-based AI is that it is really helping us find and understand lung problems. When it comes to lung cancer these new computer programs called Deep Learning and radiomics are getting better at finding nodules figuring out how bad they are and determining the stage of the cancer(Chantzi et al., 2025). For people with lung disease AI is helping doctors classify the type of disease they have and measure how much scarring is, in their lungs(Mei et al., 2023). For pulmonary embolism these computer programs can even alert doctors to blood clots in the lungs when they are looking at routine scans. All of these tools are making it possible for doctors to read CT scans faster and more accurately which is a deal when it comes to lung disease and CT-based AI(*Deep Learning-Based Algorithm for Automatic Detection of Incidental Pulmonary Embolism on Contrast-Enhanced CT: A Multicenter Multivendor Study | Radiology Advances | Oxford Academic*, n.d.).

4. QUANTIFICATION OF EMPHYSEMA, FIBROSIS, AND AIRWAY REMODELING

Artificial intelligence helps doctors see lung tissue changes on pictures that they would not be able to see. Artificial intelligence does this by finding things in the pictures that can show how a disease is progressing. This means that doctors can use intelligence to monitor what is happening with the disease and figure out what might happen to the patient. Artificial intelligence is really good at measuring these changes in lung tissue, which's very helpful, for doctors.

Emphysema, which is a type of COPD can be seen on a CT scan. The computer can automatically look at the lung tissue. Calculate how much of it is damaged. This damaged tissue is called tissue. Recent studies have shown that computers can use programs to accurately measure how bad the emphysema is(Sait & Shaikh, 2025). These programs can even find problems in the airways that can make it hard to breathe. For example computers can look at pictures of the lungs taken when a person is breathing in. This can help doctors see how the emphysema is getting worse, over time. It can also help doctors predict if the persons lung function will get worse or if they are more likely to die from COPD. Emphysema is a part of COPD and it is important for doctors to be able to measure it accurately. Artificial Intelligence can also look at the shape of the airway tree. The algorithms check how thick the airway walls are and how wide the bronchial tubes are at levels. This gives us biomarkers of airway remodelling(Sait & Shaikh, 2025).

These metrics, such as the amount of emphysema and the size of the airway wall area give us measures to track how bad the Chronic Obstructive Pulmonary Disease is, over time. The airway tree geometry and the airway wall thickness are things to consider when looking at Chronic Obstructive Pulmonary Disease severity(Sait & Shaikh, 2025).

Pulmonary Fibrosis is a problem. It is also known as Interstitial Lung Disease or ILD for short. Doctors use computers to look at pictures of the lungs and see what is going on. These computers can find the parts of the lungs like the ground-glass opacities, reticulation and traction bronchiectasis. The computers can even measure how bad the problem is. They do this by looking at the pictures from a kind of CT scan called High-Resolution Computed Tomography or HRCT. The computers can find the regions, which are the bad parts of the lungs and figure out how big they are(Hoffmann et al., 2025). For example if someone has a disease that affects the tissue in their body like Interstitial Lung Disease the computer can measure how much of their lungs are affected. It can see how much of the lungs have something called ground-glass opacities, reticulation and high-attenuation areas which're all signs of Pulmonary Fibrosis(Hoffmann et al., 2025).

Airway Remodelling is when people have lung diseases and it affects the airways. This means the walls of the airways change. We can use computer tools to look at pictures from CT scans and see how thick the walls of the airways arc gctting and how narrow the airways are becoming(Sait & Shaikh, 2025). These computer tools can even automatically measure the size of the airway walls. See if the airways are getting too big. We are starting to use these measurements like how the walls are compared to the size of the airway to see if someone has airway remodelling. For example we used computer programs to look at CT scans. We found that people, with very bad COPD and asthma have certain patterns of thickening in their airway walls. When we look at emphysema and airway measures artificial intelligence can classify certain lung conditions like combined pulmonary fibrosis and emphysema or chronic obstructive pulmonary disease types from pictures taken with a CT scanner. This is really helpful, for understanding emphysema and chronic obstructive pulmonary disease(Sait & Shaikh, 2025).

Artificial Intelligence makes Computed Tomography a precise tool. It uses formulas to calculate things like the amount of emphysema the volume of fibrotic tissue and the condition of the airways, which can be hard for a radiologist to measure on their own(*Artificial Intelligence Detects Substantial Airway Damage on CT Scans of Children with Severe Asthma - Thirona*, n.d.). These measurements, which are called imaging biomarkers are connected to the results of physical tests and can help predict what will happen to the patient(*Artificial Intelligence Detects Substantial Airway Damage on CT Scans of Children with Severe Asthma - Thirona*, n.d.). For example the amount of fibrosis that Artificial Intelligence finds is related to how someone with idiopathic pulmonary fibrosis will live. This automatic way of measuring disease progression is more objective. Can help doctors predict the future more accurately than if they just relied on their own opinions. Artificial Intelligence and Computed Tomography are useful tools, in this process.

5. RADIOMICS AND PREDICTIVE MODELLING IN LUNG DISEASES

Radiomics is about taking pictures and getting lots of information from them like what they look like their shape and how bright or dark they are. The computer uses this information and sometimes other health information to make predictions about what might happen. When doctors look at pictures of lungs radiomics is becoming an useful tool to figure out what is wrong and what might happen to the patient so they can give them the best care possible. Radiomics is helping doctors make guesses about what will happen to patients with lung problems and that is why radiomics is so important, in pulmonary imaging(Chantzi et al., 2025).

Imaging Biomarkers are really important. Radiomics is a way to turn images into kinds of biomarkers that have a lot of details. These details are not something we can see with our eyes(Chantzi et al., 2025). When we look at the pieces of data from a CT or X-ray image we can use radiomics to understand things like how different the tissue is, how irregular a nodule is and what the blood vessels look like. These details are, like markers that are not based on personal opinions(Arshad et al., 2025).

For example when we are looking at ILD, the patterns of fibrosis that show up on a CT scan can tell us what might happen to the patient in the future(Lee et al., 2020).

Radiomics can take these patterns. Turn them into numbers, which is really useful. In lung cancer we can look at things like the texture or shape of a tumor to figure out how likely it is to be bad. This is called signatures(Pan et al., 2023). It is really useful because it can even tell us things, about the genetics of the tumor. Radiomics is a way to take pictures that doctors normally take and turn them into lots of information that computers can understand. One doctor said that radiomic signatures help us learn more about what lung tissue looks like and how it works, which can help us understand what is going on with the disease, how it will progress and how it will respond to treatment(Lee et al., 2020).

The real strength of radiomics is in models that can predict things. When you combine information from radiomics with information about a patient like what their doctor says or what is going on in their body you can use artificial intelligence to guess what will happen to them and make a treatment plan that is just right for them(Lee et al., 2020)(Pan et al., 2023). For people with lung cancer models that use intelligence and look at lots of different things, like pictures and information about the patient are really good at predicting if the cancer will come back and if the patient will survive(Lee et al., 2020).

For example some models that use a kind of artificial intelligence called deep learning are better at predicting what will happen to a patient than the usual ways of guessing. These models can also help reduce the number of answers when doctors are checking patients, for cancer. In the case of ILD it turns out that special computer programs that look at pictures from CT scans can tell us something about how people will live. One study found that these computer programs can find patterns in the pictures that're very good at predicting what will happen to the patient(Dixon et al., n.d.)(Mei et al., 2023).

So basically these computer programs that look at pictures can help doctors give each patient the care that's right for them. For example they can look at a spot on the lung. Say if it is bad or not or they can tell if the patients lung function will get worse over time or they can even predict if a certain treatment will work for the patient, which helps the doctor make a plan that is just right, for that person(Pan et al., 2023)(Arshad et al., 2025).

Lung images are turned into a lot of data that the computer can understand. This is done by radiomics. Radiomics helps us get information from these lung images. This information is used to help the doctor figure out what is wrong with the patient what might happen to the patient and how to treat the patient. Many people are still working on making this system. Radiomics and lung images have a lot of potential to help doctors make good decisions and give the right treatment to people, with lung disease. Lung images and radiomics can really help with this(Lee et al., 2020)(Chantzi et al., 2025).

6. INTEGRATION OF AI INTO RADIOLOGY WORKFLOWS

Translating AI into clinical practice requires thoughtful workflow integration, standardized data exchange, and collaboration between radiologists and AI tools.

Figure 2. AI touch points in the pulmonary imaging workflow.

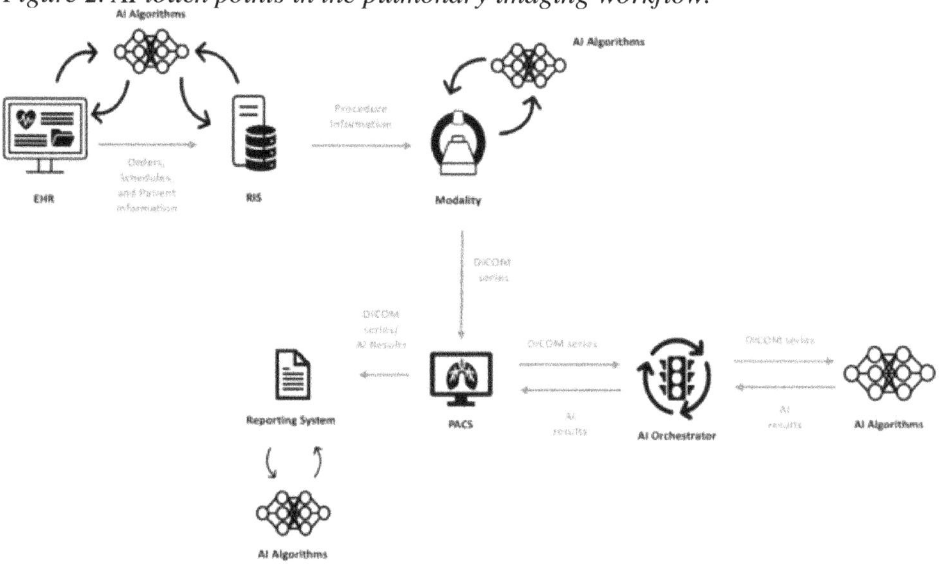

This is a diagram that shows how AI algorithms can be used at every stage of the process. It starts from when a doctor orders an imaging test and goes all the way to storing the images. The diagram, which is, from Cook et al. helps us understand how AI touch points work(Tejani et al., 2024). AI touch points can do a lot of things as find lung nodules automatically make CT protocols better and help generate reports. AI touch points can also do things to make the pulmonary imaging workflow easier(Tejani et al., 2024)

Artificial intelligence can help radiologists at different stages of the imaging process. For instance when a computerized tomography scan is loaded, a system that uses intelligence might automatically point out suspicious nodules or infiltrates and then the radiologist has to confirm these findings(Tejani et al., 2024).

Other artificial intelligence tools might look at the patients records to suggest what imaging tests should be done or they might sort the list of cases so that the ones that are most likely to be serious are looked at first. This could mean cases with large effusions or bilateral pneumonia. Artificial intelligence can make the work of radiologists easier at stages, from looking at the images to deciding what tests to do next. Using intelligence as a tool to help make decisions is a good way to integrate it into our work(Tejani et al., 2024). The doctor who looks at the pictures the radiologist, is still, in charge. Makes the final decision. They look at the notes that the artificial intelligence system has made and they decide if they want to use them or change them. This way of working with intelligence, which is called the "AI-augmented" model has been shown to help doctors find more of the things they are looking for, like nodules and not miss as many. It does this without taking the doctor out of the process, which's a good thing(Tejani et al., 2024).

Standards and interoperability are really important. Radiology AI systems need to be able to share information with systems like PACS and RIS and EHR(Tejani et al., 2024). The Integrating the Healthcare Enterprise initiative is helping with this. They have guides that show how to do it. For example the output, from Radiology AI systems can be put into a format that PACS and other systems can understand, like DICOM Structured Reports or HL7 FHIR resources(Hoffmann et al., 2025). This means that notes and measurements can be automatically added to the PACS viewer or the radiology report. Using these standards is an idea because it stops people from having to create their own custom connections, which can make a big mess of the workflow(Tejani et al., 2024). Radiology AI systems and PACS and RIS and EHR all need to work together. So one review really points out that standards-based interoperability is very important to use Artificial Intelligence across different tools and websites. When we actually do this the people, in charge of radiology departments have to get their IT team, legal team and clinical team to work together to make Artificial Intelligence work: they have to think about how to keep data private figure out who is responsible if something goes wrong and make sure the doctors and other clinicians understand what the Artificial Intelligence is telling them(Hoffmann et al., 2025)(Adam Essa, 2025).

New tools that use intelligence are being added to the process of making reports. These tools can understand language and turn pictures into text so they can help write reports about radiology. Some studies have shown that reports made by intelligence can be correct and consistent and they can point out the most important things(Mamdouh et al., 2025). This can help reduce the amount of work that radiologists have to do. For example some models that use intelligence have made draft reports about chest x-rays and computerized tomography scans that are almost as good, as reports written by experts. Radiologists can then edit these reports of having to write them from the beginning. So pulmonary radiology is really changing because of integration(Mamdouh et al., 2025). This integration goes from automated pre-reading to helping with reports. When we design these systems correctly the artificial intelligence systems work with us. The artificial intelligence systems help us do things faster they help us make mistakes and they do the routine work. Meanwhile the radiologists are, in charge they check everything. They use their clinical judgment. The artificial intelligence systems and pulmonary radiology are working together to make things better. The artificial intelligence systems are helping radiology in many ways(Mamdouh et al., 2025)(Megat Ramli et al., 2025)(Gotta et al., 2025).

7. EMERGING FRONTIERS IN AI PULMONARY IMAGING: FUTURE DIRECTIONS

Figure 3. Emerging frontiers in artificial intelligence for pulmonary imaging. The four pillars include federated learning, explainable AI (XAI), multimodal foundation models, and precision medicine integration

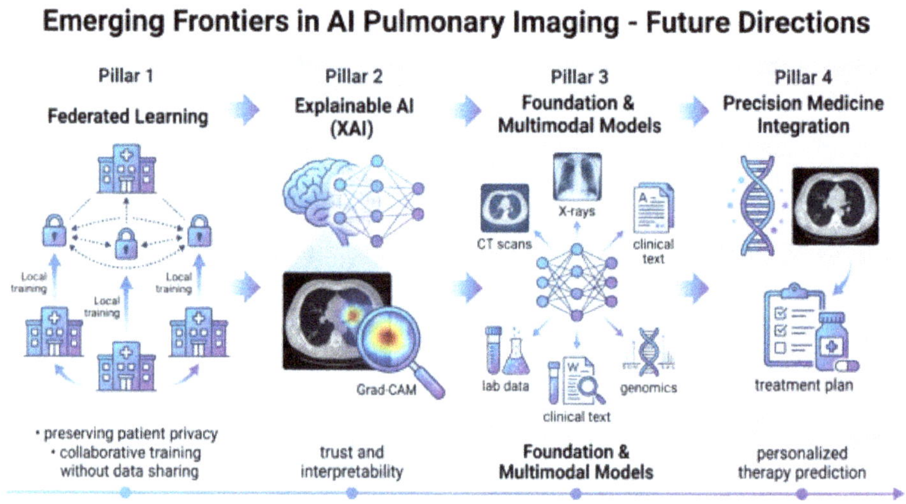

Pillar 1: Federated Learning – Privacy-Preserving Collaboration

The first pillar focuses on federated learning which enables secure joint research work between different organizations. The system of federated learning allows multiple parties to train their machine learning models through cooperative efforts without sharing their confidential data(Li et al., 2019). The traditional AI systems need to gather all patient imaging data into one central database which creates issues with protecting patient privacy and following legal requirements and institutional security protocols. Researchers can use federated learning to create institutional machine learning models which protect their data security by sending only model weights to the main server (Rieke et al., 2020).

The field of pulmonary imaging needs this technology for its applications in:

- Multi-center CT lung cancer screening
- Rare interstitial lung diseases
- Tuberculosis detection in resource-limited settings

Federated learning establishes a framework which allows researchers to develop models through their collaborative work without needing to share their complete datasets because it permits them to work together through data protection methods(Sheller et al., 2019). The system improves model performance through better generalization and cross-scanner and cross-population testing ability and helps to achieve ethical AI applications. This pillar establishes a global network which maintains user privacy while supporting worldwide research activities.

Pillar 2: Explainable AI (XAI) – Trust and Interpretability

The deep learning models demonstrate high accuracy in diagnostic testing but they operate as "black box" systems(Holzinger et al., 2017; Ribeiro et al., 2016). The purpose of Explainable AI (XAI) is to create algorithmic decision-making processes which both become understandable to users and develop healthcare professionals can comprehend.

The Grad-CAM method creates heatmaps which show chest CT and X-ray image sections that have the highest impact on a model's prediction(*Grad-CAM: Visual Explanations from Deep Networks via Gradient-Based Localization | IEEE Conference Publication | IEEE Xplore*, n.d.).

In pulmonary imaging this technology enables:

- The display of pneumonia consolidation areas
- The identification of pulmonary nodules
- The demonstration of fibrotic patterns in interstitial lung disease
- The process of explainability improves:
- The trust that radiologists display
- The process of regulatory bodies approving products
- The process of medical professionals facing legal responsibility
- The process of medical practitioners accepting new technologies

Future AI systems are expected to incorporate inherently interpretable architectures rather than relying solely on post-hoc visualization methods.

Pillar 3: Foundation & Multimodal Models – Beyond Imaging Alone

The third pillar shows a revolutionary change in foundation models and multimodal learning systems. Foundation models train on extensive diverse datasets which allow their use in multiple tasks through model training(Moor et al., 2023).

The multimodal models used in pulmonary imaging research combine(Huang et al., 2020):

- CT and X-ray imaging
- Clinical text data which includes EHR patient notes
- Laboratory test results
- Genomic information
- Results from pulmonary function assessments

Combining HRCT fibrosis patterns with autoantibody panels shows potential to enhance ILD subtype classification accuracy. The combination of CT nodule radiomics with smoking history data and genomic signatures results in improved lung cancer risk predictions(Azizi et al., 2021).

The multimodal AI systems will work to achieve three goals which include:

- Improving diagnostic precision
- Predicting disease trajectory
- Enabling holistic patient modeling

The transition from image-centric AI to patient-centric AI represents the current development.

Pillar 4: Precision Medicine Integration – Personalized Treatment Prediction

The primary objective of artificial intelligence in pulmonary imaging research goes beyond detecting diseases because it aims to provide treatment recommendations. Precision medicine integration uses quantitative imaging biomarkers together with predictive modeling to create personalized treatment plans(*Topol, E.J. (2019) Deep Medicine How Artificial Intelligence Can Make Healthcare Human Again. Basic Books. - References - Scientific Research Publishing*, n.d.).

The following applications exist for this technology:

- The system predicts how patients will respond to antifibrotic medication in IPF.

- The system identifies lung cancer patients who will benefit from immunotherapy.
- The system assesses COPD patients to determine their eligibility for biologic treatments.
- The system calculates how pulmonary embolism patients will advance through their medical condition.

The system uses AI technology as a clinical decision support system which functions within radiology operations to convert imaging data into treatment recommendations.

8. SUMMARY

Artificial intelligence is getting better and better at looking at pictures of lungs which helps doctors find problems and make decisions faster. When doctors look at chest X-rays computer programs can point out things like pneumonia, tuberculosis and nodules(Anderson et al., 2024)(Togunwa et al., 2025). They are usually right. These computer programs are like having another doctor look at the pictures to make sure nothing is missed. Artificial intelligence also helps with scans called CT scans, where it can find and describe nodules figure out what is going on with lung diseases and even spot blood clots in the lungs(Hoffmann et al., 2025)(Sait & Shaikh, 2025). Artificial intelligence is really good, at looking at lung pictures and finding lung cancer. It helps doctors do their jobs better. When we look at the numbers Artificial Intelligence can measure how emphysema is, how much fibrosis is present and the changes in airways on a CT scan. This helps create imaging biomarkers that are connected to how the lungs are working and what might happen in the future(Guo et al., 2018)(*Deep Learning-Based Algorithm for Automatic Detection of Incidental Pulmonary Embolism on Contrast-Enhanced CT: A Multicenter Multivendor Study | Radiology Advances | Oxford Academic*, n.d.).

Artificial Intelligence and other models can also combine imaging with clinical data to predict what will happen to patients and help guide the best treatment, for each person(Khalifa & Albadawy, 2024).

The thing is, we need to make sure these tools are used in life by being part of the radiology workflow: we need to use Artificial Intelligence when we take the images or when we review them we need to follow standards so everything works together and we need to make sure radiologists are still involved in the process. When doctors work with computers that use math to look at data they can find out what is wrong with peoples lungs faster and more correctly. This means they can also watch the disease closely and take better care of the patients. The combination of expertise and AI-driven analytics is very helpful, for pulmonary diagnoses and patient care(Tejani et al., 2024).

REFERENCES

Adam Essa, M. E. (2025). Diagnostic accuracy of AI in chest radiography for pneumonia and lung cancer: A meta-analysis. *European Journal of Radiology Open, 15*, 100701. DOI: 10.1016/j.ejro.2025.100701 PMID: 41278429

Anderson, P. G., Tarder-Stoll, H., Alpaslan, M., Keathley, N., Levin, D. L., Venkatesh, S., Bartel, E., Sicular, S., Howell, S., Lindsey, R. V., & Jones, R. M. (2024). Deep learning improves physician accuracy in the comprehensive detection of abnormalities on chest X-rays. *Scientific Reports, 14*(1), 25151. DOI: 10.1038/s41598-024-76608-2 PMID: 39448764

Arshad, M. F., Chowdhury, A. T., Sharif, Z., Islam, M., Sumon, M. S. I., Mohammedkasim, A., Chowdhury, M. E. H., & Pedersen, S. (2025). Artificial Intelligence and Machine Learning in Lung Cancer: Advances in Imaging, Detection, and Prognosis. *Cancers (Basel), 17*(24), 3985. DOI: 10.3390/cancers17243985 PMID: 41463234

Artificial Intelligence detects substantial airway damage on CT scans of children with severe asthma—Thirona. (n.d.). Retrieved January 31, 2026, from https://thirona.eu/blog/artificial-intelligence-detects-substantial-airway-damage-on-ct-scans-of-children-with-severe-asthma/

Azizi, S., Mustafa, B., Ryan, F., Beaver, Z., Freyberg, J., Deaton, J., Loh, A., Karthikesalingam, A., Kornblith, S., Chen, T., Natarajan, V., & Norouzi, M. (2021). Big Self-Supervised Models Advance Medical Image Classification. *2021 IEEE/CVF International Conference on Computer Vision (ICCV)*, 3458–3468. https://doi.org/DOI: 10.1109/ICCV48922.2021.00346

Chantzi, S. L., Kosvyra, A., & Chouvarda, I. (2025). Radiomics and Artificial Intelligence in Pulmonary Fibrosis. *Journal of Imaging Informatics in Medicine, 38*(5), 2779–2792. DOI: 10.1007/s10278-024-01377-3 PMID: 39762544

Deep learning-based algorithm for automatic detection of incidental pulmonary embolism on contrast-enhanced CT: a multicenter multivendor study | Radiology Advances | Oxford Academic. (n.d.). Retrieved January 31, 2026, from https://academic.oup.com/radadv/article/2/4/umaf021/8171918?login=false

Dixon, D., Sattar, H., Moros, N., Kesireddy, S. R., Ahsan, H., Lakkimsetti, M., Fatima, M., Doshi, D., Sadhu, K., & Junaid Hassan, M. (2024, May 9). (n.d.). Unveiling the Influence of AI Predictive Analytics on Patient Outcomes: A Comprehensive Narrative Review. *Cureus, 16*(5), e59954. DOI: 10.7759/cureus.59954 PMID: 38854327

Gotta, J., Grünewald, L. D., Koch, V., Mahmoudi, S., Bernatz, S., Höhne, E., Biciusca, T., Gökduman, A., Wolfram, C., Booz, C., Scholtz, J.-E., Martin, S., Eichler, K., Gruber-Rouh, T., Bucher, A., Yel, I., Vogl, T. J., & Reschke, P. (2025). Implementation of AI in radiology: The perspective of referring physicians. *Insights Into Imaging*, *16*(1), 238. DOI: 10.1186/s13244-025-02120-4 PMID: 41174325

Grad-CAM: Visual Explanations from Deep Networks via Gradient-Based Localization | IEEE Conference Publication | IEEE Xplore. (n.d.). Retrieved March 2, 2026, from https://ieeexplore.ieee.org/document/8237336

Guo, F., Capaldi, D., Kirby, M., Sheikh, K., Svenningsen, S., McCormack, D. G., Fenster, A., & Parraga, G. (2018). Development of a pulmonary imaging biomarker pipeline for phenotyping of chronic lung disease. *Journal of Medical Imaging (Bellingham, Wash.)*, *5*(2), 026002. DOI: 10.1117/1.JMI.5.2.026002 PMID: 29963580

Hoffmann, T., Teichgräber, U., Lassen-Schmidt, B., Renz, D., Brüheim, L. B., Weise, T., Krämer, M., Böttcher, J., Güttler, F., Wolf, G., & Pfeil, A. (2025). AI-based HRCT quantification reveals DLCO and TLC as key determinants of ILD severity in connective tissue diseases. *RMD Open*, *11*(4), e005963. DOI: 10.1136/rmdopen-2025-005963 PMID: 41151842

Holzinger, A., Biemann, C., Pattichis, C., & Kell, D. (2017). *What do we need to build explainable AI systems for the medical domain?* https://doi.org//arXiv.1712.09923DOI: 10.48550

Hosny, A., Parmar, C., Quackenbush, J., Schwartz, L. H., & Aerts, H. J. W. L. (2018). Artificial intelligence in radiology. *Nature Reviews. Cancer*, *18*(8), 500–510. DOI: 10.1038/s41568-018-0016-5 PMID: 29777175

Huang, S.-C., Pareek, A., Seyyedi, S., Banerjee, I., & Lungren, M. P. (2020). Fusion of medical imaging and electronic health records using deep learning: A systematic review and implementation guidelines. *NPJ Digital Medicine*, *3*(1), 136. DOI: 10.1038/s41746-020-00341-z PMID: 33083571

Jiang, W., Zhang, H., Li, Z., Jiang, X., Shao, J., Yang, X., Xiong, J., Zhou, P., Zhang, H., Wang, H., Yu, J., Su, X., Wang, Y., Liu, J., & Li, Z. (2025). AI-Powered Chest X-Ray for Diagnosing Pulmonary Tuberculosis in County and Township Health Care Facilities in Yichang: Retrospective, Real-World Study. *Journal of Medical Internet Research*, *27*, e83041. DOI: 10.2196/83041 PMID: 41328508

Khalifa, M., & Albadawy, M. (2024). Artificial Intelligence for Clinical Prediction: Exploring Key Domains and Essential Functions. *Computer Methods and Programs in Biomedicine Update*, *5*, 100148. DOI: 10.1016/j.cmpbup.2024.100148

Lambin, P., Rios-Velazquez, E., Leijenaar, R., Carvalho, S., van Stiphout, R. G. P. M., Granton, P., Zegers, C. M. L., Gillies, R., Boellard, R., Dekker, A., & Aerts, H. J. W. L. (2012). Radiomics: Extracting more information from medical images using advanced feature analysis. *European Journal of Cancer*, *48*(4), 441–446. DOI: 10.1016/j.ejca.2011.11.036 PMID: 22257792

Lee, G., Park, H., Bak, S. H., & Lee, H. Y. (2020). Radiomics in Lung Cancer from Basic to Advanced: Current Status and Future Directions. *Korean Journal of Radiology*, *21*(2), 159–171. DOI: 10.3348/kjr.2019.0630 PMID: 31997591

Li, W., Milletari, F., Xu, D., Rieke, N., Hancox, J., Zhu, W., Baust, M., Cheng, Y., Ourselin, S., Cardoso, M. J., & Feng, A. (2019). *Privacy-Preserving Federated Brain Tumour Segmentation.*, DOI: 10.1007/978-3-030-32692-0_16

Litjens, G., Kooi, T., Bejnordi, B. E., Setio, A. A. A., Ciompi, F., Ghafoorian, M., van der Laak, J. A. W. M., van Ginneken, B., & Sánchez, C. I. (2017). A survey on deep learning in medical image analysis. *Medical Image Analysis*, *42*, 60–88. DOI: 10.1016/j.media.2017.07.005 PMID: 28778026

Mamdouh, D., Attia, M., Osama, M., Mohamed, N., Lotfy, A., Arafa, T., Rashed, E. A., & Khoriba, G. (2025). Advancements in Radiology Report Generation: A Comprehensive Analysis. *Bioengineering (Basel, Switzerland)*, *12*(7), 693. DOI: 10.3390/bioengineering12070693 PMID: 40722385

Megat Ramli, P. N., Aizuddin, A. N., Ahmad, N., Abdul Hamid, Z., & Ismail, K. I. (2025). A Systematic Review: The Role of Artificial Intelligence in Lung Cancer Screening in Detecting Lung Nodules on Chest X-Rays. *Diagnostics (Basel)*, *15*(3), 246. DOI: 10.3390/diagnostics15030246 PMID: 39941176

Mei, X., Liu, Z., Singh, A., Lange, M., Boddu, P., Gong, J. Q. X., Lee, J., DeMarco, C., Cao, C., Platt, S., Sivakumar, G., Gross, B., Huang, M., Masseaux, J., Dua, S., Bernheim, A., Chung, M., Deyer, T., Jacobi, A., & Yang, Y. (2023). Interstitial lung disease diagnosis and prognosis using an AI system integrating longitudinal data. *Nature Communications*, *14*(1), 2272. DOI: 10.1038/s41467-023-37720-5 PMID: 37080956

Moor, M., Banerjee, O., Abad, Z. S. H., Krumholz, H. M., Leskovec, J., Topol, E. J., & Rajpurkar, P. (2023). Foundation models for generalist medical artificial intelligence. *Nature*, *616*(7956), 259–265. DOI: 10.1038/s41586-023-05881-4 PMID: 37045921

Pan, F., Feng, L., Liu, B., Hu, Y., & Wang, Q. (2023). Application of radiomics in diagnosis and treatment of lung cancer. *Frontiers in Pharmacology*, *14*, 1295511. Advance online publication. DOI: 10.3389/fphar.2023.1295511 PMID: 38027000

Pesapane, F., Codari, M., & Sardanelli, F. (2018). Artificial intelligence in medical imaging: Threat or opportunity? Radiologists again at the forefront of innovation in medicine. *European Radiology Experimental, 2*(1), 35. DOI: 10.1186/s41747-018-0061-6 PMID: 30353365

Ribeiro, M. T., Singh, S., & Guestrin, C. (2016). "Why Should I Trust You?": Explaining the Predictions of Any Classifier. *Proceedings of the 22nd ACM SIGKDD International Conference on Knowledge Discovery and Data Mining. KDD : Proceedings / International Conference on Knowledge Discovery & Data Mining. International Conference on Knowledge Discovery & Data Mining, 16*, 1135–1144. DOI: 10.1145/2939672.2939778

Rieke, N., Hancox, J., Li, W. *et al.* (2020). The future of digital health with federated learning. *npj Digit. Med. 3*, 119. https://doi.org/10.1038/s41746-020-00323-1

Sait, A. R. W., & Shaikh, M. A. (2025). Artificial Intelligence-Powered Chronic Obstructive Pulmonary Disease Detection Techniques—A Review. *Diagnostics (Basel), 15*(20), 2562. DOI: 10.3390/diagnostics15202562 PMID: 41153235

Sheller, M. J., Reina, G. A., Edwards, B., Martin, J., & Bakas, S. (2019). Multi-Institutional Deep Learning Modeling Without Sharing Patient Data: A Feasibility Study on Brain Tumor Segmentation. *Brainlesion: Glioma, Multiple Sclerosis, Stroke and Traumatic Brain Injuries. Lecture Notes in Computer Science, 11383*, 92–104. DOI: 10.1007/978-3-030-11723-8_9 PMID: 31231720

Tejani, A. S., Cook, T. S., Hussain, M., Sippel Schmidt, T., O'Donnell, K. P., & Arzen, S. (2024). Integrating and Adopting AI in the Radiology Workflow: A Primer for Standards and Integrating the Healthcare Enterprise (IHE) Profiles. *Radiology, 311*(3), e232653. DOI: 10.1148/radiol.232653 PMID: 38888474

Togunwa, T. O., Babatunde, A. O., Fatade, O. E., Olatunji, R., Ogbole, G., & Falade, A. (2025). Detection of pneumonia in children through chest radiographs using artificial intelligence in a low-resource setting: A pilot study. *PLOS Digital Health, 4*(9), e0000713. DOI: 10.1371/journal.pdig.0000713 PMID: 40991626

Topol, E.J. (2019) Deep Medicine How Artificial Intelligence Can Make Healthcare Human Again. Basic Books. - References—Scientific Research Publishing. (n.d.-a). Retrieved March 2, 2026, from https://www.scirp.org/reference/referencespapers?referenceid=3758241

Chapter 10

Machine Learning Applications in Asthma and COPD Management: Prediction, Monitoring, and Outcomes

Naima Khan
Department of Computer Science and IT, Cholistan University of Veterinary and Animal Sciences, Bahawalpur, Pakistan

Hira Fatima
Department of Zoology, Division of Science and Technology, University of Education, Lahore, Pakistan

Iqra Rafique
Government College University, Faisalabad, Pakistan

Imrana Amir
http://orcid.org/0000-0001-7304-2816
Department of Zoology, University of Mianwali, Mianwali, Pakistan

Saima Nousheen
Department of Zoology, University of Mianwali, Mianwali, Pakistan

Zainab Abid
University of Managaement and Technology, Lahore, Pakistan

Adnan Afzal
http://orcid.org/0009-0001-4359-5695
Government College University, Faisalabad, Pakistan

ABSTRACT

Machine learning is increasingly transforming the management of asthma and chronic obstructive pulmonary disease (COPD) by enabling data-driven prediction, continuous monitoring, and outcome optimization. This chapter examines how machine learning models leverage clinical records, digital inhalers, wearable

DOI: 10.4018/979-8-3373-7759-9.ch010

devices, and environmental data to predict exacerbations, assess disease control, and support personalized interventions. It highlights the impact of these approaches on clinical outcomes, healthcare utilization, and value-based care, while addressing challenges related to validation, interpretability, ethics, and equity. By exploring emerging research directions and implementation considerations, the chapter underscores the potential of machine learning to advance proactive and patient-centered respiratory care.

1. INTRODUCTION TO MACHINE LEARNING IN ASTHMA AND COPD MANAGEMENT

Two commonly occurring chronic respiratory diseases in the world are asthma and chronic obstructive pulmonary disease (COPD), which have significant burden to patients, healthcare, and societies (May and Li, 2015). Both illnesses are defined by the airflow obstruction, frequent symptoms, and exacerbations that have a major impact on the quality of life and long-term health outcomes (Upadhyay & Ahlawat, 2022). Although pharmacological treatment and clinical guidelines have improved, asthma and COPD are still difficult to manage because of the heterogeneity of the diseases, uncertain progression and the impact of environmental and behavioral determinants (Nici et al., 2020). It is these difficulties that have led to increased attention to data-driven methods, especially machine learning, to aid in more accurate, proactive and personalized disease management (Strielkowski et al., 2023). Conventionally, asthma and COPD treatment has been based on intermittent clinical evaluation, self-reported signs and symptoms and population-based treatment guidelines, which have not been effective in the dynamic and personal care of respiratory illness. The exacerbations can occur quickly, symptoms can vary over time and reaction to treatment is different in various patients. Consequently, clinicians are often uncertain about how the disease will develop, which patients are at the highest risk of exacerbation, and/or which interventions will be most effective (Afroz et al., 2020). To overcome these limitations, machine learning can provide new possibilities to detect complex patterns in large and diverse data. Machine learning is a collection of computational methods through which systems acquire knowledge of data and become better at it without having to explicitly program them with rules (Zhou et al., 2017). The machine learning models in the context of asthma and COPD will be able to work with high-dimensional data that consists of various sources, such as electronic health records, pulmonary function tests, imaging, biomarkers, environmental exposure data, and patient-generated health data (Goto et al., 2018). With the learning of relationships between these variables, models can be used to aid in prediction, monitoring, and optimization of outcomes on a level of granularity that is not attainable through the traditional methods of statistics. The increased access to healthcare data is one of the major facilitators of machine learning in respiratory medicine (Slavakis et al., 2014). Electronic health records will include longitudinal data about diagnoses, drug use, exacerbations, and health care use (Swinckels et al., 2024). The recent developments in digital health technologies, including smart inhalers, wearables, and mobile health applications, produce continuous symptom and medication adherence and physiological data (Kasoju et al., 2023). Environmental data of air pollution and allergens, weather conditions also add an extra layer of information to the data, especially in asthma where environmental stimulants are central. Machine learning algorithms are ideal in combining these nonhomogenous streams of data to aid real-time and predictive observations (Shamji et al., 2023).

Figure 1. Machine learning–enabled data integration and predictive approaches supporting personalized management of asthma and COPD

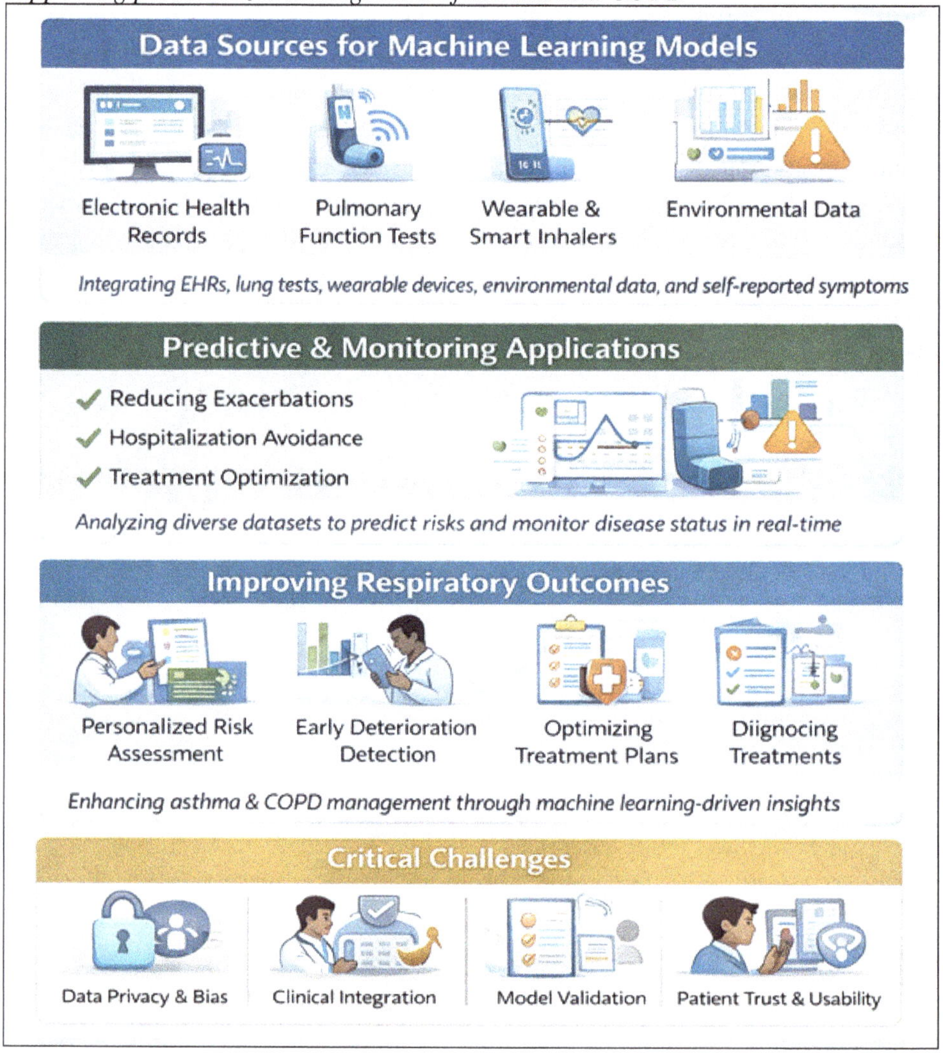

One of the most promising fields of machine learning application in the field of asthma and COPD management is prediction. The analysis of the past and real-time information may help predict the probability of the future exacerbation, hospital admission, or disease progression by use of predictive models. A timely intervention is possible by identifying the high-risk patients early, which can involve adjusting treatment, providing specific education, or monitoring patients more closely, which can help avoid serious consequences (Sanchez-Morillo et al., 2016).

Table 1.

Study	Disease Focus	ML Method	Data Source	Key Findings	Limitation
Finkelstein & Jeong (2017)	Asthma	ML prediction	EHR + symptoms	Early exacerbation prediction	Small sample
Kaplan et al. (2021)	Asthma/ COPD	AI/ML review	Clinical data	Improved diagnosis	Clinical integration issues
Molfino et al. (2024)	Asthma	Predictive ML	Longitudinal data	Better exacerbation prediction	Generalizability

Unlike conventional risk scores, machine learning models can adjust to nonlinearity and nonlinearity in the relationship and interaction between variables to enhance the quality of prediction and individualization (Steyerberg et al., 2014). Being a crucial aspect of machine learning-enabled care, monitoring is another crucial aspect of it. Periodic clinic visits may be insufficient to show the full picture of managing the disease because continuous or frequent symptom, lung, and medication monitoring can show its use (Bai et al., 2025). Monitoring data algorithm analysis can identify abnormalities or deviations of individual baselines in order to indicate loss of control or exacerbation in progress. These systems also facilitate proactive management of the disease and also shared decision-making between the patient and the medical provider. The end outcome of machine learning application in asthma and COPD management is improved clinical outcomes. Machine learning has the potential to reduce exacerbation, enhance symptom control, and optimize the use of healthcare resources by making it possible to detect deterioration earlier, stratify risks, and individualize treatment plans (Peng et al., 2020). Such benefits are especially relevant to COPD, which is typically linked to the progressive deterioration and elevated hospitalization rates, and severe or inadequately managed asthma, where the outcomes of an attack can be fatal. However, the risk of machine learning application in asthma and COPD care also presents some significant concerns (Halpin et al., 2017). The models have to be tested on a wide base of people in order to be reliable and just. The necessity to be integrated into clinical working processes is to be carefully designed not to overload clinicians (Nahar et al., 2024). Trust: Patients need to have confidence that their data will not be misused or violated; Privacy: Data needs to be kept private and should be interpreted only by patients; Interpretability: Patients need to know that predictions are not going to be used against them. These factors indicate a necessity of responsible and evidence-based implementation (Susilo & Rahman, 2025). Overall, machine learning is an effective and developing instrument toward solving the old issues in asthma and COPD treatment. Machine learning can support the transition to more personalized and proactive respiratory medicine by making it able to predict and constantly monitor data and provide outcome-driven care. The first step to realizing the potential and success of these approaches in bettering the lives of people living with the chronic respiratory disease is in understanding the underpinnings of these approaches.

2. DATA SOURCES AND DIGITAL HEALTH ECOSYSTEMS IN ASTHMA AND COPD

The quality, diversity, and integration of the sources of data in the digital health ecosystem are the key elements underlying the efficacy of machine learning in asthma and COPD management (Z. Chen et al., 2025). Contrary to the traditional care models which are based mainly on episodic clinical interactions, the contemporary respiratory care is becoming more dependent on the continuous and real-life data that are produced in a variety of clinical, behavioral, and environmental levels. These highly valuable data ecosystems allow the machine learning models to learn disease dynamics more effectively and allow prediction, monitoring, and optimization of outcomes (Price et al., 2015). Machine learning applications in asthma and COPD use electronic health records (EHRs) as a central source of data. Longitudinal clinical data provided by EHRs include diagnoses, spirometry findings, drug prescriptions, exacerbation history, comorbidities and history of healthcare utilization. This semi-structured and formalized information enables models to acquire patterns that relate severity of diseases, response to treatment and hospitalization risk. Nevertheless, EHR data can be incomplete, heterogeneous, and dependent on documentation practices, which makes it necessary to carefully preprocess and feature engineer them to guarantee reliability. Another essential part of the data ecosystem is the data on pulmonary function testing according to the measured values of forced expiratory volume and peak expiratory flow. These objective measures give information about obstruction of the airways and the development of the disease. Longitudinal analysis of the trends in pulmonary functioning can either indicate premature damage or loss of control (Budiarto et al., 2023). These measures together with symptoms and treatment information can be combined in machine learning models to better predict exacerbations and long-term outcomes. Practically, the variability of the frequency/method of testing serves as a challenge that the models should consider (Martinez-Garcia and Hernández-Lemus, 2022). New technologies that help to monitor compliance and digital inhalers have become helpful sources of patient-generated data. Smart inhalers are in a position to capture the time and a frequency of taking the medications and they can give objective data on adherence, which is frequently challenging to obtain through self-report. Poor control and exacerbation in asthma and COPD are largely caused by poor compliance. The patterns of inhaler use can be analyzed using machine learning models that define nonadherence, inefficient technique, or excessive use of rescue medication, providing the opportunity to intervene and educate specific patients. Wearable gadgets and mobile health apps further increase the data volume by recording the continuous physiological and behavioral data (Matthew, 2025). The daily impact of the disease and the level of functional status are estimated by activity levels, sleeping patterns, heart rate, and reports of symptoms measured using smartphones. Physical activity in COPD can be a predictor of deterioration of the disease or imminent exacerbation, whereas in asthma, nocturnal symptoms and activity restrictions may be the signs of poor control. Machine learning algorithms are especially most applicable in identifying meaningful patterns in these high-frequency streams of data (Bentley et al., 2020).

Table 2. Data sources and digital health ecosystems in asthma and COPD management

Data Source	Type of Data	Clinical Value	Role in Machine Learning	Key Challenges
Electronic Health Records (EHRs)	Diagnoses, spirometry, medications, exacerbations	Longitudinal view of disease severity and care use	Risk prediction, treatment response modeling	Incomplete data, heterogeneity
Pulmonary Function Tests	FEV_1, peak expiratory flow	Objective assessment of airway obstruction	Trend analysis, early decline detection	Irregular testing, technique variability
Digital / Smart Inhalers	Medication timing and frequency	Objective adherence and usage patterns	Detection of nonadherence and overuse	Access and device adoption
Wearables & mHealth Apps	Activity, sleep, heart rate, symptoms	Daily functional status and early warning signs	High-frequency pattern recognition	Data noise, user engagement
Environmental & Biomarker Data	Air quality, pollen, imaging, biomarkers	Contextual risk and disease phenotyping	Personalized, context-aware predictions	Interoperability, data integration

Both environmental and contextual data have a distinct significance in asthma treatment and a growing significance in COPD. The symptoms and exacerbations can be triggered by the air pollution level, the amount of pollen, the temperature, the humidity, and the variability of the weather (D'amato et al., 2015). By combining the environmental exposure data with the personal health data, the machine learning models are able to estimate a personalized risk depending on location and time. This integration facilitates context-based predictions and preventive measures, including the recommendation of patients to reduce activities or medication during the period of high risk (Holt, 2025). Additionally, imaging and biomarker data are also used in advanced machine learning applications and are especially useful in specialized care settings (Ahmed et al., 2020). The observation of the chest imaging, blood eosinophil levels, and other inflammatory indicators are added to the dimensions of the disease phenotyping and the stratification of treatment (Sweatt et al., 2019). Precision respiratory medicine can be supported by machine learning models that can merge these data with clinical and behavioral data to determine subgroups of patients with unique disease mechanisms and therapeutic requirements (Beitler et al., 2022). Different data sources need a powerful digital health infrastructure and interoperability to integrate them. Information tends to be stored in different disconnected systems, in disparate formats and standards. The interoperability absence suppresses the possibility to design the comprehensive datasets and impedes the generalizability of the models (Canali et al., 2022). The successful deployment of machine learning thus requires data integration platforms that synchronize temporal, semantic and context-based data and retain data quality and security (Korostin, 2025). Equity and representativeness is the consideration that occurs in digital health ecosystems. The digital tools like smart inhalers and wearables are not accessible to all because of differences in socioeconomic status, age, and digital literacy (Eze et al., 2025). Such differences affect the availability of data and can cause bias in machine learning models unless they are handled. The aspects of inclusive design, equitable access programs, and attentive assessment of the performance of models in difference populations are crucial to ensure that the current health disparity is further increased (Hanna et al., 2025). To conclude, machine learning applications in asthma and COPD management rely on the data sources and the digital health ecosystems. The combination of clinical records, patient-generated data, and environmental data in these ecosystems allows to have a holistic dynamic perspective of respiratory disease. To achieve all the potential of machine learning to enhance prediction, monitoring, and outcome in chronic respiratory care, it is important to build on reliable, interoperable, and equitable data infrastructures.

Table 3.

Clinical Task	Suitable ML Method	Why Suitable
Exacerbation Prediction	Random Forest, Gradient Boosting	Structured clinical data aur nonlinear relationships handle karte hain
Time-series Monitoring	LSTM / RNN	Symptoms aur wearable data longitudinal hote hain
Phenotyping	Clustering (K-means)	Patient subgroups identify karta hai
Treatment Adherence	Decision Trees, SVM	Medication patterns analyze karte hain
Personalized Risk Prediction	Ensemble Models	High accuracy aur adaptability

3. MACHINE LEARNING MODELS FOR EXACERBATION PREDICTION

Exacerbations are a major driver of morbidity, mortality, and healthcare utilization in both asthma and chronic obstructive pulmonary disease (COPD). Acute worsening of symptoms often leads to emergency visits, hospitalizations, and accelerated disease progression. Predicting exacerbations before they occur is therefore a central goal of modern respiratory care (Nguyen et al., 2021). Machine learning models have emerged as powerful tools for exacerbation prediction, offering the ability to analyze complex, multidimensional data and identify early warning signals that may not be apparent through traditional clinical assessment (Molfino et al., 2024). Traditional exacerbation risk assessment relies on simple clinical indicators, such as prior exacerbation history, symptom scores, lung function measurements, and medication use. While these factors are informative, they do not fully capture the dynamic and individualized nature of disease exacerbations (MacLeod et al., 2021).

Equitable implementation of machine learning in respiratory care requires addressing disparities in digital access, socioeconomic status, and technological literacy. Limited access to smart inhalers, wearables, or internet-enabled healthcare may reduce data representativeness and introduce algorithmic bias, thereby affecting prediction accuracy in underserved populations.

Figure 2. Machine learning models and multi-source data streams used for predicting asthma and COPD exacerbations and enabling early clinical intervention

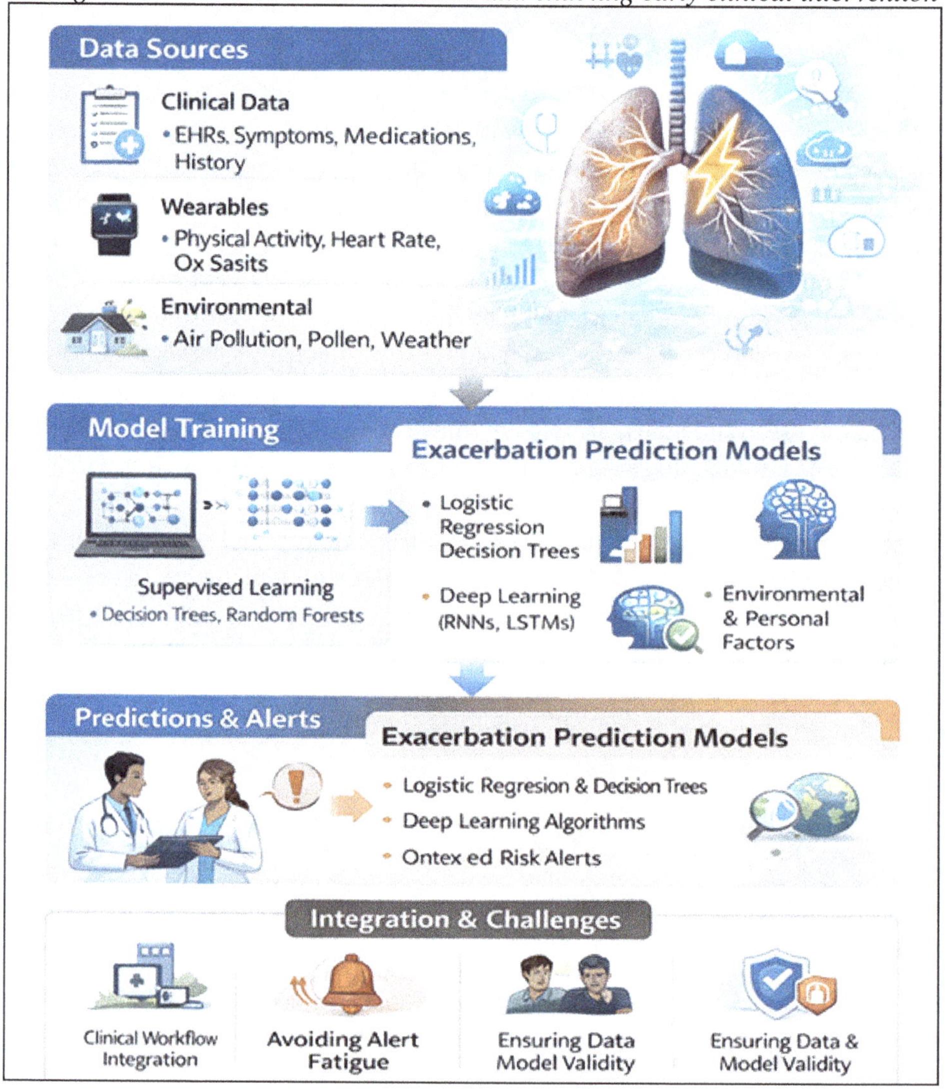

Machine learning models can incorporate a broader range of variables, including longitudinal trends, interactions among features, and real-time data streams, to generate more accurate and personalized risk predictions. Supervised learning approaches are commonly used for exacerbation prediction. These models are trained on historical data labeled with exacerbation outcomes and learn to associate specific patterns with increased risk (Sheetal et al., 2023). Algorithms such as logistic regression, decision trees, random forests, and gradient boosting machines have been widely applied due to their ability to handle structured clinical data and nonlinear relationships. These models can generate individualized risk scores that update over time as new data become available, supporting proactive intervention (Daghistani & Alshammari, 2020). Deep learning models have gained increasing attention for their ability to capture temporal patterns in longitudinal data (Lai et al., 2018). Recurrent neural networks and long short-term memory architectures are particularly well suited for modeling time-series data, such as daily symptoms, inhaler use, or physiological signals from wearables. These models can identify subtle changes and trends that precede exacerbations, enabling earlier detection than static risk assessments (Kim & Chung, 2019). In COPD, declines in physical activity or changes in heart rate patterns may signal impending exacerbation, while in asthma, increasing rescue inhaler use and nocturnal symptoms are often early indicators. Environmental and contextual data enhance the predictive power of machine learning models, especially in asthma. Air pollution, pollen levels, weather conditions, and seasonal factors interact with individual susceptibility to trigger exacerbations (Gershkovich, 2023). Machine learning models can integrate these external data with personal health information to generate context-aware predictions. For example, a patient's exacerbation risk may increase during periods of high pollution or allergen exposure, particularly if combined with poor medication adherence or declining lung function (Evans & Emma, 2024).

Personalization is a defining advantage of machine learning–based exacerbation prediction. Rather than relying on population averages, models can learn individual baselines and sensitivity to triggers (Finkelstein & Jeong, 2017). Adaptive and online learning approaches allow models to update predictions as new data are collected, improving relevance over time (Feroz Khan & Samad, 2024). This personalization is especially important given the heterogeneity of asthma and COPD, where exacerbation drivers and disease trajectories vary widely across patients. Despite their promise, exacerbation prediction models face important challenges. Data quality and completeness remain key limitations, as missing or noisy data can affect model performance (Aliyu et al., 2024). Exacerbations are relatively infrequent events, leading to class imbalance that complicates model training and evaluation (Turcatel et al., 2025). Robust validation across diverse populations and care settings is essential to ensure generalizability and avoid bias. Additionally, predictive accuracy must be balanced against clinical usability, as overly sensitive models may generate excessive alerts and contribute to alert fatigue. Integration into clinical workflows is critical for translating prediction into improved outcomes (Labarere et al., 2014). Risk scores and alerts must be presented in a clear and actionable manner, with guidance on appropriate responses. Collaboration between clinicians, data scientists, and patients is necessary to define thresholds, intervention strategies, and responsibilities. Without effective integration, even highly accurate models may fail to influence care (Peberdy et al., 2007). In summary, machine learning models offer significant potential to improve exacerbation prediction in asthma and COPD by leveraging diverse and longitudinal data sources. Through personalized, context-aware risk assessment, these models support earlier intervention and proactive disease management. Continued refinement, validation, and integration into care pathways are essential to realizing their full clinical impact.

4. MONITORING DISEASE CONTROL AND TREATMENT ADHERENCE USING MACHINE LEARNING

In order to manage asthma and chronic obstructive pulmonary disease (COPD), patients have to be continuously assessed in terms of disease control and adherence to prescribed therapies. The significant contributors to exacerbations, poor quality of life and high healthcare use are poor symptom control and suboptimal medication adherence. Conventional methods of surveillance are based on self-report and regular clinical evaluations of the patient that might not be very accurate in indicating the actual disease state and medication adherence in the long term (Sanchez-Morillo et al., 2016). Machine learning provides fresh possibilities of improving monitoring, analyzing objective and real-time data and detecting the patterns which indicate loss of control and noncompliance. The monitoring systems based on machine learning rely on various data sources such as smart inhalers, wearable devices, mobile health apps, as well as clinical records. Smart inhalers deliver objective information about the time and frequency of medication intake, which allows to determine adherence and inhaler technique (Mitta, 2021). An analysis of these data by machine learning models can help to differentiate intentional nonadherence, accidental missed doses, and behavior patterns indicative of poor technique or excessive use of rescue medication. These findings justify the need to develop specific and personalized interventions instead of general adherence counselling (Wu et al., 2020). Another important use of machine learning in the treatment of asthma and COPD is symptom monitoring. Patients can regularly report the symptoms, triggers, and quality-of-life measurements with the help of mobile applications and digital diaries (Tsang et al., 2022). In conjunction with physiological and behavioral data, e.g. activity rates and sleep cycles, machine learning models will be able to provide a more detailed image of disease control (Farrahi & Rostami, 2024). As an example, the deterioration of control in COPD or deterioration of nocturnal symptoms in asthma could be indicated even prior to the patients seeking the care (Agusti et al., 2011). Machine learning algorithms are able to detect these minor variations and warn of early review or treatment modification. Wearable devices add the new dimensions to the disease monitoring (Olyanasab & Annabestani, 2024). Respiratory health and functional status is indicated by continuous monitoring of physical activity, heart rate, and sleep (Nicolo et al., 2020). Exacerbations and hospitalizations are frequently preceded by decreases in the number of steps taken per day or greater inactivity in COPD. Machine learning algorithms are able to learn baseline patterns of individuals and detect variations that are indicators of deteriorating health. Independent monitoring can provide proactive care and reduce the number of unnecessary alerts (Aguilaniu et al., 2021).

Table 4. Machine learning–based monitoring of disease control and treatment adherence in asthma and COPD

Monitoring Aspect	Data Sources	Machine Learning Application	Clinical Benefits	Key Challenges
Medication Adherence	Smart inhalers, EHRs	Identify nonadherence patterns and poor technique	Reduced exacerbations, targeted interventions	Device use consistency, access
Symptom Monitoring	mHealth apps, digital diaries	Detect early loss of disease control	Timely treatment adjustment	Self-report reliability
Physiological & Behavioral Signals	Wearables (activity, sleep, heart rate)	Individual baseline modeling and deviation detection	Early exacerbation prediction	Data noise, missing data
Treatment Response Evaluation	Integrated clinical, symptom, and usage data	Assess effectiveness of prescribed therapies	Optimized treatment pathways	Model interpretability
Patient Engagement & Self-Management	Personalized feedback systems	Tailored reminders and insights	Improved self-management and adherence	Alert fatigue, anxiety

Machine learning analysis is also useful in treatment response monitoring. Models can evaluate the performance of the patient in relation to expected responses to prescribed treatment by combining consumption of medication, trends in symptoms, and physiological data (Bica et al., 2021). The absence of improvement or worsening of the situation despite seemingly appropriate adherence may indicate the necessity to intensify treatment, use other interventions, or conduct additional diagnosis. The insights are also especially significant in asthma to determine candidates of biologic therapies or specialist referral (May et al., 2020). Monitoring systems which are based on machine learning can be used to facilitate patient engagement and self-management. The model outputs provided to patients as personalized feedback, reminders, and visualizations can assist patients in knowing their patterns of diseases and how their behaviors affect them (Du et al., 2025). These tools should be designed in such a way that they allow the patient to actively manage his/her condition and the behavior that can positively influence health. Caution should however be taken in order to prevent information overload or anxiety due to too many alerts or complicated feedbacks (Alpay et al., 2011). Although these are the benefits, there are various challenges that should be overcome in order to make sure that monitoring is effective. Patient involvement and regular use of devices are required to achieve data completeness and accuracy but may differ with time (Joeris et al., 2023). The models should be resilient to the lack of data and flexible to behavioral or technological changes. Privacy and data security are also a major concern, because constant surveillance produces sensitive data regarding daily habits and health condition (Addae et al., 2019).

Clinical integration is one factor that has continued to be decisive. Output monitoring should have its presentation in a manner that supports clinical workflow and decision-making procedures. Clinicians and patients need clear thresholds, escalation pathways, and roles that enable the insights to cause the right action (Jayaratne et al., 2019). Absence of integration would leave the monitoring systems as mere data warehouses instead of practical mechanisms of enhancing care (Triantafyllidis et al., 2012). To conclude, machine learning improves the monitoring of asthma and COPD disease control and treatment adherence monitors with the help of objective and continuous data and personal analysis. The strategies help in early detection of loss of control, directed adherence interventions, and a more responsive treatment strategy. Machine learning-based monitoring can have a profound impact on the long-term outcomes of the chronic respiratory disease management when properly planned and offered.

5. CLINICAL OUTCOMES, HEALTHCARE UTILIZATION, AND VALUE-BASED CARE

One of the key goals in asthma and chronic obstructive pulmonary disease (COPD) management is the improvement of clinical outcomes and the decrease in unwarranted use of healthcare facilities. The proportion of the economic and societal burden of these conditions is substantial in regard to exacerbations, emergency department visits, and hospital admissions. Machine learning-based solutions can address the creation of additional opportunities to promote outcomes improvement and value-based care due to earlier intervention, decision-making treatment that is more accurate, and effective distribution of healthcare resources (van Boven et al., 2024). Machine learning models help to achieve better clinical outcomes in the context of timely risk stratification and personalized care. Predictive systems can help clinicians treat patients earlier or educate or follow-up more closely through identifying patients at high risk of exacerbation or poor control and support the optimization of treatment. Early intervention was linked to fewer and less serious exacerbations, better symptom management, and an increased quality of lung functionality over the years (Finkelstein and Jeong, 2017). This means better quality of life, fewer disruptions of day to day functions, and increased self-confidence in the ability to manage their disease, among patients. The decreases in the use of healthcare are another significant effect of machine learning-enabled care. Predictive and monitoring systems can be used to avert unnecessary emergency visits and hospitalizations through mitigating deterioration at an early stage. Asthma and COPD both have a small percentage of patients who frequently contribute a substantial portion of healthcare expenditures because of frequent attacks and hospitalizations (May and Li, 2015). The machine learning models have the ability to recognize such patients with high utilization and assist in managing the care programs that are specific to the patient, such as intensive follow-up, home monitoring, or multidisciplinary interventions (Seyam, 2025). Machine learning can further assist in more efficient utilization of healthcare resources by influencing clinical decision-making and care paths. One such example is that models can be used to identify those patients with the highest likelihood of experiencing an effective specialist referral, advanced therapies, or pulmonary rehabilitation (Adlung et al., 2021). In asthma, machine learning-based phenotyping can be used to identify the patients who could be sensitive to biologic therapy, so that expensive treatments are applied in the proper manner. Predictive tools can assist in COPD to make discharge readiness decisions or the necessity of post-acute support, which will decrease readmissions and length of stay (Kaplan et al., 2021).

Figure 3. Clinical impact of machine learning on respiratory outcomes, healthcare utilization, and value-based care in asthma and COPD management

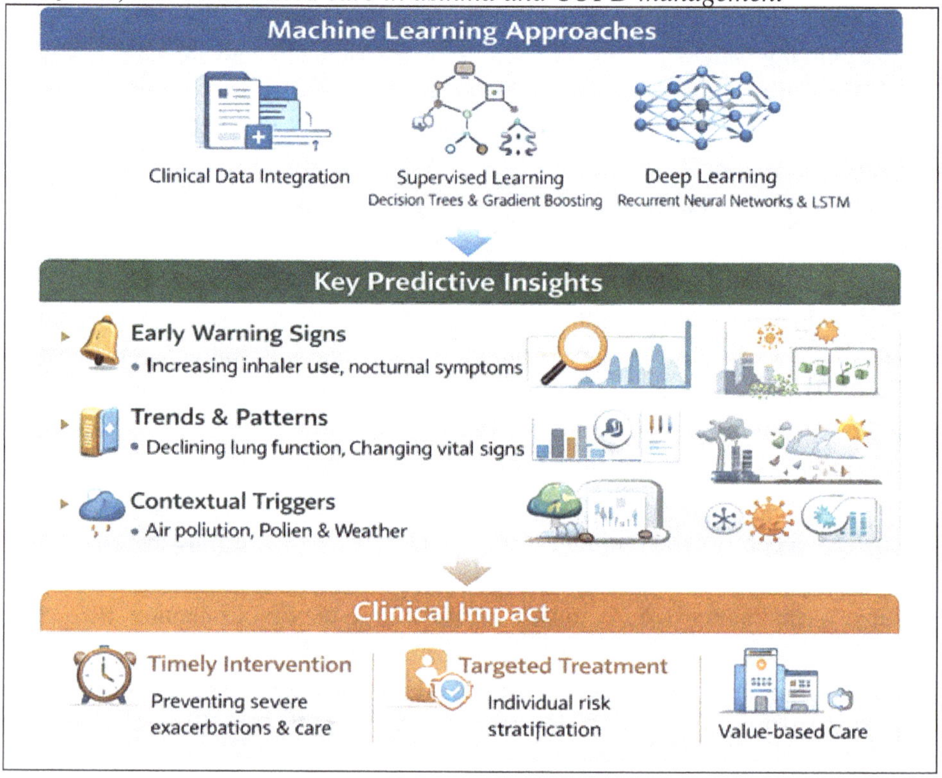

6. MODEL VALIDATION, INTERPRETABILITY, AND CLINICAL IMPLEMENTATION

To achieve real-world impact of machine learning use in asthma and COPD management, it is necessary that the model is closely validated, interpreted and implemented with proper consideration of clinical application. The predictive accuracy is not enough when models cannot be trusted by the populations and be comprehended by the clinicians and patients or be incorporated into the care pathways without any complications. These dimensions define the level of trust, adoption and eventual efficiency of machine learning tools in enhancing the outcome of respiratory health (Mahmood et al., 2025). One of the requirements of clinical use is model validation. There are several machine learning models that have shown good results on retrospective or development data sets and not as consistent with new populations or care settings (Maleki et al., 2020). The diseases of asthma and COPD are heterogeneous factors that depend on age, comorbidities, environmental exposures, and access to healthcare that vary among different populations (Levy et al., 2018). Strong validation thus involves that models need to be tested on other datasets, multiple institutions and on different demographical groups. It is especially important that prospective validation be carried out in real-world clinical practice, as it records the data quality, workflow limitations, and other behavioral variables that are usually not covered in the controlled studies (Bin Rafiq et al., 2020). Temporal validation is instrumental in the management of chronic respiratory diseases also. Models have to be correct with time as the patient behavior, treatment guidelines, and environmental conditions vary. The constant checking of model performance will identify data drift or degradation which may affect safety and effectiveness. The provision of model updating, revalidation and version control processes is critical towards providing long-term reliability in clinical practice. Meaning Making is key which contributes to clinician trust and adoption. The respiratory clinicians that are engaged should be aware of the reasons why a model has a high exacerbation risk or low control in order to act accordingly to what it advises (Sanchez-Morillo et al., 2016). Black-box predictions made in an unexplainable manner can either be dismissed or the converse is true, such as blind faith in them. Machine learning techniques that can be interpreted, like feature importance analysis, rule-based models, or graphical summaries of key risk drivers and so on, are useful in putting predictions into perspective and making informed decisions (Kanchepu, 2025). Explanations that can be broken down to understandable clinical concepts, e.g. medication adherence, symptom patterns, or environmental exposure, especially come in handy in asthma and COPD management. Interpretability facing the patient is also important. As machine learning systems provide patients with alerts or feedback, well-explained and understandable answers are likely to reduce anxiety and enable interactions. When patients become aware of how their behaviors like the use of inhaler and the level of activity affect disease control, they will be more likely to comply with their recommendations. Accessible and supportive explanations therefore are a major factor to successful implementation (George and Bender, 2019).

7. ETHICAL, PRIVACY, AND EQUITY CONSIDERATIONS IN RESPIRATORY MACHINE LEARNING APPLICATIONS

The machine learning use to manage asthma and chronic obstructive pulmonary disease (COPD) brings up critical ethical, privacy, and equity issues, which must be considered in tandem with technical and clinical problems. Such circumstances also tend to be demanding of long-term surveillance and data gathering which makes the volume and sensitivity of health information more sensitive and larger. Proper employment of machine learning in respiratory care, thus, requires the protection of patient rights, fairness, and trust between patients, clinicians, and health systems (Graña-Castro et al., 2024). One of the core issues of machine learning-based respiratory care is privacy. The applications are based on continuous or near-continuous data of smart inhalers, wearable technologies, mobile applications, and sensors placed in the environment (Al-Anazi et al., 2024). Such data can show not only health status, but also day-to-day activities, location trends and behaviors. Data protection will be needed as the key to maintaining confidentiality, which may involve secure data transmission, data encryption, access control, and a clear data storage and sharing policy (Abouelmehdi et al., 2018). Patients should also be assured that their information will not be abused or used by third parties, especially when the monitoring goes beyond the clinical context to the daily life (Jaime et al., 2023). There is further complexity of informed consent. Patients can consent to the use of their data in clinical care without having sufficient knowledge of how machine learning models process their data or provide prediction (Abouelmehdi et al., 2018). Besides, the information gathered today can be used in the coming days to retrain the model or to conduct research. Ethical practice implies clear communication regarding the way data are processed, what kind of predictions are made, and what kind of actions can be taken based on the predictions (Mathrani et al., 2021). There is a possible solution in long-term respiratory care with the use of dynamic consent models, where patients can change preferences over time (Budin-Ljøsne et al., 2017). The essential concern during asthma and COPD machine learning use is equity and fairness. The digital health technologies are not equally accessible to everyone regarding socioeconomic status, age, education level, and geographical location (Z. Chen et al., 2025). Patients who cannot use smart inhalers, smartphones, or have a well-established internet connection can be left out of the data-driven care, which constrains the representative power of training datasets (Matthew, 2025). Consequently, machine learning models can be more suitable to digitally connected groups and provide fewer accurate predictions to underserved groups. This is a very worrying risk considering that the burden of asthma and COPD is greater in the disadvantaged communities (Pleasants et al., 2016).

8. FUTURE DIRECTIONS AND RESEARCH OPPORTUNITIES IN MACHINE LEARNING–ENABLED RESPIRATORY CARE

Machine learning in the context of managing asthma and chronic obstructive pulmonary disease (COPD) has a promising future in the possibility to transform the use of these tools into a fully integrated and learning-based part of respiratory care systems. With the maturity of the digital health technologies and the spread of data, machine learning is set to increasingly take a more central role in assisting in precision, prevention and long-term disease management. To achieve this potential, methodological, infrastructure, and clinical integration, as well as policy, advances are needed. The creation of increasingly personal and adaptable models is one of the main tendencies in the future (S. Chen et al., 2025). Both asthma and COPD are very heterogeneous, and triggers, progression, and treatment response vary significantly (Feng et al., 2021). It is possible that future machine learning systems will involve online and adaptive learning methods that can continually update predictions depending on patient-specific information (Gligorea et al., 2023). These models have the potential to acquire personal baselines, sensitivity to environmental exposures, and behavioral patterns which allows predicting and monitoring risks and doing it on an individual population level instead of just estimating it the way it happens in populations (Chapizanis et al., 2021). Combination of multimodal information will also promote predictive and clinical usefulness. In the future, clinical records, smart inhaler information, wearables, imaging, biomarkers, genomics, and environmental exposures will be used together to form single analytical frameworks (Hao et al., 2025). Such a multimodal combination will aid in more sophisticated disease phenotyping and categorization of isolated subsets in asthma and COPD. Better phenotyping is especially significant in informing tailored interventions, such as biologic treatment of asthma, or individualized rehabilitation programs or pharmacological treatments of COPD. Another direction that can be considered promising is edge computing and real-time analytics (Luo et al., 2024). Reducing latency and enhancing privacy, as well as facilitating timely intervention, can be achieved by processing data nearer to the collection location e.g. smartphone or integrated inhaler. These strategies can be applied particularly to the case of early exacerbation identification and real-time adherence guidance. The development of efficient and lightweight models that can be deployed at the side of the edge will be crucial to the development of scalable and responsive respiratory care solutions (Matthew, 2025).

CONCLUSION

Machine learning can be regarded as a strong concept of resolving the chronic issues related to managing asthma and COPD, especially the necessity to predict conditions early, monitor them, and ensure better clinical results. As explained in this chapter, machine learning models have the capacity to incorporate various data types such as electronic health records, smart inhalers, wearable sensors, as well as environmental exposures with the aim of capturing the dynamicity and heterogeneity of chronic respiratory disease. These functions aid in improving predictive accuracy of exacerbation, improved evaluation of disease control and customized therapeutic approaches beyond more traditional episodic model of care. Machine learning is also clinically useful because it not only offers more predictive power but also helps to proactively and value-based care. Machine learning-based systems can decrease the number of exacerbations, hospitalizations, and the total cost of healthcare and increase the quality of life of the patients as they can identify high-risk patients earlier in life and apply specific measures to them. Follow-up of compliance and response to treatment enhances long-term disease control even more, and decision-making between patients and clinicians. Nevertheless, to achieve these benefits, it is necessary to pay special attention to validation, interpretability, and clinical integration. There should also be strict assessment of models in a wide range of populations and care environments as a way of guaranteeing safety, generalizability, and equity. Both clear and explainable outputs and easier integration in clinical paths are required to develop trust in clinicians and patients, as well as to alchemize predictions into action. The fundamental aspect of responsible deployment continues to focus on ethical issues, such as protection of privacy, an informed consent, and equitable access to digital health technologies. Going forward, there is a need to further and further research and development to provide personalized, multimodal, and real-time machine learning solutions in respiratory care. Machine learning can be used to revolutionise results with careful management and an inclusive approach and can enhance patient-centred and more predictive management of COPD and asthma.

REFERENCES

Abouelmehdi, K., Beni-Hessane, A., & Khaloufi, H. (2018). Big healthcare data: Preserving security and privacy. *Journal of Big Data*, *5*(1), 1–18. DOI: 10.1186/s40537-017-0110-7

Addae, J. H., Sun, X., Towey, D., & Radenkovic, M. (2019). Exploring user behavioral data for adaptive cybersecurity. *User Modeling and User-Adapted Interaction*, *29*(3), 701–750. DOI: 10.1007/s11257-019-09236-5

Adlung, L., Cohen, Y., Mor, U., & Elinav, E. (2021). Machine learning in clinical decision making. *Med (New York, N.Y.)*, *2*(6), 642–665. PMID: 35590138

Afroz, N., Gutzwiller, F. S., Mackay, A. J., Naujoks, C., Patalano, F., & Kostikas, K. (2020). Patient-reported outcomes (PROs) in COPD clinical trials: Trends and gaps. *International Journal of Chronic Obstructive Pulmonary Disease*, *15*, 1789–1800. DOI: 10.2147/COPD.S235845 PMID: 32801678

Aguilaniu, B., Hess, D., Kelkel, E., Briault, A., Destors, M., Boutros, J., Zhi Li, P., & Antoniadis, A. (2021). A machine learning approach to predict extreme inactivity in COPD patients using non-activity-related clinical data. *PLoS One*, *16*(8), e0255977. DOI: 10.1371/journal.pone.0255977 PMID: 34411121

Agusti, A., Hedner, J., Marin, J., Barbé, F., Cazzola, M., & Rennard, S. (2011). Night-time symptoms: A forgotten dimension of COPD. *European Respiratory Review : an Official Journal of the European Respiratory Society*, *20*(121), 183–194. DOI: 10.1183/09059180.00004311 PMID: 21881146

Ahmed, Z., Mohamed, K., Zeeshan, S., & Dong, X. (2020). Artificial intelligence with multi-functional machine learning platform development for better healthcare and precision medicine. *Database : The Journal of Biological Databases and Curation*, *2020*, baaa010. DOI: 10.1093/database/baaa010 PMID: 32185396

Al-Anazi, S., Al-Omari, A., Alanazi, S., Marar, A., Asad, M., Alawaji, F., & Alwateid, S. (2024). Artificial intelligence in respiratory care: Current scenario and future perspective. *Annals of Thoracic Medicine*, *19*(2), 117–130. DOI: 10.4103/atm.atm_192_23 PMID: 38766378

Aliyu, D. A., Akhir, E. A. P., Osman, N. A., Yahaya, S., Adamu, S., & Mamman, H. (2024). A Conceptual Framework for Personalized Early Prediction of Asthma Exacerbation Attacks Using Proximal Policy Optimization. *JOIV: International Journal on Informatics Visualization*, *8*(4), 2462–2471. DOI: 10.62527/joiv.8.4.2944

Alpay, L., van der Boog, P., & Dumaij, A. (2011). An empowerment-based approach to developing innovative e-health tools for self-management. *Health Informatics Journal, 17*(4), 247–255. DOI: 10.1177/1460458211420089 PMID: 22193825

Bai, Y., Gu, B., & Tang, C. (2025). Enhancing real-time patient monitoring in intensive care units with deep learning and the internet of things. *Big Data*, big.2024.0113. DOI: 10.1089/big.2024.0113 PMID: 39819048

Beitler, J. R., Thompson, B. T., Baron, R. M., Bastarache, J. A., Denlinger, L. C., Esserman, L., Gong, M. N., LaVange, L. M., Lewis, R. J., Marshall, J. C., Martin, T. R., McAuley, D. F., Meyer, N. J., Moss, M., Reineck, L. A., Rubin, E., Schmidt, E. P., Standiford, T. J., Ware, L. B., & Calfee, C. S. (2022). Advancing precision medicine for acute respiratory distress syndrome. *The Lancet. Respiratory Medicine, 10*(1), 107–120. DOI: 10.1016/S2213-2600(21)00157-0 PMID: 34310901

Bentley, C. L., Powell, L., Potter, S., Parker, J., Mountain, G. A., Bartlett, Y. K., Farwer, J., O'Connor, C., Burns, J., Cresswell, R. L., Dunn, H. D., & Hawley, M. S. (2020). The use of a smartphone app and an activity tracker to promote physical activity in the management of chronic obstructive pulmonary disease: Randomized controlled feasibility study. *JMIR mHealth and uHealth, 8*(6), e16203. DOI: 10.2196/16203 PMID: 32490838

Bica, I., Alaa, A. M., Lambert, C., & Van Der Schaar, M. (2021). From real-world patient data to individualized treatment effects using machine learning: Current and future methods to address underlying challenges. *Clinical Pharmacology and Therapeutics, 109*(1), 87–100. DOI: 10.1002/cpt.1907 PMID: 32449163

Bin Rafiq, R., Modave, F., Guha, S., & Albert, M. V. (2020). Validation methods to promote real-world applicability of machine learning in medicine. Proceedings of the 2020 3rd International Conference on Digital Medicine and Image Processing, Budiarto, A., Tsang, K. C., Wilson, A. M., Sheikh, A., & Shah, S. A. (2023). Machine learning–based asthma attack prediction models from routinely collected electronic health records: Systematic scoping review. *JMIR AI, 2*, e46717.

Budin-Ljøsne, I., Teare, H. J., Kaye, J., Beck, S., Bentzen, H. B., Caenazzo, L., Collett, C., D'Abramo, F., Felzmann, H., Finlay, T., Javaid, M. K., Jones, E., Katić, V., Simpson, A., & Mascalzoni, D. (2017). Dynamic consent: A potential solution to some of the challenges of modern biomedical research. *BMC Medical Ethics, 18*(1), 4. DOI: 10.1186/s12910-016-0162-9 PMID: 28122615

Canali, S., Schiaffonati, V., & Aliverti, A. (2022). Challenges and recommendations for wearable devices in digital health: Data quality, interoperability, health equity, fairness. *PLOS Digital Health*, *1*(10), e0000104. DOI: 10.1371/journal.pdig.0000104 PMID: 36812619

Chapizanis, D., Karakitsios, S., Gotti, A., & Sarigiannis, D. A. (2021). Assessing personal exposure using Agent Based Modelling informed by sensors technology. *Environmental Research*, *192*, 110141. DOI: 10.1016/j.envres.2020.110141 PMID: 32956655

Chen, S., Xing, S., Zhang, G., & Qiu, F. (2025). Innovative Applications and Challenges of Artificial Intelligence in the Whole-Course Management of Chronic Obstructive Pulmonary Disease. *International Journal of Chronic Obstructive Pulmonary Disease*, •••, 1–18. PMID: 41859017

D'amato, G., Vitale, C., De Martino, A., Viegi, G., Lanza, M., Molino, A., Sanduzzi, A., Vatrella, A., Annesi-Maesano, I., & D'amato, M. (2015). Effects on asthma and respiratory allergy of Climate change and air pollution. *Multidisciplinary Respiratory Medicine*, *10*(1), 1–8. PMID: 26697186

Daghistani, T., & Alshammari, R. (2020). Comparison of statistical logistic regression and random forest machine learning techniques in predicting diabetes. *Journal of Advances in Information Technology*, *11*(2), 78–83. DOI: 10.12720/jait.11.2.78-83

Du, Y., Yang, P., Liu, Y., Deng, C., & Li, X. (2025). Artificial intelligence in chronic disease self-management: Current applications and future directions. *Frontiers in Public Health*, *13*, 1689911. DOI: 10.3389/fpubh.2025.1689911 PMID: 41358250

Evans, M., & Emma, O. (2024). Enhancing Patient Outcomes through Context-Aware Healthcare Systems: A Comprehensive Study of Adaptive Technologies in Chronic Disease Management.

Eze, V. I., Eboh, N. A., Abdulkareem, M. O., Jimoh, T. S., Olufemi, T. D., Nwekeoma, C. O., & Bejide, V. O. (2025). The Equity Impact of Digital Health and Artificial Intelligence Tools on Health Outcomes in Underserved Populations: A Narrative Review and Conceptual Model. *Journal of Life Science and Public Health*, *1*(2), 90–102. DOI: 10.69739/jlsph.v1i2.1340

Farrahi, V., & Rostami, M. (2024). Machine learning in physical activity, sedentary, and sleep behavior research. *Journal of Activity, Sedentary and Sleep Behaviors*, *3*(1), 5. DOI: 10.1186/s44167-024-00045-9 PMID: 40217437

Feng, Y., Wang, Y., Zeng, C., & Mao, H. (2021). Artificial intelligence and machine learning in chronic airway diseases: Focus on asthma and chronic obstructive pulmonary disease. *International Journal of Medical Sciences*, *18*(13), 2871–2889. DOI: 10.7150/ijms.58191 PMID: 34220314

Feroz Khan, A., & Samad, S. (2024). Evaluating online learning adaptability in students using machine learning-based techniques: A novel analytical approach. *Educ. Sci. Manag*, *2*(1), 25–34. DOI: 10.56578/esm020103

Finkelstein, J., & Jeong, I. C. (2017). Machine learning approaches to personalize early prediction of asthma exacerbations. *Annals of the New York Academy of Sciences*, *1387*(1), 153–165. DOI: 10.1111/nyas.13218 PMID: 27627195

George, M., & Bender, B. (2019). New insights to improve treatment adherence in asthma and COPD. *Patient Preference and Adherence*, *13*, 1325–1334. DOI: 10.2147/PPA.S209532 PMID: 31534319

Gershkovich, D. (2023). *Acute exacerbation of asthma*. University of Zagreb. School of Medicine.

Gligorea, I., Cioca, M., Oancea, R., Gorski, A.-T., Gorski, H., & Tudorache, P. (2023). Adaptive learning using artificial intelligence in e-learning: A literature review. *Education Sciences*, *13*(12), 1216. DOI: 10.3390/educsci13121216

Goto, T., Camargo, C. A.Jr, Faridi, M. K., Yun, B. J., & Hasegawa, K. (2018). Machine learning approaches for predicting disposition of asthma and COPD exacerbations in the ED. *The American Journal of Emergency Medicine*, *36*(9), 1650–1654. DOI: 10.1016/j.ajem.2018.06.062 PMID: 29970272

Graña-Castro, O., Izquierdo, E., Piñas-Mesa, A., Menasalvas, E., & Chivato-Pérez, T. (2024). Assessing the impact of new technologies on managing chronic respiratory diseases. *Journal of Clinical Medicine*, *13*(22), 6913. DOI: 10.3390/jcm13226913 PMID: 39598056

Graña-Castro, O., Izquierdo, E., Piñas-Mesa, A., Menasalvas, E., & Chivato-Pérez, T. (2024). Assessing the impact of new technologies on managing chronic respiratory diseases. *Journal of Clinical Medicine*, *13*(22), 6913. DOI: 10.3390/jcm13226913 PMID: 39598056

Halpin, D. M., Miravitlles, M., Metzdorf, N., & Celli, B. (2017). Impact and prevention of severe exacerbations of COPD: A review of the evidence. *International Journal of Chronic Obstructive Pulmonary Disease*, *12*, 2891–2908. DOI: 10.2147/COPD.S139470 PMID: 29062228

Hanna, M. G., Pantanowitz, L., Jackson, B., Palmer, O., Visweswaran, S., Pantanowitz, J., Deebajah, M., & Rashidi, H. H. (2025). Ethical and bias considerations in artificial intelligence/machine learning. *Modern Pathology*, *38*(3), 100686. DOI: 10.1016/j.modpat.2024.100686 PMID: 39694331

Hao, Y., Cheng, C., Li, J., Li, H., Di, X., Zeng, X., Jin, S., Han, X., Liu, C., Wang, Q., Luo, B., Zeng, X., & Li, K. (2025). Multimodal integration in health care: Development with applications in disease management. *Journal of Medical Internet Research*, *27*, e76557. DOI: 10.2196/76557 PMID: 40840463

Holt, K. L. (2025). Predictive Modeling of Occupational Exposure Using Machine Learning and Environmental Sensor Data. *Journal of Exceptional Multidisciplinary Research*, *2*(1), 82–89. DOI: 10.69739/jemr.v2i1.617

Jaime, F. J., Muñoz, A., Rodríguez-Gómez, F., & Jerez-Calero, A. (2023). Strengthening privacy and data security in biomedical microelectromechanical systems by IoT communication security and protection in smart healthcare. *Sensors (Basel)*, *23*(21), 8944. DOI: 10.3390/s23218944 PMID: 37960646

Jayaratne, M., Nallaperuma, D., De Silva, D., Alahakoon, D., Devitt, B., Webster, K. E., & Chilamkurti, N. (2019). A data integration platform for patient-centered e-healthcare and clinical decision support. *Future Generation Computer Systems*, *92*, 996–1008. DOI: 10.1016/j.future.2018.07.061

Joeris, A., Zhu, T. Y., Lambert, S., Wood, A., & Jayakumar, P. (2023). Real-world patient data: Can they support decision making and patient engagement? *Injury*, *54*, S51–S56. DOI: 10.1016/j.injury.2021.12.012 PMID: 34949460

Kanchepu, N. (2025). Unveiling the Black Box: The Crucial Role of Interpretability in Machine Learning Models. In *Cutting-Edge Solutions for Advancing Sustainable Development: Exploring Technological Horizons for Sustainability-Part 1* (pp. 22-44). Bentham Science Publishers.

Kaplan, A., Cao, H., FitzGerald, J. M., Iannotti, N., Yang, E., Kocks, J. W., Kostikas, K., Price, D., Reddel, H. K., Tsiligianni, I., Vogelmeier, C. F., Pfister, P., & Mastoridis, P. (2021). Artificial intelligence/machine learning in respiratory medicine and potential role in asthma and COPD diagnosis. *The Journal of Allergy and Clinical Immunology. In Practice*, *9*(6), 2255–2261. DOI: 10.1016/j.jaip.2021.02.014 PMID: 33618053

Kasoju, N., Remya, N., Sasi, R., Sujesh, S., Soman, B., Kesavadas, C., Muraleedharan, C., Varma, P. H., & Behari, S. (2023). Digital health: Trends, opportunities and challenges in medical devices, pharma and bio-technology. *CSI Transactions on ICT*, *11*(1), 11–30. DOI: 10.1007/s40012-023-00380-3

Kim, J.-C., & Chung, K. (2019). Prediction model of user physical activity using data characteristics-based long short-term memory recurrent neural networks. [TIIS]. *KSII Transactions on Internet and Information Systems, 13*(4), 2060–2077.

Korostin, O. (2025). Optimising machine learning integration in real-time text analytics platforms: Technical approaches and performance criteria. *COMPUTER-INTEGRATED TECHNOLOGIES: EDUCATION, SCIENCE. Production*, (58), 38–45.

Labarere, J., Bertrand, R., & Fine, M. J. (2014). How to derive and validate clinical prediction models for use in intensive care medicine. *Intensive Care Medicine, 40*(4), 513–527. DOI: 10.1007/s00134-014-3227-6 PMID: 24570265

Lai, G., Chang, W.-C., Yang, Y., & Liu, H. (2018). Modeling long-and short-term temporal patterns with deep neural networks. The 41st international ACM SIGIR conference on research & development in information retrieval, Levy, J. I., Quirós-Alcalá, L., Fabian, M. P., Basra, K., & Hansel, N. N. (2018). Established and emerging environmental contributors to disparities in asthma and chronic obstructive pulmonary disease. *Current Epidemiology Reports, 5*(2), 114–124. PMID: 30319934

Luo, X., Zeng, W., Tang, J., Liu, W., Yang, J., Chen, H., Jiang, L., Zhou, X., Huang, J., Zhang, S., Du, L., Shen, X., Chi, H., & Wang, H. (2024). Multi-modal transcriptomic analysis reveals metabolic dysregulation and immune responses in chronic obstructive pulmonary disease. *Scientific Reports, 14*(1), 22699. DOI: 10.1038/s41598-024-71773-w PMID: 39349929

MacLeod, M., Papi, A., Contoli, M., Beghé, B., Celli, B. R., Wedzicha, J. A., & Fabbri, L. M. (2021). Chronic obstructive pulmonary disease exacerbation fundamentals: Diagnosis, treatment, prevention and disease impact. *Respirology (Carlton, Vic.), 26*(6), 532–551. DOI: 10.1111/resp.14041 PMID: 33893708

Mahmood, S., Hasan, R., Hussain, S., & Adhikari, R. (2025). An Interpretable and Generalizable Machine Learning Model for Predicting Asthma Outcomes: Integrating AutoML and Explainable AI Techniques. *WORLD (Oakland, Calif.), 6*(1), 15. DOI: 10.3390/world6010015

Maleki, F., Muthukrishnan, N., Ovens, K., Reinhold, C., & Forghani, R. (2020). Machine learning algorithm validation: From essentials to advanced applications and implications for regulatory certification and deployment. *Neuroimaging Clinics of North America, 30*(4), 433–445. DOI: 10.1016/j.nic.2020.08.004 PMID: 33038994

Martínez-García, M., & Hernández-Lemus, E. (2022). Data integration challenges for machine learning in precision medicine. *Frontiers in Medicine, 8*, 784455. DOI: 10.3389/fmed.2021.784455 PMID: 35145977

Mathrani, A., Susnjak, T., Ramaswami, G., & Barczak, A. (2021). Perspectives on the challenges of generalizability, transparency and ethics in predictive learning analytics. *Computers and Education Open*, *2*, 100060. DOI: 10.1016/j.caeo.2021.100060

Matthew, B. (2025). Smart Inhalers and Respiratory IoTs for Asthma Management Gene.

May, C., Myall, M., Lund, S., Campling, N., Bogle, S., Dace, S., & Richardson, A. (2020). Managing patient preferences and clinical responses in acute pathophysiological deterioration: What do clinicians think treatment escalation plans do? *Social Science & Medicine*, *258*, 113143. DOI: 10.1016/j.socscimed.2020.113143 PMID: 32599414

May, S. M., & Li, J. T. (2015). Burden of chronic obstructive pulmonary disease: healthcare costs and beyond. Allergy and asthma proceedings, Mitta, N. R. (2021). AI-Based Personalized Therapeutic Monitoring Systems in Chronic Disease Management: Leveraging Machine Learning for Patient Adherence Prediction, Medication Optimization, and Real-Time Intervention. *Los Angeles Journal of Intelligent Systems and Pattern Recognition*, *1*, 190–228.

Molfino, N. A., Turcatel, G., & Riskin, D. (2024). Machine learning approaches to predict asthma exacerbations: A narrative review. *Advances in Therapy*, *41*(2), 534–552. DOI: 10.1007/s12325-023-02743-3 PMID: 38110652

Nahar, K., Hossain, M. Z., Islam, R., Khan, M. M., & Hossain, M. S. (2024). Operationalizing Predictive Modeling in Clinical Workflows: Design, Integration, and Validation of Decision Support Mechanisms within US Healthcare Infrastructure. *Frontiers in Computer Science and Artificial Intelligence*, *3*(2), 37–45. DOI: 10.32996/fcsai.2022.1.2.8

Nguyen, P. L., Uddin, M. M., Mir, T., Khalil, A., Regmi, N., Pervaiz, A., Hussain, T., Babu, M. A., Ullah, I., Patel, P., Lohia, P., Saydain, G., Koul, P. A., & Soubani, A. O. (2021). Trends in incidence, and mortality of acute exacerbation of chronic obstructive pulmonary disease in the United States Emergency Department (2010–2018). *COPD*, *18*(5), 567–575. DOI: 10.1080/15412555.2021.1979500 PMID: 34530662

Nici, L., Mammen, M. J., Charbek, E., Alexander, P. E., Au, D. H., Boyd, C. M., Criner, G. J., Donaldson, G. C., Dreher, M., Fan, V. S., Gershon, A. S., Han, M. L. K., Krishnan, J. A., Martinez, F. J., Meek, P. M., Morgan, M., Polkey, M. I., Puhan, M. A., Sadatsafavi, M., & Aaron, S. D. (2020). Pharmacologic management of chronic obstructive pulmonary disease. An official American Thoracic Society clinical practice guideline. *American Journal of Respiratory and Critical Care Medicine*, *201*(9), e56–e69. DOI: 10.1164/rccm.202003-0625ST PMID: 32283960

Nicolò, A., Massaroni, C., Schena, E., & Sacchetti, M. (2020). The importance of respiratory rate monitoring: From healthcare to sport and exercise. *Sensors (Basel), 20*(21), 6396. DOI: 10.3390/s20216396 PMID: 33182463

Olyanasab, A., & Annabestani, M. (2024). Leveraging machine learning for personalized wearable biomedical devices: A review. *Journal of Personalized Medicine, 14*(2), 203. DOI: 10.3390/jpm14020203 PMID: 38392636

Peberdy, M. A., Cretikos, M., Abella, B. S., DeVita, M., Goldhill, D., Kloeck, W., Kronick, S. L., Morrison, L. J., Nadkarni, V. M., Nichol, G., Nolan, J. P., Parr, M., Tibballs, J., van der Jagt, E. W., & Young, L. (2007). Recommended guidelines for monitoring, reporting, and conducting research on medical emergency team, outreach, and rapid response systems: an Utstein-style scientific statement: a scientific statement from the International Liaison Committee on Resuscitation (American Heart Association, Australian Resuscitation Council, European Resuscitation Council, Heart and Stroke Foundation of Canada, InterAmerican Heart Foundation, Resuscitation Council of Southern Africa, and the New Zealand Resuscitation Council); the American Heart Association Emergency Cardiovascular Care Committee; the Council on Cardiopulmonary, Perioperative, and Critical Care; and the Interdisciplinary Working Group on Quality of Care and Outcomes Research. *Circulation, 116*(21), 2481–2500. DOI: 10.1161/CIRCULATIONAHA.107.186227 PMID: 17993478

Peng, J., Chen, C., Zhou, M., Xie, X., Zhou, Y., & Luo, C.-H. (2020). A machine-learning approach to forecast aggravation risk in patients with acute exacerbation of chronic obstructive pulmonary disease with clinical indicators. *Scientific Reports, 10*(1), 3118. DOI: 10.1038/s41598-020-60042-1 PMID: 32080330

Pleasants, R. A., Riley, I. L., & Mannino, D. M. (2016). Defining and targeting health disparities in chronic obstructive pulmonary disease. *International Journal of Chronic Obstructive Pulmonary Disease*, 2475-2496. Martínez-García, M., & Hernández-Lemus, E. (2022). Data integration challenges for machine learning in precision medicine. *Frontiers in medicine*, *8*, 784455.

Price, D., Brusselle, G., Roche, N., Freeman, D., & Chisholm, A. (2015). Real-world research and its importance in respiratory medicine. *Breathe (Sheffield, England), 11*(1), 26–38. DOI: 10.1183/20734735.015414 PMID: 26306101

Sanchez-Morillo, D., Fernandez-Granero, M. A., & Leon-Jimenez, A. (2016). Use of predictive algorithms in-home monitoring of chronic obstructive pulmonary disease and asthma: A systematic review. *Chronic Respiratory Disease, 13*(3), 264–283. DOI: 10.1177/1479972316642365 PMID: 27097638

Seyam, E. A. (2025). Predicting High-Cost Healthcare Utilization Using Machine Learning: A Multi-Service Risk Stratification Analysis in EU-Based Private Group Health Insurance. *Risks*, *13*(7), 133. DOI: 10.3390/risks13070133

Shamji, M. H., Ollert, M., Adcock, I. M., Bennett, O., Favaro, A., Sarama, R., Riggioni, C., Annesi-Maesano, I., Custovic, A., Fontanella, S., Traidl-Hoffmann, C., Nadeau, K., Cecchi, L., Zemelka-Wiacek, M., Akdis, C. A., Jutel, M., & Agache, I. (2023). EAACI guidelines on environmental science in allergic diseases and asthma–leveraging artificial intelligence and machine learning to develop a causality model in exposomics. *Allergy*, *78*(7), 1742–1757. DOI: 10.1111/all.15667 PMID: 36740916

Sheetal, A., Jiang, Z., & Di Milia, L. (2023). Using machine learning to analyze longitudinal data: A tutorial guide and best-practice recommendations for social science researchers. *Applied Psychology*, *72*(3), 1339–1364. DOI: 10.1111/apps.12435

Slavakis, K., Giannakis, G. B., & Mateos, G. (2014). Modeling and optimization for big data analytics:(statistical) learning tools for our era of data deluge. *IEEE Signal Processing Magazine*, *31*(5), 18–31. DOI: 10.1109/MSP.2014.2327238

Steyerberg, E. W., van der Ploeg, T., & Van Calster, B. (2014). Risk prediction with machine learning and regression methods. *Biometrical Journal. Biometrische Zeitschrift*, *56*(4), 601–606. DOI: 10.1002/bimj.201300297 PMID: 24615859

Strielkowski, W., Vlasov, A., Selivanov, K., Muraviev, K., & Shakhnov, V. (2023). Prospects and challenges of the machine learning and data-driven methods for the predictive analysis of power systems: A review. *Energies*, *16*(10), 4025. DOI: 10.3390/en16104025

Susilo, Y. K. B., & Rahman, S. A. (2025). Revolutionizing COPD and Asthma Management with Artificial Intelligence. medRxiv, 2025.2003. 2018.25324219. DOI: 10.1101/2025.03.18.25324219

Sweatt, A. J., Hedlin, H. K., Balasubramanian, V., Hsi, A., Blum, L. K., Robinson, W. H., Haddad, F., Hickey, P. M., Condliffe, R., Lawrie, A., Nicolls, M. R., Rabinovitch, M., Khatri, P., & Zamanian, R. T. (2019). Discovery of distinct immune phenotypes using machine learning in pulmonary arterial hypertension. *Circulation Research*, *124*(6), 904–919. DOI: 10.1161/CIRCRESAHA.118.313911 PMID: 30661465

Swinckels, L., Bennis, F. C., Ziesemer, K. A., Scheerman, J. F., Bijwaard, H., de Keijzer, A., & Bruers, J. J. (2024). The use of deep learning and machine learning on longitudinal electronic health records for the early detection and prevention of diseases: Scoping review. *Journal of Medical Internet Research*, *26*, e48320. DOI: 10.2196/48320 PMID: 39163096

Triantafyllidis, A. K., Koutkias, V. G., Chouvarda, I., & Maglaveras, N. (2012). A pervasive health system integrating patient monitoring, status logging, and social sharing. *IEEE Journal of Biomedical and Health Informatics*, *17*(1), 30–37. DOI: 10.1109/TITB.2012.2227269 PMID: 23193318

Tsang, K. C., Pinnock, H., Wilson, A. M., & Shah, S. A. (2022). Application of machine learning algorithms for asthma management with mHealth: A clinical review. *Journal of Asthma and Allergy*, *15*, 855–873. DOI: 10.2147/JAA.S285742 PMID: 35791395

Turcatel, G., Xiao, Y., Caveney, S., Gnacadja, G., Kim, J., & Molfino, N. A. (2025). Predicting asthma exacerbations using machine learning models. *Advances in Therapy*, *42*(1), 362–374. DOI: 10.1007/s12325-024-03053-y PMID: 39556295

Upadhyay, P., & Ahlawat, P. (2022). Improvement in Quality of Life of Survivors of Chronic Obstructive Pulmonary Disease with Minimal Interventions. *Journal of Palliative Care & Medicine*, *12*(440), 2.

van Boven, J. F., Lavorini, F., Agh, T., Sadatsafavi, M., Patino, O., & Muresan, B. (2024). Cost-effectiveness and impact on health care utilization of interventions to improve medication adherence and outcomes in asthma and chronic obstructive pulmonary disease: A systematic literature review. *The Journal of Allergy and Clinical Immunology. In Practice*, *12*(5), 1228–1243. DOI: 10.1016/j.jaip.2023.12.049 PMID: 38182099

Wu, X.-W., Yang, H.-B., Yuan, R., Long, E.-W., & Tong, R.-S. (2020). Predictive models of medication non-adherence risks of patients with T2D based on multiple machine learning algorithms. *BMJ Open Diabetes Research & Care*, *8*(1), e001055. DOI: 10.1136/bmjdrc-2019-001055 PMID: 32156739

Zhou, L., Pan, S., Wang, J., & Vasilakos, A. V. (2017). Machine learning on big data: Opportunities and challenges. *Neurocomputing*, *237*, 350–361. DOI: 10.1016/j.neucom.2017.01.026

Chapter 11
AI-Driven Innovations in Pulmonary Medicine: Promise, Pitfalls, and the Road Ahead

Shaik Aminabee
http://orcid.org/0000-0001-9256-0897
V.V. Institute of Pharmaceutical Sciences, Gudlavalleru, India

ABSTRACT

Pulmonary medicine is changing at an alarming rate due to the use of Artificial intelligence (AI) to improve the diagnosis of a disease, prediction, monitoring, and even the implementation of a personalized treatment plan. Innovative machine learning and deep learning models are being used in imaging analyses, pulmonary function test interpretation and clinical decision support systems and predict respiratory diseases, including chronic obstructive pulmonary disease, asthma, interstitial lung diseases, and lung cancer, earlier. Remote patient monitoring, tele-pulmonology, and precision medicine approaches are also aided with the help of AI innovations and enhance healthcare accessibility and outcomes. In spite of such promising innovations, there are still a number of challenges, such as the privacy of data, bias in algorithms, insufficient standardized regulatory frameworks, and inadequate clinical validation in practice. Clinician training, development of infrastructure and ethical governance are also important to integrate AI in regular pulmonary practice.

1. INTRODUCTION

Pulmonary medicine is a distinct field of clinical medicine, which deals with prevention, diagnosis, and treatment of the respiratory system diseases. In recent

DOI: 10.4018/979-8-3373-7759-9.ch011

decades, fast technological progress in the fields of biomedical technology, digital health, and data science have greatly changed the provision of healthcare. Among such developments, Artificial Intelligence (AI) may be considered one of the most potent instruments that can enhance the accuracy of the diagnosis, increase clinical decision-making and provide personalized patient care (Ferkol & Schraufnagel, 2014). The recognition of the increased burden of respiratory diseases and the necessity of innovative technological solutions to enhance the results of early detection and treatment are stressed by global health organizations like the World Health Organization. Pulmonary medicine is one of the fields where the introduction of AI can be especially relevant due to the need to identify respiratory diseases at the earliest stage, monitor them, and treat them over time. Large datasets may be analyzed and new patterns of a disease, as well as assist clinicians in providing quicker and more accurate treatment, can be identified with the help of AI-driven tools. With the shift towards digital transformation of healthcare systems, it can be argued that AI will become one of the key factors in the future of respiratory care (Soriano et al., 2020).

1.1 Overview of Pulmonary Medicine

Pulmonary medicine is concerned with the diseases of lungs and respiratory system such as chronic obstructive lung disease (COPD), asthma, pulmonary fibrosis, pneumonia, tuberculosis, lung cancer. The conditions cause serious morbidity and mortality in the world and demand the multidisciplinary approach to their management that includes diagnostics, pharmacotherapy, rehabilitation, and the long-term follow-up (Salvi, 2014). The current approach in pulmonary care engages imaging technologies, pulmonary functioning tests, bronchodoscopy, and molecular diagnostics in the correct identification of disease pathology. Respiratory diseases constitute a significant healthcare burden in the world, with millions of people being affected by the disease and burdening the health infrastructure to a considerable extent. The importance of early diagnosis and proper treatment is essential in enhancing survival and life quality of patients. Nevertheless, traditional diagnosis methods can be time-intensive and require a great deal of specialist knowledge, which is why more advanced computational techniques that would assist clinicians with comprehending intricate clinical information should be considered (Zemanick et al., 2010).

1.2 Emergence of Artificial Intelligence in Healthcare

Artificial Intelligence is another concept that has emerged as a growing phenomenon in the contemporary healthcare system in a short period of time. Nowadays, AI technologies, including machine learning, deep learning, and natural language processing, are used in the field of disease diagnosis, treatment planning, drug discovery and optimization of hospital workflow. Research shows that the use of AI in the healthcare field has significantly grown with numerous hospitals utilizing AI in the fields of diagnostic imaging, predictive analytics, and clinical decision support systems (MacLeod et al., 2021). The use of AI within healthcare is growing with an estimated 85% of healthcare organizations having used AI in at least one clinical application. Medical imaging is one of the fields where AI is most powerful, and as radiological data is often large and sometimes hard to analyze, it can be processed in significantly less time and can be more precise than other techniques. It has been reported that AI-assisted imaging systems have the potential to minimize diagnostic errors and enhance the speed of detection that can assist clinicians to make timely decisions. Also, the usage of AI tools on the global level is continually growing, and their application in the field of predictive analytics, in patient triage, and in individual treatment plans in healthcare facilities become increasingly frequent (Labaki et al., 2017).

1.3 Need for AI Integration in Respiratory Care

The respiratory diseases tend to have complicated clinical progressions that need to be identified in time and followed-up. The conventional diagnostic methods might not help diagnosing the disease at its initial stages or even subtle pathology. Imaging data, respiratory sounds, electronic health records, and wearable device data can be analyzed by the use of AI-based tools to identify abnormalities at earlier stages, allowing the latter to be proactively treated. The introduction of AI is necessary to solve the issue of healthcare accessibility as well since access to healthcare in the resources-limited environment is scarce, and specialists are few (Trivedi et al., 2017; National Academies of Sciences, Engineering, and Medicine, 2023). Telemedicine and remote monitoring systems are based on AI, which enables patients to be assessed continuously without being in the hospital, enhancing treatment compliance and disease management. Studies indicate that AI-based monitoring and predictive analytics will have a significant impact on patient interaction and clinical outcomes, since it will detect the progression of the disease earlier. Moreover, the growing amount of medical information makes the manual interpretation of the data challenging. AI systems have the capability to process big data in a cost-effective manner, assist with evidence-based clinical decision-making, and relieve clinicians of workload. This is especially applicable in pulmonary medicine, in which images, physiological, and clinical history should be combined, in order to draw reasonable diagnoses (Figure 1).

Figure 1. AI integration in respiratory care: Addressing key challenges

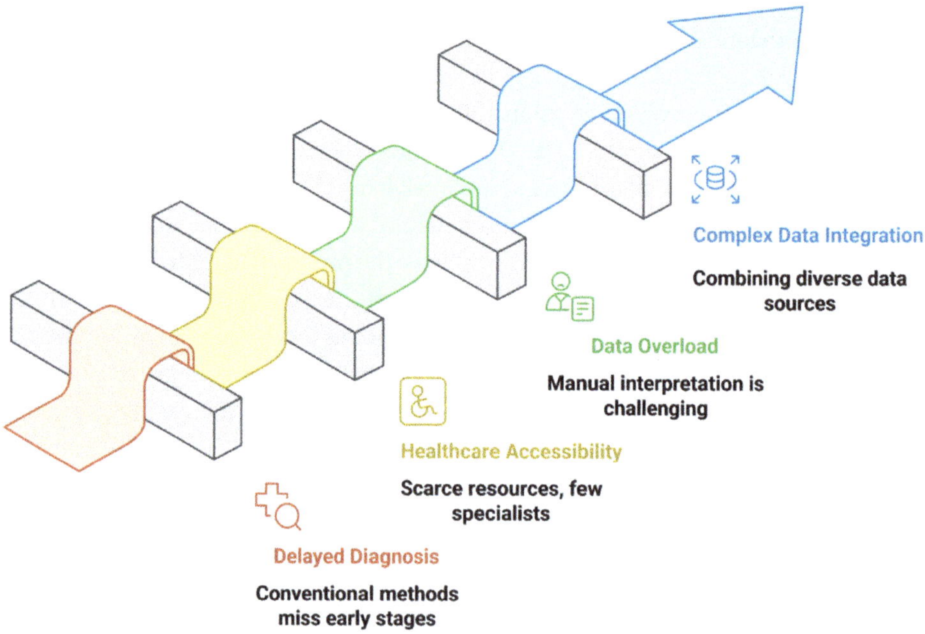

1.4 Scope and Objectives of the Chapter

The given chapter is going to offer the complete picture of the AI-based innovations in pulmonary medicine and their usage, the development, and the prospects. It discusses how AI is involved in diagnosing, tracking diseases, treatment plans tailored to an individual, and researches into the lungs. Besides, the chapter also focuses on ethical issues, regulatory issues, and barriers to implementation related to the adoption of AI in respiratory healthcare. The aim is to critically assess the potential and drawbacks of AI in pulmonary medicine and give an idea of responsible and sustainable implementation (Zhang et al., 2022). This chapter aims to pay attention to how AI may assist healthcare professionals and at the same time guarantee patient safety, data privacy, and fair access to healthcare innovations by examining technological changes and clinical demands.

2. FUNDAMENTALS OF ARTIFICIAL INTELLIGENCE IN HEALTHCARE

Artificial Intelligence (AI) can be defined as a way of using calculations of intelligible software and algorithms to simulate human intelligence into accomplishing activities like learning, reasoning, problem-solving, and decision-making. AI is changing the traditional ways of practicing healthcare since it will assist in processing of large quantities of data faster, enhance diagnostic accuracy, and assist in making evidence-based clinical judgments (Vliegenthart et al., 2022). The growing access to electronic health records, imaging databases, genomic data, and outputs of wearable devices has provided a situation in which AI can be much more supportive of healthcare delivery. Pulmonary medicine and other clinical specialties are some of the fields in which AI systems help in identifying the disease, predicting their prognosis, optimising treatment and monitoring them. Understanding the basic principles of AI is essential for healthcare professionals to effectively adopt and utilize these technologies in clinical practice.

2.1 Definition and Types of Artificial Intelligence

It is possible to broadly define Artificial Intelligence as the imitation of human thoughts with the help of computer-based systems. AI systems are created to process medical information of high complexity, extract patterns, and generate predictive or diagnostic information in healthcare. There are generally three broad categories of AI technologies, which are determined by its capability and functionality. The first one is Narrow or Weak AI, which is developed to solve a particular task, like image analyses in medicine or interpretation of clinical data. It is the most common type of AI applied to healthcare nowadays. The second is General AI which is theoretically capable of doing any intellectual task that a human can do though it is being developed (Zhou et al., 2015). Super AI is the third category that means AI systems, which are more intelligent than humans, but it is only more of a concept. In a clinical practice environment, the majority of currently implemented AI applications fall under the category of narrow AI and are utilized in applications like radiology imaging interpretation, prediction of diseases, and automated clinical documentation (Table 1).

Table 1. Types of artificial intelligence in healthcare

Type of AI	Description	Healthcare Example
Narrow AI	Performs specific predefined tasks	Medical image analysis, symptom checker tools
General AI	Can perform multiple human-like cognitive tasks (still theoretical)	Advanced clinical decision systems (future concept)
Super AI	Surpasses human intelligence (conceptual stage)	Not currently used in healthcare

2.2 Machine Learning and Deep Learning Concepts

Machine Learning (ML) is a branch of AI that will allow computers to learn through data without being programmed. ML algorithms ask questions of data and derive answers to those questions through the usage of patterns. ML finds applications in the predictive models of diseases, risk stratification of patients, and prediction of treatment outcomes in healthcare. Deep Learning (DL) is a branch of machine learning that applies multi-layered artificial neural networks to work on data of high complexity. Deep learning has been especially useful in the analysis of medical images, speech signals, and unstructured clinical text data. Deep learning models are widely applied in the field of pulmonary medicine when it comes to identifying lung abnormalities in X-rays and evaluating patterns of respiratory sound (Kole et al., 2023). ML, as well as DL, uses a large amount of high-quality datasets. These models are subject to the performance that is based on the data diversity, accuracy and size. Bad data or subjective information may result in false forecasts, which is why it is necessary to verify data and ensure the transparency of models (Table 2).

Table 2. AI technologies used in pulmonary medicine

Technology	Function	Pulmonary Application
Machine Learning	Pattern recognition from data	Disease prediction models
Deep Learning	Image and signal analysis	Chest X-ray and CT scan interpretation
Natural Language Processing	Text and speech analysis	Clinical documentation, chatbot interaction

2.3 Role of Big Data in Healthcare AI

Big Data can be described as very large and complicated data that can not be handled according to the traditional data analysis procedures. There are several sources of big data in healthcare such as electronic health records, diagnostic imaging, laboratory results, genomic sequencing, wearable devices, and remote monitoring systems. Big data is instrumental in the training of AI models since the larger the dataset the more accurate and predictive is the algorithm. Big data can be used in pulmonary healthcare to identify the trends of diseases, predict disease outbreaks, and create individualized treatment plans. It also assists in population health management because it aids clinicians in identifying high-risk groups of patients. The application of big data in the healthcare setting, however, brings up certain difficulties associated with data security, privacy of data, and sharing of ethical information (He et al., 2022). There should be appropriate data governance structures to enable the responsible utilization of healthcare data without violating patient privacy.

2.4 AI Workflow in Clinical Practice

The use of AI in clinical practice is a systematic process. The initial step would be the collection of data using different sources of healthcare information including patient records, imaging systems, and diagnostic equipment. Preprocessing of data is the second step, which involves cleaning of raw data, standardization, and analysis preparation. The third procedure is model training, which is carried out through AI algorithms that learn based on past information to recognize patterns. The fourth step will be validation and testing where the performance of the model will be tested against new datasets. The last step includes their implementation in the clinical setting, where AI systems would aid clinicians in decision-making. Clinicians, data scientists, and healthcare administrators have to work together to achieve the implementation of AI successfully (Liang et al., 2015). The accuracy and clinical reliability of AI models should be maintained by continuous monitoring and updating. It should also be able to be integrated with the current healthcare infrastructure to achieve a smooth adoption (Figure 2).

Figure 2. AI workflow in clinical practice

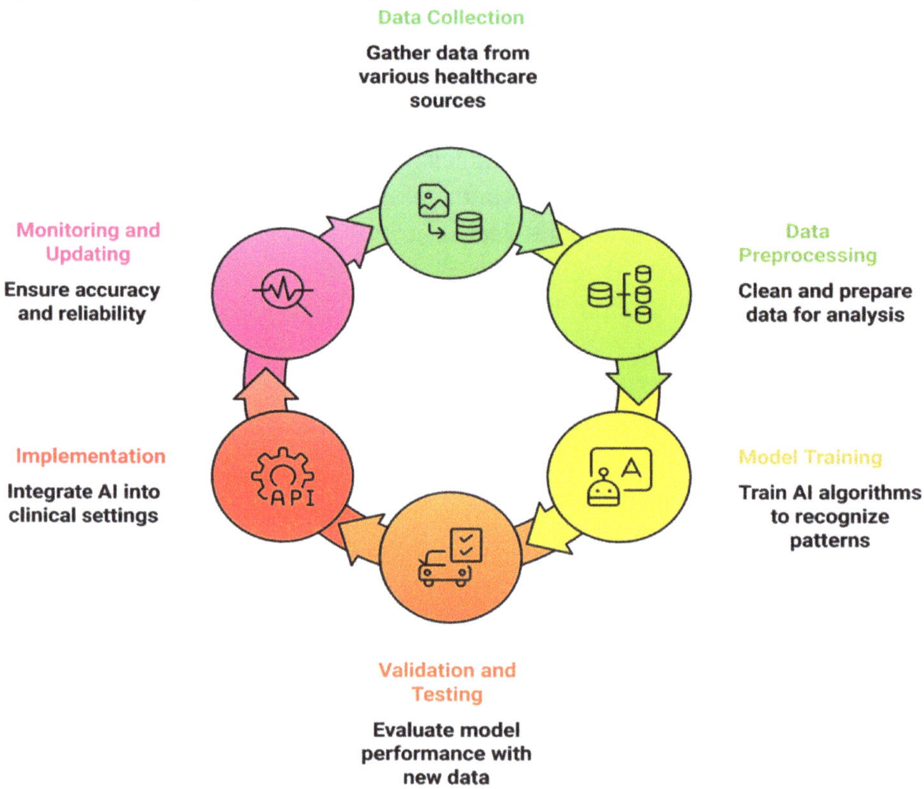

3. BURDEN OF PULMONARY DISEASES: A GLOBAL PERSPECTIVE

Respiratory diseases constitute one of the most important Burdens of morbidity and mortality as well as of health care spending in the world. The World Health Organization has agreed that chronic respiratory diseases, including chronic obstructive pulmonary disease (COPD), asthma, and lung cancer continue to be significant problems in the lives of the people of the world. The increasing levels of air pollution, smoking, work exposures, and ageing populations have only been added to the increasing pulmonary disorder burden across the world (Pilcer & Amighi, 2010). Such diseases not only impact on survival of patients, but also low quality of life and productivity, which is why respiratory health is an important health issue in the world.

3.1 Epidemiology of Major Respiratory Diseases

Epidemiological implications of respiratory diseases are expansive and related to be on the increase in most areas. COPD in itself is among the most common causes of death in the world, and the disease claims around 3.5 million lives in 2021 and approximately 5 percent of the total worldwide mortality. Approximately 90% of COPD-related deaths in persons under the age of 70 years is experienced in low- and middle-income countries, which emphasize significant disparities in health care. The estimated number of COPD prevalence across the globe in 2021 is over 213 million individuals, which brings a big part to disability-adjusted life years (DALYs) and long-term healthcare delivery (Patton et al., 2004). Another significant respiratory illness that is experienced by children and adults globally is asthma. It is a significant contributor to disease burden in the world, and each year hundreds of thousands of people die, and millions of individuals have persistent symptoms that cause them to have a negative impact on their daily lives. The prevalence of asthma-associated mortalities is more than 80 percent in low- and lower-middle-income nations because of restricted access to medical care and drugs. Disability and mortality Disability and mortality caused by chronic respiratory diseases in the world remain at the forefront of the causes of such diseases. According to reports made by world health organizations and respiratory specialists, including the European Respiratory Society, respiratory diseases remain either underdiagnosed and undervalued, which leads to late treatment and poor clinical results (Table 3).

Table 3. Global burden of major pulmonary diseases

Disease	Global Impact	Major Risk Factors
COPD	Leading cause of global mortality	Smoking, pollution, occupational exposure
Asthma	High global prevalence	Allergens, pollution, genetics
Lung Cancer	High mortality rate	Smoking, environmental toxins
Tuberculosis	High burden in developing countries	Infection transmission, poor living conditions

3.2 Socioeconomic and Healthcare Burden

In addition to clinical effects, pulmonary diseases create a significant socio-economic burden to the individual, healthcare systems, and countries. The chronic respiratory diseases result in repeated hospitalization, chronic drug usage as well as low productivity of employees. Economic studies indicate that respiratory diseases may cause billions of dollars every year in the direct medical cost and indirect costs of lost productivity (Gonda, 2000). The weight of the burden is disproportionately more in the developing nations because of the lack of proper healthcare infrastructure, lack of healthcare facilities for the diagnosis, and exposure to environmental risk factors including biomass fuel smoke in the home and air pollution outside. In the world, smoking is still considered as one of the leading causes of respiratory illnesses, with occupational sources and environmental toxicants coming second and third. Long-term social issues that arise due to respiratory diseases are disability, diminished quality of life, and dependency on healthcare systems. The impact which is experienced in the economy is not only healthcare costs but also social care costs, loss of income and also the diminished productivity of the nation (Lavorini et al., 2017).

3.3 Need for Early Diagnosis and Predictive Tools

Early pulmonary disease diagnosis is instrumental in lessening mortality and enhancing treatment results. Numerous respiratory diseases are not diagnosed until later on as their initial signs are mild or non-specific. Inadequate availability of diagnostic resources in most areas like spirometry and imaging also adds to late diagnosis. Predictive devices and sophisticated screening measures are becoming more significant in detection of high risk individuals prior to disease development. Early diagnosis provides an opportunity to start treatment early, lower hospitalization, and increase the survival rates in the long term. Moreover, predictive healthcare models may be used to track the progression of the disease and predict the acute exacerbation so that the clinical management could be implemented in advance. The increasing rate of pulmonary diseases points to the necessity to implement enhanced diagnostic services, enhanced healthcare availability, and the use of predictive digital tools (Atkins, 2024). The presence of these factors is crucial to minimizing the burden of diseases in the world and enhancing patient outcomes in respiratory medicine.

4. AI APPLICATIONS IN PULMONARY DISEASE DIAGNOSIS

Due to Artificial Intelligence, the diagnosis of pulmonary disease is changing, making it increasingly more accurate, shorter, and making it possible to detect respiratory diseases at an earlier stage. With the conventional diagnostic approaches, clinicians frequently have to be based on their experience and hand scoring of complicated datasets. The AI systems can however analyze huge amounts of medical data such as imaging, physiological measurement and clinical records so that intricate disease trends can be detected otherwise. International health organizations like the World Health Organization have been highlighting the need to detect and integrate technology at an early stage to curb the burden caused by respiratory diseases in the world (Daivd et al., 2020). Radiology, pulmonary functioning tests and infectious disease detection systems are also being integrated with AI-based diagnostic software which enhances clinical efficiency and patient outcomes.

4.1 AI in Medical Imaging (Chest X-ray, CT Scan Analysis)

One of the most developed and used fields of AI implementation in pulmonary medicine is medical imaging. Training AI algorithms, especially deep learning models, on massive amounts of chest X-rays and chest CT scans identifies the presence of abnormalities, including lung nodules, fibrosis, consolidation, and airway obstruction. The AI-assisted imaging can assist radiologists with automatic image analysis, suspicious regions, and prioritized cases. AI has the potential to identify early signs of pneumonia, tuberculosis, and lung cancer in the analysis of the chest x-ray. The AI models can analyze the structure of the lungs in detail in CT scan analysis which allows proper evaluation of the disease severity and progression. Moreover, AI imaging systems can be used to minimize inter-observer error, which means that diagnostic results should be consistent (Qureshi et al., 2023). The tools should be especially applicable in areas with a shortage of radiology specialists since AI may aid in quicker and more efficient screening.

4.2 AI in Pulmonary Function Test Interpretation

A spirometer test and lung volume assessment (pulmonary function tests, PFTs) are fundamental tests that are used to diagnose restrictive and obstructive lung diseases. Nonetheless, PFT results need an expert interpretation and may occasionally cause a discrepancy in clinical reasoning. Respiratory disorders may be accurately classified by AI systems, which will examine spirometry curves, airflow patterns, and lung volume information. Machine learning models are able to detect minor functional alterations before clinical conditions escalate to serious levels. PFT interpretation tools based on AI can also help clinicians to distinguish between asthma and chronic obstructive pulmonary disease. They also allow automatic report creation and longitudinal follow-ups on patients to assist clinicians monitor the progression of the diseases and response to the treatment in a more effective way (Deng et al., 2022).

4.3 AI in Early Detection of Lung Cancer

Lung cancer has been among the major causes of deaths due to cancer in the global society largely attributed to late diagnosis. AI is essential in early detection through detection of small nodules in the lungs and the minor tissue subtle alterations during imaging scans. AI algorithms have the potential to screen low-dose CT scans to identify suspicious nodules earlier in life and increase the efficiency of screening and decrease false-positive rates. AI models may also forecast the risk of malignancy with the help of the characteristics of imaging, patient history, and genetic information, which favors individual diagnostic plans. Early AI-assisted detection proves to be a significant improvement in terms of enhancing survival rates due to the ability to intervene in a timely manner and plan specific treatment (Jayatunga et al., 2022). AI is also used to track the progress of tumors and determine the treatment response as the therapy progresses.

4.4 AI in Tuberculosis and Infectious Lung Disease Detection

AI is also having a significant role in the diagnosis of infectious respiratory diseases particularly tuberculosis, which is a significant problem to the population of most developing states. Artificial intelligence (AI) computing could be used to analyze chest X-ray images quickly to identify tuberculosis-related pathologies and enhance prompt diagnosis and minimize diagnostic delays. In the event of an epidemic of infectious diseases, AI systems can facilitate mass screening, contact tracing, and surveillance of the disease. AI models can also examine clinical signs, laboratory reports, and imaging results and help to identify the rapid diagnosis of infectious lung diseases. AI-driven diagnostic devices can be deployed in the mobile healthcare setup of resources-limited environments, where they can screen the population and manage diseases at the initial stage (Chan et al., 2019). It is especially necessary to ensure the transmission of infectious diseases is controlled and the population health improved (Table 4).

Table 4. AI applications in pulmonary disease diagnosis

Diagnostic Area	AI Role	Clinical Benefit
Medical Imaging	Automated image analysis	Early disease detection
Pulmonary Function Tests	Data pattern recognition	Accurate disease classification
Cancer Detection	Nodule detection and malignancy prediction	Early treatment planning
Infectious Disease Detection	Rapid screening	Early outbreak control

5. AI IN DISEASE MONITORING AND PROGNOSIS

Artificial Intelligence is profoundly changing disease monitoring and prognosis in pulmonary medicine by providing an opportunity to evaluate the patient on a continuous basis, identify the early symptoms of disease progression and tailor treatment. In contrast to the previous systems of episodic healthcare services, AI-based systems enable real-time monitoring and predictive analysis, which is significant especially in the case of chronic respiratory illnesses which necessitate long-term management (Wang et al., 2021). The development of new digital health technologies, remote monitoring systems, and smart analytics have helped healthcare providers shift their focus on reactive treatment methods towards proactive disease treatment. Regulatory agencies including the U.S. Food and Drug Administration are also assessing and certifying medical software and digital monitoring devices based on AI, which is facilitating the safe use of these technologies in the clinical setting.

5.1 Remote Patient Monitoring Systems

Remote patient monitoring (RPM) systems allow tracking the health status of patients outside hospitals with the help of AI-based platforms. They are systems that monitor the respiratory rate, oxygen saturation, heart rate, and activity levels using medical devices that are connected to them and relay the data to the healthcare providers in real-time. AI complements RPM since it actively analyzes patient data in real-time and notices the early symptoms of disease aggravation. As an illustration, AI algorithms could identify subtle changes in the breathing patterns of chronic obstructive pulmonary disease or asthma patients and intervene before it is too late and decrease the number of hospital admissions (Vora et al., 2023). Remote monitoring can be especially useful in treating chronic respiratory illnesses, as well as home-based care. It also enhances healthcare access among the patients with rural or resource-constrained conditions whereby specialist pulmonary care might not be easily accessible.

5.2 Wearable Technologies and Smart Sensors

Biosensors and wearable technologies are becoming mainly applied in the monitoring of respiratory diseases. Such gadgets have the ability to monitor physiological parameters like breathing rate, physical workouts, sleep quality, and oxygenation. Large technological corporations like Apple and Fitbit have come up with wearable gadgets capable of gathering information on health-related aspects, which can be incorporated in AI-based medical check-ups. The devices are known to allow constant health monitoring and prompt detection of abnormal physiological patterns (Bao et al., 2023). Sensors that are built into the smart inhalers can also serve to track the pattern of medication use and adherence to medication, and can thus assist the clinician to maximize treatment regimens. Pulmonary medicine Wearable monitoring can be applied in managing the disease by early detection of exacerbations and long-term care strategies.

5.3 Predictive Analytics for Disease Progression

Predictive analytics involves the applications of AI algorithms that analyze both past and current patient data to forecast the development of a disease and its clinical outcomes. The inputs of the models include imaging data, tests of pulmonary functions, laboratory findings, data on environmental exposures, and lifestyle information of the patient. Predictive models have been used in pulmonary medicine to predict disease exacerbation, probability of hospitalization, and response to treatment. This enables clinicians to tailor treatment plans to the risks of the patients. Predictive analytics is especially effective in chronic respiratory illnesses where the development of the disease in individuals differs significantly (Bannigan et al., 2021). Predictive technologies that are powered by AI can also facilitate population health management, helping to define the high-risk groups of patients and implement targeted preventive healthcare plans.

5.4 AI in ICU and Critical Respiratory Care

Artificial intelligence (AI) gains a bigger role in the intensive care units (ICUs), especially in the management of patients with severe cases of respiratory failure, acute respiratory distress syndrome, and ventilator dependency. AI systems have the capability to search the extensive amounts of patient data, such as ventilator settings, blood gas, and vitals, to guide clinical decision-making. Philips is one of the healthcare technology firms that are creating artificial intelligence-based monitoring frameworks to help clinicians optimize ventilator settings and forecast patient deterioration (Jiang et al., 2022). Early signs of sepsis, respiratory distress, and organ failure may also be identified by AI-based ICU systems and increase the chances of survival. In intensive respiratory care, AI aids the individualized control of the ventilator, decreased the clinical workload, and improved patient safety by analyzing the data in real time and providing predictive alerts (Table 5).

Table 5. AI tools in disease monitoring and prognosis

Technology	Monitoring Parameter	Clinical Use
Remote Monitoring Systems	Oxygen saturation, respiratory rate	Chronic disease management
Wearable Devices	Activity, sleep, breathing pattern	Early exacerbation detection
Predictive Analytics	Risk prediction	Preventive treatment planning
ICU AI Systems	Ventilator and vital data analysis	Critical care optimization

6. AI IN PERSONALIZED AND PRECISION PULMONARY MEDICINE

Personalized and precision medicine is focused on defining the medical treatment to individual patient features, such as genetic profile, environmental exposure, lifestyle, and disease phenotype. Artificial Intelligence is taking on a radical position in facilitating accuracy pulmonary medicine by assessing mass clinical, genomic, and molecular data. AI can assist in recognizing the individual disease pattern, predicting the response to treatment, and optimizing the treatment and ultimately enhance the outcomes of treatment and reduce adverse drug reactions. The rising trend to precision medicine is reinforced by international health research programs and regulatory paradigms advocated by the organizations like the National Institutes of Health, which focuses on custom-made healthcare methods that depend on genetic and molecular information (Aliper et al., 2023). AI-based precision approaches have become a trend in pulmonary medicine and finding their way to the management of chronic respiratory diseases, lung cancer, and rare pulmonary conditions.

6.1 Individualized Treatment Planning

AI can assist with treating patients individually by examining various parameters about the patient, including clinical history, imaging, pulmonary function testing, biomarker profiles, or genetic data. Machine learning technologies can be used to determine which patients have a higher probability of responding to particular treatment which can then be used to choose and administer the most effective treatment plan by the clinician. When used in pulmonary diseases like asthma and chronic obstructive pulmonary disease, AI can be used to categorize patients into disease subtypes depending on their inflammation patterns, genetic susceptibility and the environment. This enables the clinicians to decide on specific therapies instead of treating them in a general manner (Harrer et al., 2019). AI-driven decision support systems are also useful in optimizing drug doses, forecasting complications surrounding treatment, and keeping track of the treatment outcomes. One-on-one treatment planning enhances the patient outcomes by minimizing errors in prescribing, and ensures that negative drug reactions are minimized.

6.2 Pharmacogenomics and AI

Pharmacogenomics is a research field focused on the analysis of the impact of genetic variations on drug response. Genomic datasets have become a chosen subject of AI applications that can be used to discover gene-drug interactions that influence drug metabolism, efficacy, and toxicity. Pharmacogenomics is also a useful concept in pulmonary medicine especially in the treatment of lung cancer where mutations in genes are used to define the choice of the treatment. AI has the ability to study tumor genome and predict response to targeted therapy and immunotherapy. This assists clinicians to make a choice of the best treatment that is least toxic (Chen et al., 2021). The AI is also used in the detection of genetic biomarkers that can be used to predict disease predisposition and response to treatment. Using genomic data with clinical data, AI assists in enhancing individual respiratory therapy plans and enhancing the long-term disease management results.

6.3 AI in Drug Discovery for Respiratory Disorders

AI is transforming the process of drug discovery by speeding up the process of target discovery, compound screening, and optimization of clinical trials. The conventional methods of drug discovery are time consuming and costly in that it may take over ten years before a drug is in the market. Molecular structures can be analyzed, drug-target interfaces predicted, and drugs-target identified far quicker using AI-based drug discovery platforms. AI is being applied in pharmaceutical companies like Insilico Medicine that are designing novel therapeutic molecules to treat different diseases including respiratory diseases. AI models can also forecast the drug toxicity, optimize the molecular design, and define the repurposing opportunities of the existing drugs. AI-enabled drug discovery in respiratory medicine is used in designing treatments of pulmonary fibrosis, asthma, chronic obstructive pulmonary disease, and lung cancer (Zhou et al., 2020). Clinical trial design Clinical trials can also be optimized with the assistance of AI, who identifies appropriate patients and predicts outcomes of treatment, which increases the success rate of new drug development (Figure 3).

Figure 3. AI in pulmonary medicine

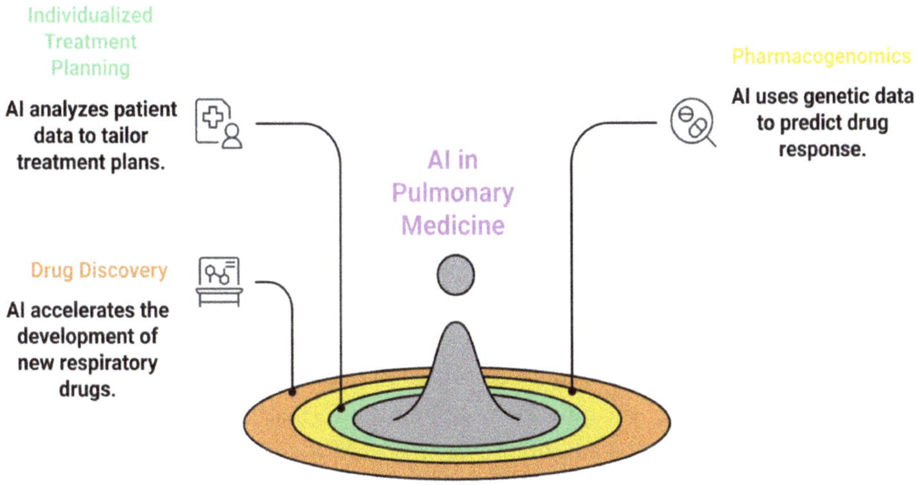

7. AI IN PULMONARY RESEARCH AND CLINICAL TRIALS

AI is transforming pulmonary research and clinical trials, making them more efficient, less expensive, and more accurate because of clinical outcomes. Conventional clinical trials can be time consuming, costly and constrained by the problem of recruiting patients and complex data. Optimization of clinical trials, finding qualified subjects, interpreting massive amounts of data, and forecasting the results of treatment are now being optimized using AI technologies. International regulatory and research agencies like the world health organization have highlighted why there is a need to develop innovative ways of research so that drugs development can be accelerated and that drugs can be made more accessible (Banat et al., 2023). The AI-initiated clinical research can potentially revolutionize the field of pulmonary medicine, as it can create new treatments of respiratory diseases much faster.

7.1 AI in Patient Recruitment

One of the hardest and time consuming in clinical trials is to recruit patients. It has been observed that many trials become delayed because of the inability to find eligible participants, who meet the rigorous inclusion and exclusion criteria. Electronic health records, genome data, imaging and clinical histories can be analyzed through AI to quickly find potential trial participants. The AI-driven recruitment systems are used to find the right clinical trial to match the patient to the disease stage, biomarker profile, and treatment history. Portals associated with databases of research like the ClinicalTrials.gov allow automatic patient eligibility screening, which enhances the efficiency of recruitment. AI is also useful in ensuring diversity in clinical trials, as it can be used to identify underrepresented groups, enhance the reliability and generalizability of the results of clinical trials (Newman, 2005). The accelerated recruitment lowers the time of trial and speeds up the schedule of drug development.

7.2 AI in Data Analysis and Outcome Prediction

Clinical trials yield large quantities of structured and unstructured information such as laboratory data, imaging data, genomic information and patient-reported information. These datasets can be processed by AI algorithms within a short period and patterns that would be hard to detect using normal statistical tools can be recognized. Machine learning models have the potential to forecast the outcomes of treatment, detect safety signals and assist in adapting clinical trials. AI-based analytics are also useful in predicting the treatment response through biomarkers, resulting in a more significant development of treatments. Such regulatory organizations like the U.S. Food and Drug Administration are starting to consider AI-powered device in clinical studies and drug development. Data analysis with the help of AI will enhance its accuracy, minimize the human factor, and provide the opportunity to monitor the progress of a trial in real-time (Smyth, 2003).

7.3 Virtual Clinical Trials and Digital Biomarkers

Virtual or decentralized clinical trials are those clinical trials that involve digital technologies, telemedicine platforms, and remote monitoring tools to carry out the research without frequently attending the hospital. AI is essential in the management of virtual trials by gathering and performing data analysis on the wearable, mobile, and home-based diagnostic devices on the patient. Objective physiological and behavioral data gathered using digital devices are increasingly applied in pulmonary studies, in the form of digital biomarkers. They are respiratory rate data, oxygen saturation data and activity data gathered using wearable sensors. The models of AI examine these biomarkers to track the development of the disease and assess the effectiveness of treatment. Virtual trials enhance patient engagement, minimize the increased travel load, and enable the target audience to involve patients who represent geographically different areas (Moon et al., 2019). It is anticipated that AI-enabled digital clinical trials will become a major part of the future of the pulmonary research, enhancing the accessibility and effectiveness of the trials (Table 6).

Table 6. AI in clinical trials

Clinical Trial Stage	AI Contribution	Benefit
Patient Recruitment	Automated eligibility screening	Faster recruitment
Data Analysis	Pattern detection and prediction	Improved accuracy
Virtual Trials	Remote patient participation	Increased accessibility

8. ROLE OF AI IN TELE-PULMONOLOGY AND DIGITAL HEALTH

Artificial Intelligence is also becoming crucial in the development of tele-pulmonology and digital health services, increasing access to respiratory care, improving remote diagnosis, and monitoring of patients. Tele-pulmonology is a combination of telecommunication and pulmonary care with the help of the combination of these two, clinicians can examine, diagnose and treat respiratory conditions through remote monitoring. This practice gained extra significance during the world epidemics and remains to assist in chronic illnesses management. International healthcare bodies like the World Health Organization emphasize digital health and telemedicine as one of the strategies that can enhance the quality of healthcare access, particularly in areas where there is limited supply of specialists (Fink & Stapleton, 2024). AI can simplify tele-pulmonology: it can be used to conduct automated symptom evaluation, interpret remote imaging, and predictive disease monitoring, which improves the efficiency of healthcare delivery.

8.1 Telemedicine Platforms in Respiratory Care

The telemedicine online service will enable patients who have respiratory disease to receive remote consultation, diagnosis, and follow-up treatment. Such tools allow clinicians to be informed about the symptoms of patients, analyze reported diagnostic tests, and modify treatment options without the need to visit patients personally. Telemedicine platforms are being created by healthcare technology firms like Teladoc Health that combine AI-based diagnostic support software. These platforms will enable real-time video consultation, remote vital monitoring and digital prescription management. Tele-pulmonology can be specifically helpful in the treatment of such chronic respiratory illnesses as asthma and chronic obstructive pulmonary disease, where the follow-up is the key (Jiang et al., 2023). The systems of AI-based telemedicine have the ability to analyze patient-reported symptoms and physiological data to identify the initial indications of disease upswing, and provide medical help in a timely manner.

8.2 AI Chatbots and Virtual Health Assistants

Virtual health assistants and AI chatbots are finding more applications in patient education, triaging symptoms, and in reminding people of their medications. These systems are based on natural language processing and communicate with patients and give them tailored health advice. Google and other technology firms are investing in AI-based healthcare conversational systems that can help check their symptoms and interact with their patients. AI chatbots can be useful to educate patients on the symptoms of diseases, give self-care instructions, and refer them to the relevant healthcare services when needed (Tanoli et al., 2021). AI chatbots may be used in pulmonary care to assist patients in monitoring their symptoms like breathlessness, the frequency of cough, and inhaler use. These technologies enhance patient interaction and help in the long-term management of diseases especially those related to respiratory illnesses.

8.3 AI for Rural and Resource-Limited Settings

Digital health technologies driven by AI can have a profound impact on the access to respiratory healthcare in limited and rural environments. Most of the areas have a shortage of pulmonologists, diagnostic imaging centers, and high-end laboratory services. The gap may be addressed by use of AI-based diagnostic tools that can offer automated disease screening and clinical decision support. Big Data Mobile health driven by artificial intelligence imaging analysis and remote monitoring solutions can facilitate mass respiratory disease screening. These technologies are used to identify diseases like tuberculosis and pneumonia earlier in the course of treatment and thereby enhance the treatment. Moreover, AI based digital health systems are able to lower healthcare expenses by decreasing the number of unnecessary visits to a hospital and providing care at home (Wan et al., 2025). AI as a tool in the telemedicine process allows to eliminate geographic healthcare inequalities, as well as enhances healthcare equity on the whole.

9. CHALLENGES AND PITFALLS OF AI IN PULMONARY MEDICINE

Although Artificial Intelligence can be used in pulmonary medicine in a transformative way, a number of challenges restrict its broad application and safe clinical use. Although AI has a higher diagnostic accuracy, predictive analytics, and personalized treatment plans, it presents the issues about data protection, its ethical use, regulatory control, and clinical predictability. These issues need to be tackled so that AI technologies can be safe, equitable and clinically effective. The world health and regulatory bodies like the World Health Organization have stressed that AI implementation should be done responsibly wherein there must be robust governance structures, transparency and constant monitoring to ensure the safety of the patients and the trust of the people (Dotolo et al., 2021).

9.1 Data Privacy and Security Issues

AI systems need to be connected to high amounts of healthcare data, such as electronic health records, imaging data, genomic data, and real-time monitoring data. Although this information is necessary to train and enhance AI models, it causes significant concern related to patient privacy and confidentiality of information. Sensitive patient data could be exposed in case of healthcare data breaches, which may result in ethical, legal, and social implications. Hacking, ransomware attacks, and sharing unauthorized data are some of the cybersecurity threats that can affect healthcare systems that employ AI technologies. The regulatory bodies like the U.S. Food and Drug Administration insist on the importance of safe data management procedures, encryption measures, and adherence to healthcare information protection legislation (Ahmed et al., 2022). To establish trust and adherence to the law, healthcare organizations should make sure they safely store data, control access to information, and provide clear patient consent procedures.

9.2 Algorithm Bias and Ethical Concerns

One of the most severe ethical issues in healthcare systems based on AI is algorithm bias. AI models are trained using past data, and in case the past data is incomplete or unrepresentative then the algorithms might result in biased results. In pulmonary medicine, biased algorithms can result in wrong diagnosis or treatment recommendations of certain groups of people, especially those who are underrepresented in the training set. This may increase healthcare disparities and decrease effectiveness of treatment (Elbadawi et al., 2024). Other ethical issues involve the absence of transparency in AI decision-making, so-called black box, where clinicians can poorly comprehend the AI systems to generate suggestions. The ethical development of AI should be done with clarity within its algorithm as well as multiple training sets and constant performance analysis.

9.3 Regulatory and Legal Challenges

The swift progress of the AI technologies has posed the regulatory dilemma to healthcare professionals on the global level. The current regulatory frameworks were initially created to suit the usual medical devices and might not be completely relevant in the dynamic nature of AI-based software systems. The regulatory bodies are in the process of formulating standards of AI-based medical devices, such as validation standards, risk classification, and post-market follow-up. The regulatory frameworks are being actively pursued by such agencies as European Medicines Agency to guarantee the safe and effective implementation of AI in healthcare. The liability questions are also a matter of legal concern in the situations of the AI-based diagnostic mistakes (Gates et al., 2019). The legal issue of responsibility in the software developers, health care providers, and health care institutions is still a complicated issue.

9.4 Clinical Validation and Reliability Issues

To have AI systems work in the real clinical setting, clinical validation is necessary. A significant number of AI models are trained and tested on controlled datasets and might fail to work reliably in various patient groups or medical environments. Imaging equipment, clinical procedures, and patient demographics variability may have an impact on the performance of AI. Absence of extensive real-world validation research constraints clinician trust to AI-based decision support technology (van Eck & Waltman, 2014). The AI reliability must be ensured by continuous monitoring, regular updates of the model, and clinical trials in real-world conditions. Clinicians should also be trained and supported with the infrastructure to make AI systems integration into clinical workflows possible (Table 7).

Table 7. Challenges of AI in pulmonary medicine

Challenge	Impact	Required Solution
Data Privacy Risks	Patient confidentiality issues	Strong cybersecurity systems
Algorithm Bias	Unequal healthcare outcomes	Diverse training datasets
Regulatory Limitations	Slow approval process	Updated AI regulations
Clinical Validation Gaps	Reduced clinician trust	Real-world clinical trials

10. IMPLEMENTATION CHALLENGES IN CLINICAL PRACTICE

Not only technological development is necessary to make the concept of the successful integration of Artificial Intelligence into the pulmonary medicine field feasible, but also a well-developed healthcare infrastructure, financial resources, the workforce and the willingness of clinicians and patients. Although AI tools have shown potential positive clinical outcomes, their practical application is still a maze because of operational, technical, and behavioral obstacles. These difficulties need to be overcome so that AI technologies would be safely and effectively included in the everyday clinical processes (Cao et al., 2021). Digital health implementation, according to international health policy bodies including the World Health Organization, should be facilitated by strong infrastructure, training of workforce, and patient-focused strategies of adoption to maximize healthcare effects.

10.1 Infrastructure Requirements

Implementation of AI needs high levels of digital infrastructure which includes high performance computing systems, secure data storage systems, high speed internet connection, and interoperative electronic health records systems. Still, many healthcare organizations, especially in developing countries, have paper-based or semi-digitized healthcare systems, which restricts the use of AI. Pulmonary diagnostic tools based on AI usually need to be combined with radiology imaging devices, databases of lab reports, and patient monitoring applications. The absence of interoperability between healthcare systems may cause silos of data, which decreases the effectiveness of AI. There are also other reliable cloud computing infrastructure requirements that are required to support real-time information processing and remote monitoring. To back AI-enabled clinical workflows, healthcare institutions need to invest in digital transformation, standard data format and a secure networking system (Boyack & Klavans, 2010).

10.2 Cost and Accessibility Issues

Another obstacle is the high cost of adopting AI technologies particularly on the low- and middle-income countries. To implement AI, it is necessary to invest in hardware and software, as well as cybersecurity and the training of the staff. There is also maintenance cost, software upgrading and data storage, which contribute to long-term financial expense. The other significant issue is accessibility. The high-tech AI systems tend to be concentrated in major cities in hospitals and research facilities and tend to create inequalities in access to healthcare. In rural and underserved areas, AI-based diagnostic and monitoring tools may not be beneficial given the inadequate healthcare systems. To counter the cost barrier, government funding will be needed, public- private collaboration, and creation of low-cost AI systems that will be utilized in resource-constrained healthcare environments (Su & Lee, 2010).

10.3 Training and Skill Development for Healthcare Professionals

Medical experts should be provided with the training to be able to utilize AI instruments when it comes to clinical decision making. The current state of affairs is that many clinicians do not have formal training in data science, AI interpretation, and digital health technologies. Clinicians might not be eager to base on AI-generated insights without adequate training. Basic AI literacy, knowledge of the constraints of algorithms, and interpretation of AI-generated clinical outputs should be part of the training programs. Clinicians, data scientists, and biomedical engineers must cooperate with one another in a multidisciplinary manner to ensure that AI implementation is successful. Currently, medical education systems might be required to include digital health and AI courses in the undergraduate and postgraduate healthcare programs to equip future healthcare professionals with AI-enabled clinical practice (Groneberg et al., 2003).

10.4 Acceptance by Clinicians and Patients

The user trust and acceptance are essential to the successful implementation of AI. There is the fear of over-dependence on AI, possible job loss, and absence of transparency in the process of AI decision-making that some clinicians may have. To assure clinician acceptance of AI tools, it is worthwhile to ensure that they act as decision-support systems, and not substitutes to clinical judgment. The acceptance of the patient is important as well (Aminabee et al., 2011). The patients might worry about the privacy of the data, the automatization of the decision-making process, and the decline in human interaction during the healthcare delivery process. Patient trust can be built by open communication regarding the use of AI and the protection of their data and the clinical benefits. To enhance the rate of adoption by both healthcare providers and patients, AI interfaces must be user friendly, clinicians need to be involved in the development of AI systems, and robust ethical governance systems are imperative.

11. INTEGRATION OF SUPPORTING RESEARCH EVIDENCE

11.1 Nanotechnology and Computational Drug Discovery Research

Studies in technologies in the advanced pharmaceutical have shown the increasing relevance of nanotechnology and computational drug discovery in the modern therapeutic treatments. Metal oxide nanoparticles metal oxide nanoparticles have demonstrated interesting pharmacological capabilities in experimental screening, especially in increasing drug delivery efficiency, improving bioavailability, and targeted therapy (Prasanth et al., 2020). Similar progress in the pharmacoinformatics field has allowed one to identify plant-derived bioactive molecules that could be used as an inhibitor against viral targets. The presented findings all point to the shift toward technology-aided drug discovery strategies that are in line with the wider shift towards artificial intelligence-aided therapeutic discovery in respiratory and systemic conditions (Prasanth et al., 2021; Aminabee et al., 2019).

11.2 Natural Product Pharmacology and Experimental Therapeutics

The therapeutic potential of medicinal plants has been confirmed through much experimental work on in-vitro and in-vivo models. There are pharmacological studies that have shown analgesic, antioxidant, anti-inflammatory and anthelmintic effects of various plant extracts and fractions (Aminabee et al., 2019). These studies offer scientific evidence to the traditional medicine and present fresh possibilities of creating the therapeutic agents using plants. There has been extensive use of standardized experimental protocols, animal models and biochemical assays as a means of determining safety, efficacy and mechanism of action (Aminabee et al., 2023).

11.3 Chronic Disease Management and Therapeutic Optimization

Studies that have been conducted on the chronic disease conditions have brought out the need to ensure that effective pharmacological interventions are selected in order to enhance patient outcomes (Aminabee & Lakshmana Rao, 2024). Research on the assessment of treatment options of neuropathic pain in relation to metabolic disorders has emphasized on the ability to customize treatment methods. Moreover, scientific articles about the use of natural resources in disease management have also been reviewed, which justifies the use of natural and synthetic therapeutics in medical systems (Aminabee et al., 2023).

11.4 Pharmacoeconomics and Healthcare Resource Utilization

There has been growing interest in healthcare research on economic assessment of therapeutic choices. In the comparative pharmacoeconomic analyses that have been conducted to determine the significance of cost-effectiveness analysis, advanced biological therapies and their substitutes have proven to be effective in enhancing the accessibility of treatments. Economic analyses of pharmacological treatments applied in substance use disorders have also given positive information on the management of healthcare expenditures and this has aided evidence-based policy decisions and prudent choice of drugs (Leelavati et al., 2023).

11.5 Public Health, Telehealth, and Behavioral Health Research

The studies on the healthcare delivery models have revealed the efficiency of digital health technologies in enhancing patients access and satisfaction. The healthcare delivery systems that are based on telemedicine have been found to decrease geographical barriers and enhance continuity of care. Behavioral health patterns of student populations have also been examined in a research conducted at the field of public health to provide information about lifestyle factors like substance use and their possible influence on academic performance and long-term health outcomes (Leelavati et al., 2023; Madhavi et al., 2024; KNVC, 2024).

11.6 Advanced Pharmaceutical Formulation and Drug Delivery Systems

The scientific studies of the development of the formulations have been directed at the optimization of the systems of drug delivery based on the statistical experimental design. Such strategies have been able to design controlled drug release formulations that are more stable, have better therapeutic effect and compliance by patients. These formulation strategies are specifically applicable in the management of chronic diseases where the delivery of the drug over a long period of time is needed (Leelavati et al., 2025).

11.7 Pharmaceutical Education and Ethical Healthcare Practice

The recent scholarly articles have focused on the need to have ethical decision-making skills in pharmaceutical education. Ethical education in healthcare promotes responsible clinical practice, patient safety and professional accountability. This specifically applies in the age of AI-assisted healthcare, where ethical factors in the use of data, patient privacy, and clinical decision support systems are of critical importance (Raju et al., 2024; Zeng et al., 1995).

12. FUTURE DIRECTIONS AND EMERGING TRENDS

The future of Artificial Intelligence in pulmonary medicine will be determined by the development of explainable algorithms, interrelated medical devices, integration with genomics, and cooperation among healthcare policies across the globe. With the development of AI technologies, the emphasis is changing to responsible, scalable, and patient-centred healthcare solutions rather than the experimental implementation. The new AI technologies should not only enhance the diagnostic and treatment accuracy, but also provide transparency, ethical management, and fair healthcare delivery (Mathias & Hussain, 2010). The global health organizations, including the World Health Organization, argue the critical role of global collaboration, ethical AI models, and digital health policies to fulfill the goal of making the benefits of AI reach various healthcare systems and populations.

12.1 Explainable AI in Healthcare

Explainable Artificial Intelligence(XAI) is a concept of AI systems that give clear-cut and understandable results in decision-making. Conventional AI systems, especially deep learning models, are often treated as black box systems in which the rationale of predictions is not easily seen by clinicians. Explainable AI would enhance clinician trust as it gives clear elucidations to either diagnostic or treatment suggestions. In pulmonary medicine, XAI can be used to assist clinicians in decoding why an AI system detects a nodule in the lung as malignant or at risk of becoming a disease (et al., 2016). This openness will increase clinical confidence, shared decision-making and patient safety. Also essential is explainable AI related to regulatory approval and ethical AI usage because healthcare authorities are demanding more transparency in AI-based clinical decision systems.

12.2 Integration with Internet of Medical Things (IoMT)

The Internet of Medical Things (IoMT) is a network of connected medical equipment and health-related applications sharing patient information on the digital network. When combined with IoMT, AI will allow continuously monitoring patients in real-time and perform automated health analytics. Smart inhalers, wearable respiratory monitors, and residential spirometry devices are IoMT devices that produce big data in real-time health information. This data is inputted into AI algorithms to identify the early exacerbation of the disease, treatment response, and preventive health approaches (Tang et al., 2022). It is anticipated that AI implementation in combination with IoMT will assist the personalization of healthcare delivery, decrease hospitalization, and enhance the management of chronic respiratory illnesses, as well as constant patient monitoring.

12.3 AI and Genomics in Pulmonary Medicine

Precision pulmonary medicine is anticipated to impact greatly when both AI and genomics are combined. The genomic technologies produce high volumes of data that is difficult to analyze without very complex computational software. The AI assists in determining genetic mutations and disease prone markers, as well as molecular pathways of respiratory diseases. Genomic analysis with the use of AI is specifically important in pulmonary medicine in areas such as lung cancer, rare genetic lung diseases, and inflammatory respiratory illnesses. AI has the capability of processing complicated genomic data to forecast a disease risk, how the disease will respond to treatment, and its long term outcomes (Andrade et al., 2013). The AI-based genomic research is also growing due to research efforts funded by organizations like the National Institutes of Health, which aid in the creation of specific drugs and personalized treatment approaches in the field of respiratory medicine.

12.4 Role of Policy and Global Collaboration

The effective implementation of AI in pulmonary medicine in future depends on good healthcare policies, ethical systems of governance, and transnational cooperation. The introduction of AI should be facilitated by uniform regulation policies, data-sharing policies, and international research collaboration. Global cooperation can enable us to make AI technologies evolved with the different set of data to minimize the bias of the algorithms and enhance the global applicability of healthcare. Some of the ethical issues that should be addressed by policymakers include data privacy, a transparent algorithm, and fair access to healthcare. The global digital health programs will significantly contribute to the implementation of responsible AI implementation models (Sharma et al., 2019). Both instances of joint work between healthcare organizations, governments, research centers, and technology providers will be necessary to make safe, ethical, and sustainable AI contribution to pulmonary medicine (Table 8).

Table 8. Future trends in AI pulmonary medicine

Future Trend	Expected Impact
Explainable AI	Increased clinician trust
IoMT Integration	Continuous patient monitoring
AI + Genomics	Precision medicine advancement
Global Collaboration	Standardized AI healthcare systems

13. THE ROAD AHEAD: BUILDING RESPONSIBLE AI IN PULMONARY MEDICINE

With AI-related changes to the field of pulmonary medicine, the necessity to make AI technologies responsible is growing steadily. Although artificial intelligence has much to provide in terms of diagnosing, treatment planning, and disease monitoring, ethical design, developed regulation, and cooperative healthcare innovation will be the key to its long-term success. The responsible AI development is concerned with patient safety, fairness, transparency, and clinical effectiveness and provides equitable access to advanced healthcare technologies. International healthcare leadership organizations like the World Health Organization highlight the significance of ethical governing of AI, cooperation on the international level, and sustainable strategies of digital health implementation (Mangal et al., 2017). Responsible AI structures should be created so that AI can improve the healthcare delivery without undermining the rights of patients and clinical quality.

13.1 Ethical AI Frameworks

AI ethics models are crucial in making sure the AI systems are established and implemented in a way that supports patient safety, equity, and openness. Data privacy, informed patient consent, transparency of the algorithm, and avoidance of bias in the healthcare decision-making process are ethical AI principles. Ethical AI is used in the field of pulmonary medicine to ensure that diagnostic devices deliver justifiable performance in terms of age, gender, ethnicity, and geographic location. The other approach that has been covered by ethical frameworks is the so-called human-in-the-loop approach in which the overall decision-making process remains with clinicians and AI is employed as a support mechanism. Continued check ups on the performance of the algorithms are also ethical AI governance to ensure that unintended bias or safety risks are realized. Honesty with patients about the use of

AI in healthcare decision-making is a key to preserving the trust of a population (Xiong et al., 2024).

13.2 Standardization and Regulatory Pathways

Regulatory frameworks should be standardized to bring about safety, quality, and efficacy of AI-based healthcare technologies. AI systems can also change with time, unlike traditional medical devices, which makes them difficult to regulate. The U.S. Food and Drug Administration, as one of the regulatory bodies, is working on the guidelines on how to gauge AI-based software as a medical device. These frameworks are centered on the classification of risk, clinical validation, post-market surveillance and ongoing performance monitoring. Healthcare data formats, interoperability protocols, and clinical reporting systems should also be standardized to provide smooth AI integration in healthcare institutions. There should be an international regulatory cooperation to create the globally recognized standards of AI validation (Clark, 2022).

13.3 Multidisciplinary Collaboration Models

Several stakeholders who are clinicians, data scientists, biomedical engineers, regulatory experts, and healthcare policymakers are needed to develop and implement AI in pulmonary medicine. Multidisciplinary collaboration: Multidisciplinary collaboration is a necessary requirement to guarantee the clinical relevance of AI tools, as well as their technical strength and ethical adherence. Educational institutions, health care facilities and tech firms need to collaborate to create AI models based on various and high quality datasets. Teamwork also helps to accelerate AI innovations in clinical translation into clinical practice. The organizations like National Institutes of Health encourage healthcare innovation programs, which support collaborative AI research programs that integration of clinical knowledge with modern computational technologies (Nagy et al., 2022). These collaborations are mandatory towards the rapid uptake of responsible AI in pulmonary medicine.

14. CONCLUSION

The field of pulmonary medicine is quickly changing due to the use of Artificial Intelligence, which allows detecting the disease early, enhancing the diagnostic accuracy, predicting personal treatment plans, and monitoring the disease over a long period of time. The use of artificial intelligence (AI) is transforming the process of diagnosing, treating, and preventing respiratory diseases through AI-assisted medical imaging and predictive analytics, artificial intelligence to monitor patients across distance, and digital health platforms. Such developments can greatly decrease the worldwide burden of pulmonary diseases and enhance patient outcomes in various healthcare facilities (Farkas et al., 2021). Nevertheless, AI in pulmonary medicine can be successfully integrated only with taking into account ethical, regulatory, and operational issues. The problems like data privacy, algorithm bias, clinical validation, and regulatory compliance are to be addressed to offer safe and fair implementation of AI. Even today, international health organizations like the World Health Organization are stressing the idea of responsible AI implementation by having robust governance structures, transparency, and patient-centered healthcare policies. The role of AI in respiratory medicine is likely to be further reinforced in the future due to further developments of explainable AI, integration of genomics, Internet of Medical Things (IoMT), and global digital health cooperation. A key factor that will determine safe clinical implementation of AI-based medical technology will be the establishment of uniform regulatory routes by regulatory bodies including the U.S. Food and Drug Administration. Finally, AI, when it is applied in pulmonary medicine, should be held to responsible innovation, a multidisciplinary approach, and a continuous assessment of clinical efficiency (Wang et al., 2022). Ethical healthcare practices can be transformed by technological innovations to use AI as a means to revolutionize pulmonary care and make it more predictive, customizable, accessible, and effective. The future of the road needs a collaborative approach by clinicians, researchers, policymakers, and technology developers to make sure that AI is a potent resource in the enhancement of respiratory health of patients without jeopardizing their safety and confidence.

REFERENCES

Ahmed, F., Soomro, A. M., Salih, A. R. C., Samantasinghar, A., Asif, A., Kang, I. S., & Choi, K. H. (2022). A comprehensive review of artificial intelligence and network based approaches to drug repurposing in Covid-19. *Biomedicine and Pharmacotherapy*, *153*, 113350. DOI: 10.1016/j.biopha.2022.113350 PMID: 35777222

Aliper, A., Kudrin, R., Polykovskiy, D., Kamya, P., Tutubalina, E., Chen, S., Ren, F., & Zhavoronkov, A. (2023). Prediction of clinical trials outcomes based on target choice and clinical trial design with multi-modal artificial intelligence. *Clinical Pharmacology and Therapeutics*, *114*(5), 972–980. DOI: 10.1002/cpt.3008 PMID: 37483175

Aminabee, S., Dasari, S. K., Rao, K. H., Sirisha, V., Kumari, V. A., Dasari, N., & Leelavati, T. S. (2023). Pharmacoeconomic analysis of biologic vs. biosimilar therapies in rheumatoid arthritis. *International Journal of Chemical and Biochemical Science*, *24*(4), 395–400.

Aminabee, S., Devi Mallika, K., & Lakshmana Rao, A. (2023). Natural resources in management and treatment of diseases: A review. *Pharmacy Times*, *55*(11), 7–10.

Aminabee, S., & Lakshmana Rao, A. (2024). Computational identification of selected bioactive compounds from *Cedrus deodara* as inhibitors against SARS-CoV-2 main protease: A pharmacoinformatics study. *Indian Drugs*, *61*(2), 78–91. DOI: 10.53879/id.61.02.13859

Aminabee, S., Prabhakar, M. C., Prasad, R. G. S. V., & Lakshmana Rao, A. (2011). Screening the pharmacological activity of cerium oxide nanoparticles in-vitro. *Biomedical & Pharmacology Journal*, *4*(2), 287–289. DOI: 10.13005/bpj/296

Aminabee, S., Rao, A. L., Sowmya, K., Nymisha, D., Lakshmi, K. K. N., Manikanta, K. V. N. S., & Kumar, P. P. (2019). Evaluation of Analgesic Activity of Ficus Palmata: Evaluation of Analgesic activity of Ficus palmata. *Iranian Journal of Pharmaceutical Sciences*, *15*(3), 47–60.

Aminabee, S., Rao, A. L., Sowmya, K., Nymisha, D., Lakshmi, K. K. N., Manikanta, K. V. N. S., & Kumar, P. P. (2019). Evaluation of Analgesic Activity of Ficus Palmata: Evaluation of Analgesic activity of Ficus palmata. *Iranian Journal of Pharmaceutical Sciences*, *15*(3), 47–60.

Andrade, F., Rafael, D., Videira, M., Ferreira, D., Sosnik, A., & Sarmento, B. (2013). Nanotechnology and pulmonary delivery to overcome resistance in infectious diseases. *Advanced Drug Delivery Reviews*, *65*(13-14), 1816–1827. DOI: 10.1016/j.addr.2013.07.020 PMID: 23932923

Atkins, P. J. (2024). Dry powder inhalers: An overview. *Respiratory Care*, *50*(10), 1304–1312. DOI: 10.4187/respcare.05501304 PMID: 16185366

Banat, H., Ambrus, R., & Csóka, I. (2023). Drug combinations for inhalation: Current products and future development addressing disease control and patient compliance. *International Journal of Pharmaceutics*, *643*, 643. DOI: 10.1016/j.ijpharm.2023.123070 PMID: 37230369

Bannigan, P., Aldeghi, M., Bao, Z., Häse, F., Aspuru-Guzik, A., & Allen, C. (2021). Machine learning directed drug formulation development. *Advanced Drug Delivery Reviews*, *175*, 113806. DOI: 10.1016/j.addr.2021.05.016 PMID: 34019959

Bao, Z., Bufton, J., Hickman, R. J., Aspuru-Guzik, A., Bannigan, P., & Allen, C. (2023). Revolutionizing drug formulation development: The increasing impact of machine learning. *Advanced Drug Delivery Reviews*, *202*, 115108. DOI: 10.1016/j.addr.2023.115108 PMID: 37774977

Boyack, K. W., & Klavans, R. (2010). Co-citation analysis, bibliographic coupling, and direct citation: Which citation approach represents the research front most accurately? *Journal of the American Society for Information Science and Technology*, *61*(12), 2389–2404. DOI: 10.1002/asi.21419

Cao, S., Huang, H., Xiao, M., Yan, L., Xu, W., Tang, X., Luo, X., & Zhao, Q. (2021). Research on safety in home care for older adults: A bibliometric analysis. *Nursing Open*, *8*(4), 1720–1730. DOI: 10.1002/nop2.812 PMID: 33626246

Chan, H. S., Shan, H., Dahoun, T., Vogel, H., & Yuan, S. (2019). Advancing drug discovery via artificial intelligence. *Trends in Pharmacological Sciences*, *40*(8), 592–604. DOI: 10.1016/j.tips.2019.06.004 PMID: 31320117

Chen, Z. Y., Liu, X., Hogan, W., Shenkman, E., & Bian, J. (2021). Applications of artificial intelligence in drug development using real-world data. *Drug Discovery Today*, *26*(5), 1256–1264. DOI: 10.1016/j.drudis.2020.12.013 PMID: 33358699

Clark, A. R. (2022). Half a century of technological advances in pulmonary drug delivery: A personal perspective. *Frontiers in Drug Delivery*, *2*, 871147. DOI: 10.3389/fddev.2022.871147

Deng, J., Yang, Z., Ojima, I., Samaras, D., & Wang, F. (2022). Artificial intelligence in drug discovery: Applications and techniques. *Briefings in Bioinformatics*, *23*(1), bbab430. DOI: 10.1093/bib/bbab430 PMID: 34734228

Dotolo, S., Marabotti, A., Facchiano, A., & Tagliaferri, R. (2021). A review on drug repurposing applicable to COVID-19. *Briefings in Bioinformatics*, *22*(2), 726–741. DOI: 10.1093/bib/bbaa288 PMID: 33147623

Elbadawi, M., Li, H. X., Basit, A. W., & Gaisford, S. (2024). The role of artificial intelligence in generating original scientific research. *International Journal of Pharmaceutics*, *652*, 652. DOI: 10.1016/j.ijpharm.2023.123741 PMID: 38181989

Farkas, D., Madarász, L., Nagy, Z. K., Antal, I., & Kállai-Szabó, N. (2021). Image analysis: A versatile tool in the manufacturing and quality control of pharmaceutical dosage forms. *Pharmaceutics*, *13*(5), 685. DOI: 10.3390/pharmaceutics13050685 PMID: 34068724

Ferkol, T., & Schraufnagel, D. (2014). The global burden of respiratory disease. *Annals of the American Thoracic Society*, *11*(3), 404–406. DOI: 10.1513/AnnalsATS.201311-405PS PMID: 24673696

Fink, J. B., & Stapleton, K. W. (2024). Nebulizers. *Journal of Aerosol Medicine and Pulmonary Drug Delivery*, *37*(3), 140–156. DOI: 10.1089/jamp.2024.29110.jbf PMID: 38683652

Gates, A. J., Ke, Q., Varol, O., & Barabási, A. L. (2019). Nature's reach: Narrow work has broad impact. *Nature*, *575*(7781), 32–34. DOI: 10.1038/d41586-019-03308-7 PMID: 31695218

Gonda, I. (2000). The ascent of pulmonary drug delivery. *Journal of Pharmaceutical Sciences*, *89*(7), 940–945. DOI: 10.1002/1520-6017(200007)89:7<940::AID-JPS11>3.0.CO;2-B PMID: 10861595

Groneberg, D. A., Witt, C., Wagner, U., Chung, K. F., & Fischer, A. (2003). Fundamentals of pulmonary drug delivery. *Respiratory Medicine*, *97*(4), 382–387. DOI: 10.1053/rmed.2002.1457 PMID: 12693798

Harrer, S., Shah, P., Antony, B., & Hu, J. Y. (2019). Artificial intelligence for clinical trial design. *Trends in Pharmacological Sciences*, *40*(8), 577–591. DOI: 10.1016/j.tips.2019.05.005 PMID: 31326235

He, S., Gui, J., Xiong, K., Chen, M., Gao, H., & Fu, Y. (2022). A roadmap to pulmonary delivery strategies for the treatment of infectious lung diseases. *Journal of Nanobiotechnology*, *20*(1), 101. DOI: 10.1186/s12951-022-01307-x PMID: 35241085

Jayatunga, M. K., Xie, W., Ruder, L., Schulze, U., & Meier, C. (2022). AI in small-molecule drug discovery: A coming wave. *Nature Reviews. Drug Discovery*, *21*(3), 175–176. DOI: 10.1038/d41573-022-00025-1 PMID: 35132242

Jiang, J., Lu, A., Ma, X., Ouyang, D., & Williams, R. O.III. (2023). The applications of machine learning to predict the forming of chemically stable amorphous solid dispersions prepared by hot-melt extrusion. *International Journal of Pharmaceutics: X*, *5*, 100164. DOI: 10.1016/j.ijpx.2023.100164 PMID: 36798832

Jiang, J., Ma, X., Ouyang, D., & Williams, R. O.III. (2022). Emerging artificial intelligence (AI) technologies used in the development of solid dosage forms. *Pharmaceutics, 14*(11), 2257. DOI: 10.3390/pharmaceutics14112257 PMID: 36365076

KNVC, L. (2024). FORMULATION AND EVALUATION OF PROPRANOLOL HYDROCHLORIDE FLOATING TABLETS BY 32 FACTORIAL DESIGN. *INTERNATIONAL JOURNAL, 14*(4), 1716-1721.

Kole, E., Jadhav, K., Shirsath, N., Dudhe, P., Verma, R. K., Chatterjee, A., & Naik, J. (2023). Nanotherapeutics for pulmonary drug delivery: An emerging approach to overcome respiratory diseases. *Journal of Drug Delivery Science and Technology, 81*, 104261. DOI: 10.1016/j.jddst.2023.104261

Labaki, W. W., Martinez, C. H., Martinez, F. J., Galbán, C. J., Ross, B. D., Washko, G. R., Barr, R. G., Regan, E. A., Coxson, H. O., Hoffman, E. A., Newell, J. D.Jr, Curran-Everett, D., Hogg, J. C., Crapo, J. D., Lynch, D. A., Kazerooni, E. A., & Han, M. K. (2017). The role of chest computed tomography in the evaluation and management of the patient with chronic obstructive pulmonary disease. *American Journal of Respiratory and Critical Care Medicine, 196*(11), 1372–1379. DOI: 10.1164/rccm.201703-0451PP PMID: 28661698

Lavorini, F., Pistolesi, M., & Usmani, O. S. (2017). Recent advances in capsule-based dry powder inhaler technology. *Multidisciplinary Respiratory Medicine, 12*, 1–7. DOI: 10.4081/mrm.2017.236

Leelavati, T. S.. (2023). Revolutionizing healthcare delivery: Telemedicine's influence on access and patient satisfaction. *International Journal of Chemical and Biochemical Science, 24*(5), 106–115.

Leelavati, T. S., Madhavi, S., & Aminabee, S. (2025). Fostering ethical decision-making skills in pharmaceutical education: Vital for future pharmacists. *Indian Journal of Pharmaceutical Education and Research, 59*(2), 433–440. DOI: 10.5530/ijper.20254872

Leelavati, T. S., Madhavi, S., Susmitha, K., Kumar, K. S. V., Goud, P. V. P., & Raju, K. G. (2023). Exploring university student attitudes, beliefs, and alcohol usage patterns: An investigation into alcohol and drug use within the student lifestyle. *Journal of Drug and Alcohol Research, 12*(6).

Liang, Z., Ni, R., Zhou, J., & Mao, S. (2015). Recent advances in controlled pulmonary drug delivery. *Drug Discovery Today, 20*(3), 380–389. DOI: 10.1016/j.drudis.2014.09.020 PMID: 25281854

MacLeod, M., Papi, A., Contoli, M., Beghé, B., Celli, B. R., Wedzicha, J. A., & Fabbri, L. M. (2021). Chronic obstructive pulmonary disease exacerbation fundamentals: Diagnosis, treatment, prevention and disease impact. *Respirology (Carlton, Vic.)*, *26*(6), 532–551. DOI: 10.1111/resp.14041 PMID: 33893708

Madhavi, S.. (2024). Unravelling the impact of alcohol use on college students' educational success: A systematic analysis. *Journal of Drug and Alcohol Research*, *13*(2), 1–5.

Mangal, S., Gao, W., Li, T. L., & Zhou, Q. (2017). Pulmonary delivery of nanoparticle chemotherapy for the treatment of lung cancers: Challenges and opportunities. *Acta Pharmacologica Sinica*, *38*(6), 782–797. DOI: 10.1038/aps.2017.34 PMID: 28504252

Mathias, N. R., & Hussain, M. A. (2010). Non-invasive systemic drug delivery: Developability considerations for alternate routes of administration. *Journal of Pharmaceutical Sciences*, *99*(1), 1–20. DOI: 10.1002/jps.21793 PMID: 19499570

Moon, C., Smyth, H. D. C., Watts, A. B., & Williams, R. O.III. (2019). Delivery technologies for orally inhaled products: An update. *AAPS PharmSciTech*, *20*(3), 117. DOI: 10.1208/s12249-019-1314-2 PMID: 30783904

Nagy, B., Galata, D. L., Farkas, A., & Nagy, Z. K. (2022). Application of artificial neural networks in the process analytical technology of pharmaceutical manufacturing—A review. *The AAPS Journal*, *24*(4), 74. DOI: 10.1208/s12248-022-00706-0 PMID: 35697951

National Academies of Sciences, Engineering, and Medicine. (2023). Advances in the diagnosis and evaluation of disabling physical health conditions. National Academies Press.

Newman, S. P. (2005). Principles of metered-dose inhaler design. *Respiratory Care*, *50*(9), 1177–1190. DOI: 10.4187/respcare.05501177 PMID: 16122401

Patton, J. S., Fishburn, C. S., & Weers, J. G. (2004). The lungs as a portal of entry for systemic drug delivery. *Proceedings of the American Thoracic Society*, *1*(4), 338–344. DOI: 10.1513/pats.200409-049TA PMID: 16113455

Pilcer, G., & Amighi, K. (2010). Formulation strategy and use of excipients in pulmonary drug delivery. *International Journal of Pharmaceutics*, *392*(1-2), 1–19. DOI: 10.1016/j.ijpharm.2010.03.017 PMID: 20223286

Prasanth, D. S. N. B. K., Aminabee, S. K., Rao, A. L., Guntupalli, C., Reddy, A. R., Kulandaivelu, U., Koteswara, S. N., & Rajeshwari, P. (2021). Inhibitory effects of Manosa alliacea in Freund's adjuvant arthritis on inflammatory markers and its confirmation by In-silico strategy. *Thaiphesatchasan*, *45*(6), 532–544. DOI: 10.56808/3027-7922.2535

Prasanth, D. S. N. B. K., Aminabee, S. K., Rao, A. L., Teja, N., Bhargavi, K., Monika, C., Pujitha, B., Sandhya, T., Lalitha, A., & Panda, S. P. (2020). Anthelmintic activity of Mansoa alliacea against Pheretima posthuma: In vitro and in silico approach. *Thaiphesatchasan*, *44*(3), 186–196. DOI: 10.56808/3027-7922.2451

Qureshi, R., Irfan, M., Gondal, T. M., Khan, S., Wu, J., Hadi, M. U., Heymach, J., Le, X., Yan, H., & Alam, T. (2023). AI in drug discovery and its clinical relevance. *Heliyon*, *9*(7), e17575. DOI: 10.1016/j.heliyon.2023.e17575 PMID: 37396052

Raju, K. G., Goud, P. V., Parween, S., Ramarao, M., Leelavati, T. S., Madhavi, S., & Aminabee, S. (2024). Economic Analysis of Pharmacological Interventions for Substance Use Disorders Cost-effectiveness and Market Dynamics. *Ashdin Publishing Journal of Drug and Alcohol Research, 13*(29), 01-04.

Salvi, S. (2014). Tobacco smoking and environmental risk factors for chronic obstructive pulmonary disease. *Clinics in Chest Medicine*, *35*(1), 17–27. DOI: 10.1016/j.ccm.2013.09.011 PMID: 24507834

Sharma, P., Mehta, M., Dhanjal, D. S., Kaur, S., Gupta, G., Singh, H., Thangavelu, L., Rajeshkumar, S., Tambuwala, M., Bakshi, H. A., Chellappan, D. K., Dua, K., & Satija, S. (2019). Emerging trends in the novel drug delivery approaches for the treatment of lung cancer. *Chemico-Biological Interactions*, *309*, 108720. DOI: 10.1016/j.cbi.2019.06.033 PMID: 31226287

Smyth, H. D. C. (2003). The influence of formulation variables on the performance of alternative propellant-driven metered dose inhalers. *Advanced Drug Delivery Reviews*, *55*(7), 807–828. DOI: 10.1016/S0169-409X(03)00079-6 PMID: 12842602

Soriano, J. B., Kendrick, P. J., Paulson, K. R., Gupta, V., Abrams, E. M., Adedoyin, R. A., & Moradi, M. (2020). Prevalence and attributable health burden of chronic respiratory diseases, 1990–2017: A systematic analysis for the Global Burden of Disease Study 2017. *The Lancet. Respiratory Medicine*, *8*(6), 585–596. DOI: 10.1016/S2213-2600(20)30105-3 PMID: 32526187

Su, H. N., & Lee, P. C. (2010). Mapping knowledge structure by keyword co-occurrence: A first look at journal papers in technology foresight. *Scientometrics*, *85*(1), 65–79. DOI: 10.1007/s11192-010-0259-8

Tang, J., Ouyang, Q., Li, Y., Zhang, P., Jin, W., Qu, S., Yang, F., He, Z., & Qin, M. (2022). Nanomaterials for delivering antibiotics in the therapy of pneumonia. *International Journal of Molecular Sciences*, *23*(24), 15738. DOI: 10.3390/ijms232415738 PMID: 36555379

Tanoli, Z., Vähä-Koskela, M., & Aittokallio, T. (2021). Artificial intelligence, machine learning, and drug repurposing in cancer. *Expert Opinion on Drug Discovery*, *16*(9), 977–989. DOI: 10.1080/17460441.2021.1883585 PMID: 33543671

Trivedi, A., Hall, C., Hoffman, E. A., Woods, J. C., Gierada, D. S., & Castro, M. (2017). Using imaging as a biomarker for asthma. *The Journal of Allergy and Clinical Immunology*, *139*(1), 1–10. DOI: 10.1016/j.jaci.2016.11.009 PMID: 28065276

van Eck, N. J., & Waltman, L. (2014). Visualizing bibliometric networks. In Ding, Y., Rousseau, R., & Wolfram, D. (Eds.), *Measuring scholarly impact: Methods and practice* (pp. 285–320). Springer. DOI: 10.1007/978-3-319-10377-8_13

Vliegenthart, R., Fouras, A., Jacobs, C., & Papanikolaou, N. (2022). Innovations in thoracic imaging: CT, radiomics, AI and x-ray velocimetry. *Respirology (Carlton, Vic.)*, *27*(10), 818–833. DOI: 10.1111/resp.14344 PMID: 35965430

Vora, L. K., Gholap, A. D., Jetha, K., Thakur, R. R. S., Solanki, H. K., & Chavda, V. P. (2023). Artificial intelligence in pharmaceutical technology and drug delivery design. *Pharmaceutics*, *15*(7), 1916. DOI: 10.3390/pharmaceutics15071916 PMID: 37514102

Wan, Z., Sun, X., Li, Y., Chu, T., Hao, X., Cao, Y., & Zhang, P. (2025). Applications of artificial intelligence in drug repurposing. *Advancement of Science*, *12*(14), 2411325. DOI: 10.1002/advs.202411325 PMID: 40047357

Wang, W., Feng, S., Ye, Z. Y. F., Gao, H. L., Lin, J. Z., & Ouyang, D. F. (2022). Prediction of lipid nanoparticles for mRNA vaccines by the machine learning algorithm. *Acta Pharmaceutica Sinica. B*, *12*(6), 2950–2962. DOI: 10.1016/j.apsb.2021.11.021 PMID: 35755271

Wang, W., Ye, Z., Gao, H., & Ouyang, D. (2021). Computational pharmaceutics-A new paradigm of drug delivery. *Journal of Controlled Release*, *338*, 119–136. DOI: 10.1016/j.jconrel.2021.08.030 PMID: 34418520

Xiong, L., Li, X., Lu, X., Zhang, Z., Zhang, Y., Wu, W., & Wang, C. (2024). Inhaled multilevel size-tunable, charge-reversible and mucus-traversing composite microspheres as trojan horse: Enhancing lung deposition and tumor penetration. *Chinese Chemical Letters*, *35*(9), 109384. DOI: 10.1016/j.cclet.2023.109384

Zemanick, E. T., Harris, J. K., Conway, S., Konstan, M. W., Marshall, B., Quittner, A. L., Retsch-Bogart, G., Saiman, L., & Accurso, F. J. (2010). Measuring and improving respiratory outcomes in cystic fibrosis lung disease: Opportunities and challenges to therapy. *Journal of Cystic Fibrosis*, *9*(1), 1–16. DOI: 10.1016/j.jcf.2009.09.003 PMID: 19833563

Zeng, X. M., Martin, G. P., & Marriott, C. (1995). The controlled delivery of drugs to the lung. *International Journal of Pharmaceutics*, *124*(2), 149–164. DOI: 10.1016/0378-5173(95)00104-Q

Zhang, Z., Ma, P., Ahmed, R., Wang, J., Akin, D., Soto, F., Liu, B.-F., Li, P., & Demirci, U. (2022). Advanced point-of-care testing technologies for human acute respiratory virus detection. *Advanced Materials*, *34*(1), 2103646. DOI: 10.1002/adma.202103646 PMID: 34623709

Zhou, Q. T., Leung, S. S. Y., Tang, P., Parumasivam, T., Loh, Z. H., & Chan, H. K. (2015). Inhaled formulations and pulmonary drug delivery systems for respiratory infections. *Advanced Drug Delivery Reviews*, *85*, 83–99. DOI: 10.1016/j.addr.2014.10.022 PMID: 25451137

Zhou, Y., Wang, F., Tang, J., Nussinov, R., & Cheng, F. (2020). Artificial intelligence in COVID-19 drug repurposing. *The Lancet. Digital Health*, *2*(12), e667–e676. DOI: 10.1016/S2589-7500(20)30192-8 PMID: 32984792

Compilation of References

Aberle, D. R., Black, W. C., Chiles, C., Church, T. R., Gareen, I. F., Gierada, D. S., Mahon, I., Miller, E. A., Pinsky, P. F., & Sicks, J. D. (2019). Lung cancer incidence and mortality with extended follow-up in the National Lung Screening Trial. *Journal of Thoracic Oncology*, *14*(10), 1732–1742. DOI: 10.1016/j.jtho.2019.05.044 PMID: 31260833

Abouelmehdi, K., Beni-Hessane, A., & Khaloufi, H. (2018). Big healthcare data: Preserving security and privacy. *Journal of Big Data*, *5*(1), 1–18. DOI: 10.1186/s40537-017-0110-7

Adam Essa, M. E. (2025). Diagnostic accuracy of AI in chest radiography for pneumonia and lung cancer: A meta-analysis. *European Journal of Radiology Open*, *15*, 100701. DOI: 10.1016/j.ejro.2025.100701 PMID: 41278429

Addae, J. H., Sun, X., Towey, D., & Radenkovic, M. (2019). Exploring user behavioral data for adaptive cybersecurity. *User Modeling and User-Adapted Interaction*, *29*(3), 701–750. DOI: 10.1007/s11257-019-09236-5

Adlung, L., Cohen, Y., Mor, U., & Elinav, E. (2021). Machine learning in clinical decision making. *Med (New York, N.Y.)*, *2*(6), 642–665. PMID: 35590138

Aerts, H. J. W. L., Velazquez, E. R., Leijenaar, R. T. H., Parmar, C., Grossmann, P., Carvalho, S., Bussink, J., Monshouwer, R., Haibe-Kains, B., Rietveld, D., Hoebers, F., Rietbergen, M. M., Leemans, C. R., Dekker, A., Quackenbush, J., Gillies, R. J., & Lambin, P. (2014). Decoding tumour phenotype by noninvasive imaging using a quantitative radiomics approach. *Nature Communications*, *5*(1), 4006. DOI: 10.1038/ncomms5006 PMID: 24892406

Afroz, N., Gutzwiller, F. S., Mackay, A. J., Naujoks, C., Patalano, F., & Kostikas, K. (2020). Patient-reported outcomes (PROs) in COPD clinical trials: Trends and gaps. *International Journal of Chronic Obstructive Pulmonary Disease*, *15*, 1789–1800. DOI: 10.2147/COPD.S235845 PMID: 32801678

Aguilaniu, B., Hess, D., Kelkel, E., Briault, A., Destors, M., Boutros, J., Zhi Li, P., & Antoniadis, A. (2021). A machine learning approach to predict extreme inactivity in COPD patients using non-activity-related clinical data. *PLoS One*, *16*(8), e0255977. DOI: 10.1371/journal.pone.0255977 PMID: 34411121

Agusti, A., Hedner, J., Marin, J., Barbé, F., Cazzola, M., & Rennard, S. (2011). Night-time symptoms: A forgotten dimension of COPD. *European Respiratory Review : an Official Journal of the European Respiratory Society*, *20*(121), 183–194. DOI: 10.1183/09059180.00004311 PMID: 21881146

Ahmad, P., Xu, H., Nasir, M., & Shen, L. (2024). Deep learning for lung cancer detection: A review. *Artificial Intelligence Review*, *57*(12), 3345–3390. DOI: 10.1007/s10462-024-10807-1

Ahmed, F., Soomro, A. M., Salih, A. R. C., Samantasinghar, A., Asif, A., Kang, I. S., & Choi, K. H. (2022). A comprehensive review of artificial intelligence and network based approaches to drug repurposing in Covid-19. *Biomedicine and Pharmacotherapy*, *153*, 113350. DOI: 10.1016/j.biopha.2022.113350 PMID: 35777222

Ahmed, Z., Mohamed, K., Zeeshan, S., & Dong, X. (2020). Artificial intelligence with multi-functional machine learning platform development for better healthcare and precision medicine. *Database : The Journal of Biological Databases and Curation*, *2020*, baaa010. DOI: 10.1093/database/baaa010 PMID: 32185396

Aishwarya, K. V., & Asuntha, A. (2025). A survey on comparative study of lung nodules applying machine learning and deep learning techniques. *Multimedia Tools and Applications*, *84*(5), 2127–2181. DOI: 10.1007/s11042-024-20009-0

Akgündoğdu, A., & Çelikbaş, Ş. (2025). Explainable deep learning framework for brain tumor detection: Integrating LIME, Grad-CAM, and SHAP for enhanced accuracy. *Medical Engineering & Physics*, *144*(1), 104405. DOI: 10.1016/j.medengphy.2025.104405 PMID: 40925692

Akter, L., Mondal, R. S., & Bhuiyan, M. N. A. (2025). Artificial intelligence application in public health: Advancement and associated challenges. *Journal of Primeasia*, *6*(1), 1–10. DOI: 10.25163/primeasia.6110325

Alam, R., Peden, D. B., & Lach, J. C. (2020). Wearable respiration monitoring: Interpretable inference with context and sensor biomarkers. arXiv. PMID: N/A. https://doi.org//arXiv.2007.01413DOI: 10.1101/2020.07.04.20146456

Al-Anazi, S., Al-Omari, A., Alanazi, S., Marar, A., Asad, M., Alawaji, F., & Al-wateid, S. (2024). Artificial intelligence in respiratory care: Current scenario and future perspective. *Annals of Thoracic Medicine*, *19*(2), 117–130. DOI: 10.4103/atm.atm_192_23 PMID: 38766378

Albaradei, S. (2025). AI-Driven Approaches to Utilization of Multi-Omics Data for Personalized Diagnosis and Treatment of Cancer: A Comprehensive Review. *Computer Modeling in Engineering & Sciences*, *145*(3), 2937–2970. DOI: 10.32604/cmes.2025.072584

Aliper, A., Kudrin, R., Polykovskiy, D., Kamya, P., Tutubalina, E., Chen, S., Ren, F., & Zhavoronkov, A. (2023). Prediction of clinical trials outcomes based on target choice and clinical trial design with multi-modal artificial intelligence. *Clinical Pharmacology and Therapeutics*, *114*(5), 972–980. DOI: 10.1002/cpt.3008 PMID: 37483175

Aliyu, D. A., Akhir, E. A. P., Osman, N. A., Yahaya, S., Adamu, S., & Mamman, H. (2024). A Conceptual Framework for Personalized Early Prediction of Asthma Exacerbation Attacks Using Proximal Policy Optimization. *JOIV: International Journal on Informatics Visualization*, *8*(4), 2462–2471. DOI: 10.62527/joiv.8.4.2944

Allena, N., & Khanal, S. (2023). The algorithmic lung detective: Artificial intelligence in the diagnosis of pulmonary embolism. *Cureus*, *15*(12), e51006. DOI: 10.7759/cureus.51006 PMID: 38259362

Al-Musawi, J. M., Al-Shadeedi, F., Shakir, N. A., & Ibrahim, S. Q. (2025). Epidemiological Characteristics of Lung Cancer Patients in the Middle Euphrates Region of Iraq: Retrospective Analysis from the Middle Euphrates Cancer Center (2018-2023). *Al-Rafidain Journal of Medical Sciences (ISSN 2789-3219)*, *8*(2), 63-70.

Alowais, S. A., Alghamdi, S. S., Alsuhebany, N., Alqahtani, T., Alshaya, A. I., Almohareb, S. N., Aldairem, A., Alrashed, M., Bin Saleh, K., & Badredin, H. A. (2023). Revolutionizing healthcare: The role of artificial intelligence in clinical practice. *BMC Medical Education*, *23*(1), 689. DOI: 10.1186/s12909-023-04698-z PMID: 37740191

Alpay, L., van der Boog, P., & Dumaij, A. (2011). An empowerment-based approach to developing innovative e-health tools for self-management. *Health Informatics Journal*, *17*(4), 247–255. DOI: 10.1177/1460458211420089 PMID: 22193825

American Thoracic Society Journals. (n.d.). OUP Academic. Retrieved May 28, 2026, from https://academic.oup.com/atsjournals/atsjournals

Aminabee, S., Dasari, S. K., Rao, K. H., Sirisha, V., Kumari, V. A., Dasari, N., & Leelavati, T. S. (2023). Pharmacoeconomic analysis of biologic vs. biosimilar therapies in rheumatoid arthritis. *International Journal of Chemical and Biochemical Science*, *24*(4), 395–400.

Aminabee, S., Devi Mallika, K., & Lakshmana Rao, A. (2023). Natural resources in management and treatment of diseases: A review. *Pharmacy Times*, *55*(11), 7–10.

Aminabee, S., & Lakshmana Rao, A. (2024). Computational identification of selected bioactive compounds from *Cedrus deodara* as inhibitors against SARS-CoV-2 main protease: A pharmacoinformatics study. *Indian Drugs*, *61*(2), 78–91. DOI: 10.53879/id.61.02.13859

Aminabee, S., Prabhakar, M. C., Prasad, R. G. S. V., & Lakshmana Rao, A. (2011). Screening the pharmacological activity of cerium oxide nanoparticles in-vitro. *Biomedical & Pharmacology Journal*, *4*(2), 287–289. DOI: 10.13005/bpj/296

Aminabee, S., Rao, A. L., Sowmya, K., Nymisha, D., Lakshmi, K. K. N., Manikanta, K. V. N. S., & Kumar, P. P. (2019). Evaluation of Analgesic Activity of Ficus Palmata: Evaluation of Analgesic activity of Ficus palmata. *Iranian Journal of Pharmaceutical Sciences*, *15*(3), 47–60.

Ancoli-Israel, S., Cole, R., Alessi, C., Chambers, M., Moorcroft, W., & Pollak, C. P. (2003). The role of actigraphy in the study of sleep and circadian rhythms. *Sleep*, *26*(3), 342–392. DOI: 10.1093/sleep/26.3.342 PMID: 12749557

Anderson, P. G., Tarder-Stoll, H., Alpaslan, M., Keathley, N., Levin, D. L., Venkatesh, S., Bartel, E., Sicular, S., Howell, S., Lindsey, R. V., & Jones, R. M. (2024). Deep learning improves physician accuracy in the comprehensive detection of abnormalities on chest X-rays. *Scientific Reports*, *14*(1), 25151. DOI: 10.1038/s41598-024-76608-2 PMID: 39448764

Andrade, F., Rafael, D., Videira, M., Ferreira, D., Sosnik, A., & Sarmento, B. (2013). Nanotechnology and pulmonary delivery to overcome resistance in infectious diseases. *Advanced Drug Delivery Reviews*, *65*(13-14), 1816–1827. DOI: 10.1016/j.addr.2013.07.020 PMID: 23932923

Antão, J., de Mast, J., Marques, A., Franssen, F. M. E., Spruit, M. A., & Deng, Q. (2024). Dcmystification of artificial intelligence for respiratory clinicians managing patients with obstructive lung diseases. *Expert Review of Respiratory Medicine*, *17*(12), 1207–1219. DOI: 10.1080/17476348.2024.2302940 PMID: 38270524

Anthimopoulos, M., Christodoulidis, S., Ebner, L., Christe, A., & Mougiakakou, S. (2016). Lung pattern classification for interstitial lung diseases using a deep convolutional neural network. *IEEE Transactions on Medical Imaging*, *35*(5), 1207–1216. DOI: 10.1109/TMI.2016.2535865 PMID: 26955021

Application of artificial intelligence in diagnosis of pulmonary tuberculosis | Chinese Medical Journal. (n.d.). Retrieved May 28, 2026, from https://mednexus.org/doi/full/10.1097/CM9.0000000000003018

Applications of Artificial Intelligence in Drug Repurposing—Wan—2025—Advanced Science—Wiley Online Library. (n.d.). Retrieved May 28, 2026, from https://advanced.onlinelibrary.wiley.com/doi/full/10.1002/advs.202411325

Ardila, D., Kiraly, A. P., Bharadwaj, S., Choi, B., Reicher, J. J., Peng, L., Tse, D., Etemadi, M., Ye, W., Corrado, G., Naidich, D. P., & Shetty, S. (2019). End-to-end lung cancer screening with three-dimensional deep learning on low-dose chest computed tomography. *Nature Medicine*, *25*(6), 954–961. DOI: 10.1038/s41591-019-0447-x PMID: 31110349

Arshad, M. F., Chowdhury, A. T., Sharif, Z., Islam, M., Sumon, M. S. I., Mohammedkasim, A., Chowdhury, M. E. H., & Pedersen, S. (2025). Artificial Intelligence and Machine Learning in Lung Cancer: Advances in Imaging, Detection, and Prognosis. *Cancers (Basel)*, *17*(24), 3985. DOI: 10.3390/cancers17243985 PMID: 41463234

Artificial Intelligence detects substantial airway damage on CT scans of children with severe asthma—Thirona. (n.d.). Retrieved January 31, 2026, from https://thirona.eu/blog/artificial-intelligence-detects-substantial-airway-damage-on-ct-scans-of-children-with-severe-asthma/

Ashrafi, A., Akter, Z., Modareszadeh, P., Modareszadeh, P., Berisha, E., Alemi, P. S., Chacon Castro, M. C., Deese, A. R., & Zhang, L. (2022). Current landscape of therapeutic resistance in lung cancer and promising strategies to overcome resistance. *Cancers (Basel)*, *14*(19), 4562. DOI: 10.3390/cancers14194562 PMID: 36230484

Atkins, P. J. (2024). Dry powder inhalers: An overview. *Respiratory Care*, *50*(10), 1304–1312. DOI: 10.4187/respcare.05501304 PMID: 16185366

Avanzo, M., Wei, L., Stancanello, J., Vallieres, M., Rao, A., Morin, O., Mattonen, S. A., & El Naqa, I. (2020). Machine and deep learning methods for radiomics. *Medical Physics*, *47*(5), e185–e202. DOI: 10.1002/mp.13678 PMID: 32418336

Azizi, S., Mustafa, B., Ryan, F., Beaver, Z., Freyberg, J., Deaton, J., Loh, A., Karthikesalingam, A., Kornblith, S., Chen, T., Natarajan, V., & Norouzi, M. (2021). Big Self-Supervised Models Advance Medical Image Classification. *2021 IEEE/CVF International Conference on Computer Vision (ICCV)*, 3458–3468. https://doi.org/DOI: 10.1109/ICCV48922.2021.00346

Aziz, S., Ali, A. A. M., & Aslam, H.. (2025). Wearable artificial intelligence for sleep disorders: Scoping review. *Journal of Medical Internet Research*, *27*, e65272. DOI: 10.2196/65272 PMID: 40327852

Bahado-Singh, R., Vlachos, K. T., Aydas, B., Gordevicius, J., Radhakrishna, U., & Vishwesvaraiah, S. (2022). Precision oncology: Artificial intelligence and DNA methylation analysis of circulating cell-free DNA for lung cancer detection. *Frontiers in Oncology*, *12*, 790645. DOI: 10.3389/fonc.2022.790645 PMID: 35600397

Bai, N., Cao, J., Zhang, H., Liu, X., & Yin, M. (2024). Digital cognitive behavioural therapy for patients with insomnia and depression: A systematic review and meta-analysis. *Journal of Psychiatric and Mental Health Nursing*, *31*(4), 654–667. DOI: 10.1111/jpm.13024 PMID: 38226714

Bai, Y., Gu, B., & Tang, C. (2025). Enhancing real-time patient monitoring in intensive care units with deep learning and the internet of things. *Big Data*, big.2024.0113. DOI: 10.1089/big.2024.0113 PMID: 39819048

Banat, H., Ambrus, R., & Csóka, I. (2023). Drug combinations for inhalation: Current products and future development addressing disease control and patient compliance. *International Journal of Pharmaceutics*, *643*, 643. DOI: 10.1016/j.ijpharm.2023.123070 PMID: 37230369

Bannigan, P., Aldeghi, M., Bao, Z., Häse, F., Aspuru-Guzik, A., & Allen, C. (2021). Machine learning directed drug formulation development. *Advanced Drug Delivery Reviews*, *175*, 113806. DOI: 10.1016/j.addr.2021.05.016 PMID: 34019959

Bao, Z., Bufton, J., Hickman, R. J., Aspuru-Guzik, A., Bannigan, P., & Allen, C. (2023). Revolutionizing drug formulation development: The increasing impact of machine learning. *Advanced Drug Delivery Reviews*, *202*, 115108. DOI: 10.1016/j.addr.2023.115108 PMID: 37774977

Baron, K. G., Duffecy, J., Berendsen, M. A., Cheung Mason, I., Lattie, E. G., & Manalo, N. C. (2018). Feeling validated yet? A scoping review of the use of consumer-targeted wearable and mobile technology to measure and improve sleep. *Sleep Medicine Reviews*, *40*, 151–159. DOI: 10.1016/j.smrv.2017.12.002 PMID: 29395985

Baumann, M., Krause, M., Overgaard, J., Debus, J., Bentzen, S. M., Daartz, J., Richter, C., Zips, D., & Bortfeld, T. (2016). Radiation oncology in the era of precision medicine. *Nature Reviews. Cancer*, *16*(4), 234–249. DOI: 10.1038/nrc.2016.18 PMID: 27009394

Beil, M., Proft, I., van Heerden, D., Sviri, S., & van Heerden, P. V. (2019). Ethical considerations about artificial intelligence for prognostication in intensive care. *Intensive Care Medicine Experimental*, *7*(1), 70. Advance online publication. DOI: 10.1186/s40635-019-0286-6 PMID: 31823128

Beitler, J. R., Thompson, B. T., Baron, R. M., Bastarache, J. A., Denlinger, L. C., Esserman, L., Gong, M. N., LaVange, L. M., Lewis, R. J., Marshall, J. C., Martin, T. R., McAuley, D. F., Meyer, N. J., Moss, M., Reineck, L. A., Rubin, E., Schmidt, E. P., Standiford, T. J., Ware, L. B., & Calfee, C. S. (2022). Advancing precision medicine for acute respiratory distress syndrome. *The Lancet. Respiratory Medicine*, *10*(1), 107–120. DOI: 10.1016/S2213-2600(21)00157-0 PMID: 34310901

Bellani, G., Laffey, J. G., Pham, T., Fan, E., Brochard, L., Esteban, A., Gattinoni, L., van Haren, F., Larsson, A., McAuley, D. F., Ranieri, M., Rubenfeld, G., Thompson, B. T., Wrigge, H., Slutsky, A. S., & Pesenti, A.LUNG SAFE Investigators and the ESICM Trials Group. (2016). Epidemiology, patterns of care, and mortality for patients with acute respiratory distress syndrome in intensive care units in 50 countries. *Journal of the American Medical Association*, *315*(8), 788–800. DOI: 10.1001/jama.2016.0291 PMID: 26903337

Bentley, C. L., Powell, L., Potter, S., Parker, J., Mountain, G. A., Bartlett, Y. K., Farwer, J., O'Connor, C., Burns, J., Cresswell, R. L., Dunn, H. D., & Hawley, M. S. (2020). The use of a smartphone app and an activity tracker to promote physical activity in the management of chronic obstructive pulmonary disease: Randomized controlled feasibility study. *JMIR mHealth and uHealth*, *8*(6), e16203. DOI: 10.2196/16203 PMID: 32490838

Berdahl, C. T., Baker, L., Mann, S., Osoba, O., & Girosi, F. (2023). Strategies to improve the impact of artificial intelligence on health equity: Scoping review. JMIR AI, 2, e42936. PMID: N/A. https://doi.org/DOI: 10.2196/42936

Berkhout, W. E. M., van Wijngaarden, J. J., Workum, J. D., van de Sande, D., Hilling, D. E., Jung, C., Meyfroidt, G., Gommers, D., Buijsman, S. N. R., & van Genderen, M. E. (2025). Operationalization of artificial intelligence applications in the intensive care unit. *JAMA Network Open*, *8*(7), e2522866. DOI: 10.1001/jamanetworkopen.2025.22866 PMID: 40699572

Bhatt, A., Sengupta, S., Abolhassani, A., Brower, D., Forehand, C., Keats, K., Kwon, Y., & Healy, W. J. (2025). Awakening sleep medicine: The transformative role of artificial intelligence in sleep health. *Current Sleep Medicine Reports*, *11*(1), 13. Advance online publication. DOI: 10.1007/s40675-025-00328-w

Bhuiyan, M. N. A., Mondal, R. S., & Akter, L. (2025). Advancing cancer imaging with artificial intelligence: Clinical application and challenges. *Journal of Primeasia*, *6*(1), 1–11. DOI: 10.25163/primeasia.6110322

Bica, I., Alaa, A. M., Lambert, C., & Van Der Schaar, M. (2021). From real-world patient data to individualized treatment effects using machine learning: Current and future methods to address underlying challenges. *Clinical Pharmacology and Therapeutics*, *109*(1), 87–100. DOI: 10.1002/cpt.1907 PMID: 32449163

Biesheuvel, L. A., van Workum, J. D., & Reuland, M.. (2025). Large language models in critical care. *Journal of Intensive Medicine*, *5*(2), 113–118. Advance online publication. DOI: 10.1016/j.jointm.2024.12.001 PMID: 40241839

Bilgin, G. B., Bilgin, C., Burkett, B. J., Orme, J. J., Childs, D. S., Thorpe, M. P., Halfdanarson, T. R., Johnson, G. B., Kendi, A. T., & Sartor, O. (2024). Theranostics and artificial intelligence: New frontiers in personalized medicine. *Theranostics*, *14*(6), 2367–2378. DOI: 10.7150/thno.94788 PMID: 38646652

Bin Rafiq, R., Modave, F., Guha, S., & Albert, M. V. (2020). Validation methods to promote real-world applicability of machine learning in medicine. Proceedings of the 2020 3rd International Conference on Digital Medicine and Image Processing, Budiarto, A., Tsang, K. C., Wilson, A. M., Sheikh, A., & Shah, S. A. (2023). Machine learning–based asthma attack prediction models from routinely collected electronic health records: Systematic scoping review. *JMIR AI*, *2*, e46717.

Birrer, V., Elgendi, M., Lambercy, O., Giggins, O. M., & Penders, J. (2024). Evaluating reliability in wearable devices for sleep staging. npj. *Digital Medicine*, *7*(1), 74. DOI: 10.1038/s41746-024-01016-9 PMID: 38499793

Biswal, S., Sun, H., Goparaju, B., Westover, M. B., Sun, J., & Bianchi, M. T. (2018). Expert-level sleep scoring with deep neural networks. *Journal of the American Medical Informatics Association : JAMIA*, *25*(12), 1643–1650. DOI: 10.1093/jamia/ocy131 PMID: 30445569

Borno, M. N. A., Shovon, M. S. H., Sikder, M. D., Rimi, I. F., Alahmadi, T. J., & Moni, M. A. (2025). Federated Learning with LoRA Optimized DeiT and Multiscale Patch Embedding for Secure Eye Disease Recognition. arXiv preprint arXiv:2505.06982.

Botta, M., Wenstedt, E. F. E., Tsonas, A. M., Buiteman-Kruizinga, L. A., van Meenen, D. M. P., Korsten, H. H. M., Horn, J., Paulus, F., Bindels, A. G. J. H., Schultz, M. J., & De Bie, A. J. R. (2021). Effectiveness, safety and efficacy of INTELLiVENT–adaptive support ventilation, a closed-loop ventilation mode for use in ICU patients: A systematic review. *Expert Review of Respiratory Medicine*, *15*(11), 1403–1413. DOI: 10.1080/17476348.2021.1933450 PMID: 34047244

Bouderhem, R. (2022). AI Regulation in Healthcare: New Paradigms for A Legally Binding Treaty Under the World Health Organization. *2022 14th International Conference on Computational Intelligence and Communication Networks (CICN)*, 277–281. DOI: 10.1109/CICN56167.2022.10008303

Boyack, K. W., & Klavans, R. (2010). Co-citation analysis, bibliographic coupling, and direct citation: Which citation approach represents the research front most accurately? *Journal of the American Society for Information Science and Technology*, *61*(12), 2389–2404. DOI: 10.1002/asi.21419

Bray, F., Ferlay, J., Soerjomataram, I., Siegel, R. L., Torre, L. A., & Jemal, A. (2018). Global cancer statistics 2018: GLOBOCAN estimates of incidence and mortality worldwide for 36 cancers in 185 countries. *CA: a Cancer Journal for Clinicians*, *68*(6), 394–424. DOI: 10.3322/caac.21492 PMID: 30207593

Brosch-Lenz, J., Yousefirizi, F., Zukotynski, K., Beauregard, J. M., Gaudet, V., Saboury, B., Rahmim, A., & Uribe, C. (2021). Role of artificial intelligence in theranostics: Toward routine personalized radiopharmaceutical therapies. *PET Clinics*, *16*(4), 627–641. DOI: 10.1016/j.cpet.2021.06.002 PMID: 34537133

Bubeck, S., Chandrasekaran, V., Eldan, R., Gehrke, J., Horvitz, E., Kamar, E., Lee, P., Lee, Y. T., Li, Y., Lundberg, S., Nori, H., Palangi, H., Ribeiro, M. T., & Zhang, Y. (2023). Sparks of artificial general intelligence: Early experiments with GPT 4. arXiv. PMID: N/A. https://doi.org//arXiv.2303.12712DOI: 10.48550

Budin-Ljøsne, I., Teare, H. J., Kaye, J., Beck, S., Bentzen, H. B., Caenazzo, L., Collett, C., D'Abramo, F., Felzmann, H., Finlay, T., Javaid, M. K., Jones, E., Katić, V., Simpson, A., & Mascalzoni, D. (2017). Dynamic consent: A potential solution to some of the challenges of modern biomedical research. *BMC Medical Ethics*, *18*(1), 4. DOI: 10.1186/s12910-016-0162-9 PMID: 28122615

Buess, L., Keicher, M., Navab, N., & Maier, A. (2025). From large language models to multimodal AI: A scoping review on the potential of generative AI in medicine. Biomedical Engineering / Biomedizinische Technik. Advance online publication.

Canali, S., Schiaffonati, V., & Aliverti, A. (2022). Challenges and recommendations for wearable devices in digital health: Data quality, interoperability, health equity, fairness. *PLOS Digital Health*, *1*(10), e0000104. DOI: 10.1371/journal.pdig.0000104 PMID: 36812619

Cao, S., Huang, H., Xiao, M., Yan, L., Xu, W., Tang, X., Luo, X., & Zhao, Q. (2021). Research on safety in home care for older adults: A bibliometric analysis. *Nursing Open*, *8*(4), 1720–1730. DOI: 10.1002/nop2.812 PMID: 33626246

Carvelli, L., Olesen, A. N., Brink-Kjær, A., Leary, E. B., Peppard, P. E., Mignot, E., Sørensen, H. B. D., & Jennum, P. (2020). Design of a deep learning model for automatic scoring of periodic and non-periodic leg movements during sleep validated against multiple human experts. *Sleep Medicine*, *69*, 109–119. DOI: 10.1016/j.sleep.2019.12.032 PMID: 32062037

Cecconi, M., Greco, M., Shickel, B., Angus, D. C., Bailey, H., Bignami, E., Calandra, T., Celi, L. A., Einav, S., Elbers, P., Ercole, A., Gómez, H., Gong, M. N., Komorowski, M., Liu, V., Park, S., Sarwal, A., Seymour, C. W., Zampieri, F. G., & Bihorac, A. (2025). Implementing artificial intelligence in critical care medicine: A consensus of 22. *Critical Care*, *29*(1), 29. Advance online publication. DOI: 10.1186/s13054-025-05532-2 PMID: 40629428

Champendal, M., Muller, H., Prior, J., & dos Reis, C. S. (2023). A scoping review of interpretability and explainability concerning artificial intelligence methods in medical imaging. *European Journal of Radiology*, *169*, 111159. DOI: 10.1016/j.ejrad.2023.111159 PMID: 37976760

Chan, H. S., Shan, H., Dahoun, T., Vogel, H., & Yuan, S. (2019). Advancing drug discovery via artificial intelligence. *Trends in Pharmacological Sciences*, *40*(8), 592–604. DOI: 10.1016/j.tips.2019.06.004 PMID: 31320117

Chantzi, S. L., Kosvyra, A., & Chouvarda, I. (2025). Radiomics and Artificial Intelligence in Pulmonary Fibrosis. *Journal of Imaging Informatics in Medicine*, *38*(5), 2779–2792. DOI: 10.1007/s10278-024-01377-3 PMID: 39762544

Chapizanis, D., Karakitsios, S., Gotti, A., & Sarigiannis, D. A. (2021). Assessing personal exposure using Agent Based Modelling informed by sensors technology. *Environmental Research*, *192*, 110141. DOI: 10.1016/j.envres.2020.110141 PMID: 32956655

Chatburn, R. L., & Mireles-Cabodevila, E. (2011). Closed-loop control of mechanical ventilation: Description and classification of targeting schemes. *Respiratory Care*, *56*(1), 85–102. DOI: 10.4187/respcare.00967 PMID: 21235841

Chen, B. T., Chen, Z., Ye, N., Mambetsariev, I., Fricke, J., Daniel, E., Wang, T., Wong, C. W., Rockne, R. C., Colen, R. R., Nasser, M. W., Batra, S. K., Holodny, A. I., Sampath, S., & Salgia, R. (2020). Differentiating peripherally-located small cell lung cancer from non-small cell lung cancer using a CT radiomic approach. *Frontiers in Oncology*, *10*, 593. DOI: 10.3389/fonc.2020.00593 PMID: 32391274

Chen, C., Hung, C.-M., Ko, S.-C., Cheng, K.-C., Chao, C., Sung, M.-I., Hsing, S., Wang, J.-J., Chen, C., Lai, C., Chen, C., & Chiu, C. (2022). An artificial intelligence system to predict the optimal timing for mechanical ventilation weaning for intensive care unit patients: A two-stage prediction approach. *Frontiers in Medicine*, *9*, 935366. Advance online publication. DOI: 10.3389/fmed.2022.935366 PMID: 36465940

Cheng, C. H., & Shi, S. S. (2025). Artificial intelligence in cancer: Applications, challenges, and future perspectives. *Molecular Cancer*, *24*(1), 274. DOI: 10.1186/s12943-025-02450-3 PMID: 41168799

Cheng, D. O., Khaw, C. R., Mccabe, J., Pennycuick, A., Nair, A., Moore, D. A., Janes, S. M., & Jacob, J. (2024). Predicting histopathological features of aggressiveness in lung cancer using CT radiomics: A systematic review. *Clinical Radiology*, *79*(9), 681–689. DOI: 10.1016/j.crad.2024.04.022 PMID: 38853080

Cheng, Y., Lama, N., Chen, M., Amidi, E., Ramzanpour, M., Rahman, M. A., Xiu, J., Helmstetter, A., Dickman, L., Ribeiro, J. R., Ghani, H., Oberley, M., Spetzler, D., & Sledge, G. W. (2025). Synergistic H&E and IHC image analysis by AI predicts cancer biomarkers and survival outcomes in colorectal and breast cancer. *Communications Medicine*, *5*(1), 328. DOI: 10.1038/s43856-025-01045-9 PMID: 40750675

Chen, S., Xing, S., Zhang, G., & Qiu, F. (2025). Innovative Applications and Challenges of Artificial Intelligence in the Whole-Course Management of Chronic Obstructive Pulmonary Disease. *International Journal of Chronic Obstructive Pulmonary Disease*, •••, 1–18. PMID: 41859017

Chen, Z. Y., Liu, X., Hogan, W., Shenkman, E., & Bian, J. (2021). Applications of artificial intelligence in drug development using real-world data. *Drug Discovery Today*, *26*(5), 1256–1264. DOI: 10.1016/j.drudis.2020.12.013 PMID: 33358699

Chepelev, L. L., Wang, X., Gold, B., Bonzel, C. L., Rybicki, F. J., Uyeda, J. W., & Sheikh, A. (2021). Improved appropriateness of advanced diagnostic imaging after implementation of clinical decision support mechanism. Journal of Digital Imaging, 34, 397–403. PMID: N/A. https://doi.org/DOI: 10.1007/s10278-021-00433-6

Cherezov, D., Goldgof, D., Hall, L., Gillies, R., Schabath, M., Muller, H., & Gu, Y. (2019). Revealing tumor habitats from texture heterogeneity analysis for classification of lung cancer malignancy and aggressiveness. *Scientific Reports*, *9*(1), 4500. DOI: 10.1038/s41598-019-38831-0 PMID: 30872600

Cherukuri, S. P., Kaur, A., Goyal, B., Kukunoor, H. R., Sahito, A. F., Sachdeva, P., Yerrapragada, G., Elangovan, P., Shariff, M. N., Natarajan, T., Janarthanan, J., Richard, S., Pallikaranai Venkatesaprasath, S., Karuppiah, S. S., Iyer, V. N., Helgeson, S. A., & Arunachalam, S. P. (2025). Artificial Intelligence-Enhanced Liquid Biopsy and Radiomics in Early-Stage Lung Cancer Detection: A Precision Oncology Paradigm. *Cancers (Basel)*, *17*(19), 3165. DOI: 10.3390/cancers17193165 PMID: 41097693

Chhikara, B. S., & Parang, K. (2023). Global Cancer Statistics 2022: the trends projection analysis. *Chemical biology letters, 10*(1), 451-451.

Chiu, P. K., Alberts, A. R., Venderbos, L. D. F., Bangma, C. H., Roobol, M. J., & Ng, C. F. (2017). Additional benefit of using a risk-based selection for prostate biopsy: An analysis of biopsy complications in the Rotterdam section of the European Randomized Study of Screening for Prostate Cancer. *BJU International*, *120*(3), 394–400. DOI: 10.1111/bju.13913 PMID: 28498624

Clark, A. R. (2022). Half a century of technological advances in pulmonary drug delivery: A personal perspective. *Frontiers in Drug Delivery*, *2*, 871147. DOI: 10.3389/fddev.2022.871147

Codlin, A. J., Vo, L. N. Q., Dao, T. P., Forse, R. J., Dang, H. T. M., Nguyen, L. H., Nguyen, H. B., Dinh, L. V., Annerstedt, K. S., Lundin, J., & Lönnroth, K. (2025). Comparison of different Lunit INSIGHT CXR software versions when reading chest radiographs for tuberculosis. *PLOS Digital Health*, *4*(4), e0000813. DOI: 10.1371/journal.pdig.0000813 PMID: 40233023

Computer aided detection of tuberculosis on chest radiographs: An evaluation of the CAD4TB v6 system | Scientific Reports. (n.d.). Retrieved May 28, 2026, from https://www.nature.com/articles/s41598-020-62148-y

Cooper, M., Ji, Z., & Krishnan, R. G. (2023). Machine learning in computational histopathology: Challenges and opportunities. *Genes, Chromosomes & Cancer*, *62*(9), 540–556. DOI: 10.1002/gcc.23177 PMID: 37314068

Coudray, N., Ocampo, P. S., Sakellaropoulos, T., Narula, N., Snuderl, M., Fenyö, D., Moreira, A. L., Razavian, N., & Tsirigos, A. (2018). Classification and mutation prediction from non-small cell lung cancer histopathology images using deep learning. *Nature Medicine*, *24*(10), 1559–1567. DOI: 10.1038/s41591-018-0177-5 PMID: 30224757

D'amato, G., Vitale, C., De Martino, A., Viegi, G., Lanza, M., Molino, A., Sanduzzi, A., Vatrella, A., Annesi-Maesano, I., & D'amato, M. (2015). Effects on asthma and respiratory allergy of Climate change and air pollution. *Multidisciplinary Respiratory Medicine*, *10*(1), 1–8. PMID: 26697186

Daghistani, T., & Alshammari, R. (2020). Comparison of statistical logistic regression and random forest machine learning techniques in predicting diabetes. *Journal of Advances in Information Technology*, *11*(2), 78–83. DOI: 10.12720/jait.11.2.78-83

Danker-Hopfe, H., Anderer, P., Zeitlhofer, J., Boeck, M., Dorn, H., Gruber, G., Heller, E., Loretz, E., Moser, D., Parapatics, S., Saletu, B., Schmidt, A., & Dorffner, G. (2009). Interrater reliability for sleep scoring according to the Rechtschaffen & Kales and the new AASM standard. *Journal of Sleep Research*, *18*(1), 74–84. DOI: 10.1111/j.1365-2869.2008.00700.x PMID: 19250176

Dasgupta, S. (2024). Next-generation cancer phenomics: A transformative approach to unraveling lung cancer complexity and advancing precision medicine. *OMICS: A Journal of Integrative Biology*, *28*(12), 585–595. DOI: 10.1089/omi.2024.0175 PMID: 39435580

Das, N., Happaerts, S., Gyselinck, I., Staes, M., Derom, E., Brusselle, G., Burgos, F., Contoli, M., Dinh-Xuan, A. T., Franssen, F. M. E., Gonem, S., Greening, N., Haenebalcke, C., Man, W. D.-C., Moisés, J., Peché, R., Poberezhets, V., Quint, J. K., Steiner, M. C., & Janssens, W. (2023). Collaboration between explainable artificial intelligence and pulmonologists improves the accuracy of pulmonary function test interpretation. *The European Respiratory Journal*, *61*(5), 2201720. DOI: 10.1183/13993003.01720-2022 PMID: 37080566

Davri, A., Birbas, E., Kanavos, T., Ntritsos, G., Giannakeas, N., Tzallas, A. T., & Batistatou, A. (2023). Deep learning for lung cancer diagnosis, prognosis and prediction using histological and cytological images: A systematic review. *Cancers (Basel)*, *15*(15), 3981. DOI: 10.3390/cancers15153981 PMID: 37568797

De Zambotti, M., Goldstein, C., Cook, J. D., Menghini, L., Altini, M., Cheng, P., & Robillard, R. (2023). State of the science and recommendations for using wearable technology in sleep and circadian research. *Sleep (Basel)*, *47*(4), zsad325. Advance online publication. DOI: 10.1093/sleep/zsad325 PMID: 38149978

Deep learning-based algorithm for automatic detection of incidental pulmonary embolism on contrast-enhanced CT: a multicenter multivendor study | Radiology Advances | Oxford Academic. (n.d.). Retrieved January 31, 2026, from https://academic.oup.com/radadv/article/2/4/umaf021/8171918?login=false

Demrozi, F., Borzì, L., & Olmo, G. (2023). Wearable sensors for supporting diagnosis, prognosis, and monitoring of neurodegenerative diseases. *Electronics (Basel)*, *12*(6), 1269. DOI: 10.3390/electronics12061269

Deng, J., Yang, Z., Ojima, I., Samaras, D., & Wang, F. (2022). Artificial intelligence in drug discovery: Applications and techniques. *Briefings in Bioinformatics*, *23*(1), bbab430. DOI: 10.1093/bib/bbab430 PMID: 34734228

Depeursinge, A., Vargas, A., Platon, A., Geissbuhler, A., Poletti, P. A., & Müller, H. (2012). BuInterstitial Lung Diseases in a reference multimedia database for interstitial lung diseases. *Computerized Medical Imaging and Graphics*, *36*(3), 227–238. DOI: 10.1016/j.compmedimag.2011.07.003 PMID: 21803548

Depner, C. M., Cheng, P. C., Devine, J. K., Khosla, S., De Zambotti, M., Robillard, R., Vakulin, A., & Drummond, S. P. A. (2020). Wearable technologies for developing sleep and circadian biomarkers: A summary of workshop discussions. *Sleep (Basel)*, *43*(2), zsz254. Advance online publication. DOI: 10.1093/sleep/zsz254 PMID: 31641776

Dixon, D., Sattar, H., Moros, N., Kesireddy, S. R., Ahsan, H., Lakkimsetti, M., Fatima, M., Doshi, D., Sadhu, K., & Junaid Hassan, M. (2024, May 9). (n.d.). Unveiling the Influence of AI Predictive Analytics on Patient Outcomes: A Comprehensive Narrative Review. *Cureus*, *16*(5), e59954. DOI: 10.7759/cureus.59954 PMID: 38854327

Dong, X., Li, M., Zhou, P., Deng, X., Li, S., Zhao, X., Wu, Y., Qin, J., & Guo, W. (2022). Fusing pre-trained convolutional neural networks features for multi-differentiated subtypes of liver cancer on histopathological images. *BMC Medical Informatics and Decision Making*, *22*(1), 122. DOI: 10.1186/s12911-022-01798-6 PMID: 35509058

Doshi-Velez, F., & Kim, B. (2017). Towards a rigorous science of interpretable machine learning. arXiv preprint arXiv:1702.08608. https://arxiv.org/abs/1702.08608

Dotolo, S., Marabotti, A., Facchiano, A., & Tagliaferri, R. (2021). A review on drug repurposing applicable to COVID-19. *Briefings in Bioinformatics*, *22*(2), 726–741. DOI: 10.1093/bib/bbaa288 PMID: 33147623

Du, Y., Yang, P., Liu, Y., Deng, C., & Li, X. (2025). Artificial intelligence in chronic disease self-management: Current applications and future directions. *Frontiers in Public Health*, *13*, 1689911. DOI: 10.3389/fpubh.2025.1689911 PMID: 41358250

Ebrahimian, S., Homayounieh, F., Rockenbach, M. A. B. C., Putha, P., Raj, T., Dayan, I., Bizzo, B. C., Buch, V., Wu, D., Kim, K., Li, Q., Digumarthy, S. R., & Kalra, M. K. (2021). Artificial intelligence matches subjective severity assessment of pneumonia for prediction of patient outcome and need for mechanical ventilation: A cohort study. *Scientific Reports, 11*(1), 858. DOI: 10.1038/s41598-020-79470-0 PMID: 33441578

Elbadawi, M., Li, H. X., Basit, A. W., & Gaisford, S. (2024). The role of artificial intelligence in generating original scientific research. *International Journal of Pharmaceutics, 652*, 652. DOI: 10.1016/j.ijpharm.2023.123741 PMID: 38181989

ElMoaqet, H., Eid, M., Glos, M., Ryalat, M., & Penzel, T. (2020, September 4). *Deep recurrent neural networks for automatic detection of sleep apnea from single channel respiration signals*. MDPI. https://www.mdpi.com/1424-8220/20/18/5037

Elsayed, B., Alksas, A., Shehata, M., Mahmoud, A., Zaky, M., Alghandour, R., Abdelwahab, K., Abdelkhalek, M., Ghazal, M., Contractor, S., El-Din Moustafa, H., & El-Baz, A. (2023). Exploring neoadjuvant chemotherapy, predictive models, radiomic, and pathological markers in breast cancer: A comprehensive review. *Cancers (Basel), 15*(21), 5288. DOI: 10.3390/cancers15215288 PMID: 37958461

Espie, C. A., Emsley, R., Kyle, S. D., Gordon, C., Drake, C. L., Siriwardena, A. N., Cape, J., Ong, J. C., Sheaves, B., Foster, R., Freeman, D., Costa-Font, J., Marsden, A., & Luik, A. I. (2019). Effect of digital cognitive behavioral therapy for insomnia on health, psychological well-being, and sleep-related quality of life: A randomized clinical trial. *JAMA Psychiatry, 76*(1), 21–30. DOI: 10.1001/jamapsychiatry.2018.2745 PMID: 30264137

Espie, C. A., Kyle, S. D., Williams, C., Ong, J. C., Douglas, N. J., Hames, P., & Brown, J. S. (2012). A randomized, placebo-controlled trial of online cognitive behavioral therapy for chronic insomnia disorder delivered via an automated media-rich web application. *Sleep (Basel), 35*(6), 769–781. DOI: 10.5665/sleep.1872 PMID: 22654196

Evans, M., & Emma, O. (2024). Enhancing Patient Outcomes through Context-Aware Healthcare Systems: A Comprehensive Study of Adaptive Technologies in Chronic Disease Management.

Evans, A. J., Vajpeyi, R., Henry, M., & Chetty, R. (2021). Establishment of a remote diagnostic histopathology service using whole slide imaging (digital pathology). *Journal of Clinical Pathology, 74*(7), 421–424. DOI: 10.1136/jclinpath-2020-206762 PMID: 32611763

Eze, V. I., Eboh, N. A., Abdulkareem, M. O., Jimoh, T. S., Olufemi, T. D., Nwekeoma, C. O., & Bejide, V. O. (2025). The Equity Impact of Digital Health and Artificial Intelligence Tools on Health Outcomes in Underserved Populations: A Narrative Review and Conceptual Model. *Journal of Life Science and Public Health, 1*(2), 90–102. DOI: 10.69739/jlsph.v1i2.1340

Farkas, D., Madarász, L., Nagy, Z. K., Antal, I., & Kállai-Szabó, N. (2021). Image analysis: A versatile tool in the manufacturing and quality control of pharmaceutical dosage forms. *Pharmaceutics, 13*(5), 685. DOI: 10.3390/pharmaceutics13050685 PMID: 34068724

Farrahi, V., & Rostami, M. (2024). Machine learning in physical activity, sedentary, and sleep behavior research. *Journal of Activity, Sedentary and Sleep Behaviors, 3*(1), 5. DOI: 10.1186/s44167-024-00045-9 PMID: 40217437

Fehr, J., Gunda, R., Siedner, M. J., Hanekom, W., Ndung'u, T., Grant, A., Lippert, C., & Wong, E. B. (2023). CAD4TB software updates: Different triaging thresholds require caution by users and regulation by authorities. *The International Journal of Tuberculosis and Lung Disease : the Official Journal of the International Union against Tuberculosis and Lung Disease, 27*(2), 157–160. DOI: 10.5588/ijtld.22.0437 PMID: 36853104

Felfli, M., Liu, Y., Zerka, F., Voyton, C., Thinnes, A., Jacques, S., Iannessi, A., & Bodard, S. (2023). Systematic review, meta-analysis and radiomics quality score assessment of CT radiomics-based models predicting tumor EGFR mutation status in patients with non-small-cell lung cancer. *International Journal of Molecular Sciences, 24*(14), 11433. DOI: 10.3390/ijms241411433 PMID: 37511192

Feng, Y., Wang, Y., Zeng, C., & Mao, H. (2021). Artificial intelligence and machine learning in chronic airway diseases: Focus on asthma and chronic obstructive pulmonary disease. *International Journal of Medical Sciences, 18*(13), 2871–2889. DOI: 10.7150/ijms.58191 PMID: 34220314

Ferkol, T., & Schraufnagel, D. (2014). The global burden of respiratory disease. *Annals of the American Thoracic Society, 11*(3), 404–406. DOI: 10.1513/AnnalsATS.201311-405PS PMID: 24673696

Feroz Khan, A., & Samad, S. (2024). Evaluating online learning adaptability in students using machine learning-based techniques: A novel analytical approach. *Educ. Sci. Manag, 2*(1), 25–34. DOI: 10.56578/esm020103

Finkelstein, J., & Jeong, I. C. (2017). Machine learning approaches to personalize early prediction of asthma exacerbations. *Annals of the New York Academy of Sciences, 1387*(1), 153–165. DOI: 10.1111/nyas.13218 PMID: 27627195

Fink, J. B., & Stapleton, K. W. (2024). Nebulizers. *Journal of Aerosol Medicine and Pulmonary Drug Delivery*, *37*(3), 140–156. DOI: 10.1089/jamp.2024.29110.jbf PMID: 38683652

Flaiban, E., Orhan, K., Gonçalves, B. C., Lopes, S. L. P. D. C., & Costa, A. L. F. (2025). Radiomics in Action: Multimodal Synergies for Imaging Biomarkers. *Bioengineering (Basel, Switzerland)*, *12*(11), 1139. DOI: 10.3390/bioengineering12111139 PMID: 41301095

Foguem, G. T., & Keleko, A. T. (2023). Artificial intelligence applied in pulmonary hypertension: A bibliometric analysis. *AI and Ethics*, *3*(4), 1063–1093. Advance online publication. DOI: 10.1007/s43681-023-00267-8 PMID: 37360147

Forde, P. M., Chaft, J. E., Smith, K. N., Anagnostou, V., Cottrell, T. R., Hellmann, M. D., Zahurak, M., Yang, S. C., Jones, D. R., Broderick, S., Battafarano, R. J., Velez, M. J., Rekhtman, N., Olah, Z., Naidoo, J., Marrone, K. A., Verde, F., Guo, H., Zhang, J., & Pardoll, D. M. (2018). Neoadjuvant PD-1 blockade in resectable lung cancer. *The New England Journal of Medicine*, *378*(21), 1976–1986. DOI: 10.1056/NEJMoa1716078 PMID: 29658848

Frauscher, B., Gabelia, D., Biermayr, M., Stefani, A., Hackner, H., Mitterling, T., Poewe, W., & Högl, B. (2014). Validation of an integrated software for the detection of rapid eye movement sleep behavior disorder. *Sleep (Basel)*, *37*(10), 1663–1671. DOI: 10.5665/sleep.4076 PMID: 25197814

Frauscher, B., Iranzo, A., Gaig, C., Gschliesser, V., Guaita, M., Raffelseder, V., Ehrmann, L., Sola, N., Salamero, M., Tolosa, E., Poewe, W., Santamaria, J., & Högl, B. (2012). Normative EMG values during REM sleep for the diagnosis of REM sleep behavior disorder. *Sleep (Basel)*, *35*(6), 835–847. DOI: 10.5665/sleep.1886 PMID: 22654203

Friedman, S. H., Long, K. J., Sexauer, S., Menon, A. A., & Kilb, E. F. (2024). Role of Artificial Intelligence in Assisting Pulmonary and Critical Care Clinical Decision-Making. *American Journal of Respiratory and Critical Care Medicine*, *210*(5), 662–664. DOI: 10.1164/rccm.202402-0331RR PMID: 38924771

Fu, F., Zhang, X., Wang, Z., Xie, L., Fu, M., Peng, J., Wu, J., Wang, Z., Guan, T., He, Y., Lin, J.-S., Zhu, L., & Dai, W. (2025). A pathology-attention multi-instance learning framework for multimodal classification of colorectal lesions. *Frontiers in Pharmacology*, *16*, 1592950. DOI: 10.3389/fphar.2025.1592950 PMID: 40548052

Gallifant, J., Zhang, J., Arias Lopez, M. D. P., Zhu, T., Camporota, L., Celi, L. A., & Formenti, F. (2022). Artificial intelligence for mechanical ventilation: Systematic review of design, reporting standards, and bias. *British Journal of Anaesthesia*, *128*(2), 343–351. DOI: 10.1016/j.bja.2021.09.025 PMID: 34772497

Gandrup, J., Ali, S. M., McBeth, J., van der Veer, S. N., & Dixon, W. G. (2020). Remote symptom monitoring integrated into electronic health records: A systematic review. *Journal of the American Medical Informatics Association : JAMIA*, *27*(11), 1752–1763. DOI: 10.1093/jamia/ocaa177 PMID: 32968785

Gates, A. J., Ke, Q., Varol, O., & Barabási, A. L. (2019). Nature's reach: Narrow work has broad impact. *Nature*, *575*(7781), 32–34. DOI: 10.1038/d41586-019-03308-7 PMID: 31695218

Georgakopoulou, V. E., Spandidos, D. A., & Corlateanu, A. (2025). Diagnostic tools in respiratory medicine. *Biomedical Reports*, *23*(1), 112. DOI: 10.3892/br.2025.1990 PMID: 40420977

George, M., & Bender, B. (2019). New insights to improve treatment adherence in asthma and COPD. *Patient Preference and Adherence*, *13*, 1325–1334. DOI: 10.2147/PPA.S209532 PMID: 31534319

Gershkovich, D. (2023). *Acute exacerbation of asthma*. University of Zagreb. School of Medicine.

Gillies, R. J., Kinahan, P. E., & Hricak, H. (2016). Radiomics: Images are more than pictures, they are data. *Radiology*, *278*(2), 563–577. DOI: 10.1148/radiol.2015151169 PMID: 26579733

Giri, P. C., Chowdhury, A. M., Bedoya, A., Chen, H., Lee, H. S., Lee, P., Henriquez, C., MacIntyre, N. R., & Huang, Y. C. T. (2021). Application of machine learning in pulmonary function assessment: Where are we now and where are we going? *Frontiers in Physiology*, *12*, 678540. DOI: 10.3389/fphys.2021.678540 PMID: 34248665

Gligorea, I., Cioca, M., Oancea, R., Gorski, A.-T., Gorski, H., & Tudorache, P. (2023). Adaptive learning using artificial intelligence in e-learning: A literature review. *Education Sciences*, *13*(12), 1216. DOI: 10.3390/educsci13121216

Goel, R., Moore, W., Sumer, B., Khan, S., Sher, D., & Subramaniam, R. M. (2017). Clinical practice in PET/CT for the management of head and neck squamous cell cancer. *AJR. American Journal of Roentgenology*, *209*(2), 289–303. DOI: 10.2214/AJR.17.18301 PMID: 28731808

Goldstein, C., Berry, R. B., Kent, D. T., Kristo, D. A., Seixas, A., Redline, S., & Westover, M. B. (2020). Artificial intelligence in sleep medicine: Background and implications for clinicians. *Journal of Clinical Sleep Medicine : JCSM : Official Publication of the American Academy of Sleep Medicine*, *16*(4), 609–618. DOI: 10.5664/jcsm.8388 PMID: 32065113

Gonda, I. (2000). The ascent of pulmonary drug delivery. *Journal of Pharmaceutical Sciences*, *89*(7), 940–945. DOI: 10.1002/1520-6017(200007)89:7<940::AID-JPS11>3.0.CO;2-B PMID: 10861595

Gonsard, A., Genet, M., & Drummond, D. (2024). Digital twins for chronic lung diseases. European Respiratory Review, 33(174), 240159. PMID: N/A. https://doi.org/DOI: 10.1183/16000617.0159-2024

Goto, T., Camargo, C. A.Jr, Faridi, M. K., Yun, B. J., & Hasegawa, K. (2018). Machine learning approaches for predicting disposition of asthma and COPD exacerbations in the ED. *The American Journal of Emergency Medicine*, *36*(9), 1650–1654. DOI: 10.1016/j.ajem.2018.06.062 PMID: 29970272

Gotta, J., Grünewald, L. D., Koch, V., Mahmoudi, S., Bernatz, S., Höhne, E., Biciusca, T., Gökduman, A., Wolfram, C., Booz, C., Scholtz, J.-E., Martin, S., Eichler, K., Gruber-Rouh, T., Bucher, A., Yel, I., Vogl, T. J., & Reschke, P. (2025). Implementation of AI in radiology: The perspective of referring physicians. *Insights Into Imaging*, *16*(1), 238. DOI: 10.1186/s13244-025-02120-4 PMID: 41174325

Gottlieb, D. J., & Punjabi, N. M. (2020). Diagnosis and management of obstructive sleep apnea. *Journal of the American Medical Association*, *323*(14), 1389–1400. DOI: 10.1001/jama.2020.3514 PMID: 32286648

Gould, M. K., Huang, B. Z., Tammemagi, M. C., Kinar, Y., & Shiff, R. (2021). Machine learning for early lung cancer identification using routine clinical and laboratory data. *American Journal of Respiratory and Critical Care Medicine*, *204*(4), 445–453. DOI: 10.1164/rccm.202007-2791OC PMID: 33823116

Grad-CAM: Visual Explanations from Deep Networks via Gradient-Based Localization | IEEE Conference Publication | IEEE Xplore. (n.d.). Retrieved March 2, 2026, from https://ieeexplore.ieee.org/document/8237336

Graña-Castro, O., Izquierdo, E., Piñas-Mesa, A., Menasalvas, E., & Chivato-Pérez, T. (2024). Assessing the impact of new technologies on managing chronic respiratory diseases. *Journal of Clinical Medicine*, *13*(22), 6913. DOI: 10.3390/jcm13226913 PMID: 39598056

Greenspan, H., Van Ginneken, B., & Summers, R. M. (2016). Guest editorial deep learning in medical imaging: Overview and future promise of an exciting new technique. *IEEE Transactions on Medical Imaging*, *35*(5), 1153–1159. DOI: 10.1109/TMI.2016.2553401

Groneberg, D. A., Witt, C., Wagner, U., Chung, K. F., & Fischer, A. (2003). Fundamentals of pulmonary drug delivery. *Respiratory Medicine*, *97*(4), 382–387. DOI: 10.1053/rmed.2002.1457 PMID: 12693798

Guitor, A. K., & Wright, G. D. (2018). Antimicrobial Resistance and Respiratory Infections. *Chest*, *154*(5), 1202–1212. DOI: 10.1016/j.chest.2018.06.019 PMID: 29959904

Guo, F., Capaldi, D., Kirby, M., Sheikh, K., Svenningsen, S., McCormack, D. G., Fenster, A., & Parraga, G. (2018). Development of a pulmonary imaging biomarker pipeline for phenotyping of chronic lung disease. *Journal of Medical Imaging (Bellingham, Wash.)*, *5*(2), 026002. DOI: 10.1117/1.JMI.5.2.026002 PMID: 29963580

Guo, Y., Li, T., Gong, B., Hu, Y., Wang, S., Yang, L., & Zheng, C. (2025). From Images to Genes: Radiogenomics Based on Artificial Intelligence to Achieve Non-Invasive Precision Medicine in Cancer Patients. *Advancement of Science*, *12*(2), 2408069. DOI: 10.1002/advs.202408069 PMID: 39535476

Hadweh, P., Niset, A., Salvagno, M., Al Barajraji, M., El Hadwe, S., Taccone, F. S., & Barrit, S. (2025). Machine learning and artificial intelligence in intensive care medicine: Critical recalibrations from rule-based systems to frontier models. *Journal of Clinical Medicine*, *14*(12), 4026. DOI: 10.3390/jcm14124026 PMID: 40565770

Haga, A., Takahashi, W., Aoki, S., Nawa, K., Yamashita, H., Abe, O., & Nakagawa, K. (2018). Classification of early stage non-small cell lung cancers on computed tomographic images into histological types using radiomic features: Interobserver delineation variability analysis. *Radiological Physics and Technology*, *11*(1), 27–35. DOI: 10.1007/s12194-017-0433-2 PMID: 29209915

Haixian, L., Shu, P., Zhao, L., Chunfeng, L., & Lun, L. (2025). Machine learning approaches for EGFR mutation status prediction in NSCLC: An updated systematic review. *Frontiers in Oncology*, *15*, 1576461. DOI: 10.3389/fonc.2025.1576461 PMID: 40708937

Halpin, D. M., Miravitlles, M., Metzdorf, N., & Celli, B. (2017). Impact and prevention of severe exacerbations of COPD: A review of the evidence. *International Journal of Chronic Obstructive Pulmonary Disease*, *12*, 2891–2908. DOI: 10.2147/COPD.S139470 PMID: 29062228

Handa, T. (2023). The potential role of artificial intelligence in the clinical practice of interstitial lung disease. *Respiratory Investigation*, *61*(6), 702–710. DOI: 10.1016/j.resinv.2023.08.006 PMID: 37708636

Hanif, U., Vitrac, J., Marinho, P., Jennum, P., Gozal, D., Mignot, E., & Elbaz, M. (2026). Rethinking CPAP adherence with artificial intelligence. *Sleep (Basel)*, •••, zsag097. Advance online publication. DOI: 10.1093/sleep/zsag097 PMID: 41947377

Hanna, M. G., Pantanowitz, L., Jackson, B., Palmer, O., Visweswaran, S., Pantanowitz, J., Deebajah, M., & Rashidi, H. H. (2025). Ethical and bias considerations in artificial intelligence/machine learning. *Modern Pathology*, *38*(3), 100686. DOI: 10.1016/j.modpat.2024.100686 PMID: 39694331

Hao, L., Wang, C., Che, J., Sun, M., & Wang, Y. (2025). Deep learning-based time series prediction in multispectral and hyperspectral imaging for cancer detection. *Frontiers in Medicine*, *12*, 1605865. DOI: 10.3389/fmed.2025.1605865 PMID: 40823576

Hao, Y., Cheng, C., Li, J., Li, H., Di, X., Zeng, X., Jin, S., Han, X., Liu, C., Wang, Q., Luo, B., Zeng, X., & Li, K. (2025). Multimodal integration in health care: Development with applications in disease management. *Journal of Medical Internet Research*, *27*, e76557. DOI: 10.2196/76557 PMID: 40840463

Harandi, H., Shafaati, M., Salehi, M., Roozbahani, M. M., Mohammadi, K., Akbarpour, S., Rahimnia, R., Hassanpour, G., Rahmani, Y., & Seifi, A. (2025). Artificial intelligence-driven approaches in antibiotic stewardship programs and optimizing prescription practices: A systematic review. *Artificial Intelligence in Medicine*, *162*, 103089. DOI: 10.1016/j.artmed.2025.103089 PMID: 39955846

Harrer, S., Shah, P., Antony, B., & Hu, J. Y. (2019). Artificial intelligence for clinical trial design. *Trends in Pharmacological Sciences*, *40*(8), 577–591. DOI: 10.1016/j.tips.2019.05.005 PMID: 31326235

He, K., Gkioxari, G., Dollár, P., & Girshick, R. (2020). Mask R-CNN. *IEEE Transactions on Pattern Analysis and Machine Intelligence*, *42*(2), 386–397. DOI: 10.1109/TPAMI.2018.2844175 PMID: 29994331

Hellmann, M. D., Chaft, J. E., William, W. N.Jr, Rusch, V., Pisters, K. M., Kalhor, N., Pataer, A., Travis, W. D., Swisher, S. G., & Kris, M. G. (2014). Pathological response after neoadjuvant chemotherapy in resectable non-small-cell lung cancer: Proposal for the use of major pathological response as a surrogate endpoint. *The Lancet. Oncology*, *15*(1), e42–e50. DOI: 10.1016/S1470-2045(13)70334-6 PMID: 24384493

He, S., Gui, J., Xiong, K., Chen, M., Gao, H., & Fu, Y. (2022). A roadmap to pulmonary delivery strategies for the treatment of infectious lung diseases. *Journal of Nanobiotechnology*, *20*(1), 101. DOI: 10.1186/s12951-022-01307-x PMID: 35241085

Hoffmann, T., Teichgräber, U., Lassen-Schmidt, B., Renz, D., Brüheim, L. B., Weise, T., Krämer, M., Böttcher, J., Güttler, F., Wolf, G., & Pfeil, A. (2025). AI-based HRCT quantification reveals DLCO and TLC as key determinants of ILD severity in connective tissue diseases. *RMD Open*, *11*(4), e005963. DOI: 10.1136/rmdopen-2025-005963 PMID: 41151842

Holt, K. L. (2025). Predictive Modeling of Occupational Exposure Using Machine Learning and Environmental Sensor Data. *Journal of Exceptional Multidisciplinary Research*, *2*(1), 82–89. DOI: 10.69739/jemr.v2i1.617

Hosny, A., Parmar, C., Quackenbush, J., Schwartz, L. H., & Aerts, H. J. W. L. (2018). Artificial intelligence in radiology. *Nature Reviews. Cancer*, *18*(8), 500–510. DOI: 10.1038/s41568-018-0016-5 PMID: 29777175

Huang, S. C., Pareek, A., Seyyedi, S., Banerjee, I., & Lungren, M. P. (2020). Fusion of medical imaging and electronic health records using deep learning: A systematic review and implementation guidelines. *NPJ Digital Medicine*, *3*(1), 136. DOI: 10.1038/s41746-020-00341-z PMID: 33083571

Huang, Y. Q., Liang, C. H., He, L., Tian, J., Liang, C. S., Chen, X., Ma, Z. L., & Liu, Z. Y. (2016). Development and validation of a radiomics nomogram for preoperative prediction of lymph node metastasis in colorectal cancer. *Journal of Clinical Oncology*, *34*(18), 2157–2164. DOI: 10.1200/JCO.2015.65.9128 PMID: 27138577

Huang, Y., Ai, L., Wang, X., Sun, Z., & Wang, F. (2022). Review and Updates on the Diagnosis of Tuberculosis. *Journal of Clinical Medicine*, *11*(19), 5826. DOI: 10.3390/jcm11195826 PMID: 36233689

Huang, Y., Li, Q., Chen, H., Zhou, X., Han, Q., Lu, H., Cui, N., & Cao, Q. (2025). A novel approach to integrating Vision Transformers and machine learning for robust lung nodule classification using CT imaging. *Journal of Radiation Research and Applied Sciences*, *18*(3), 101672. DOI: 10.1016/j.jrras.2025.101672

Hussain, D., Al-Masni, M. A., Aslam, M., Sadeghi-Niaraki, A., Hussain, J., Gu, Y. H., & Naqvi, R. A. (2024). Revolutionizing tumor detection and classification in multimodality imaging based on deep learning approaches: Methods, applications and limitations. *Journal of X-Ray Science and Technology*, *32*(4), 857–911. DOI: 10.3233/XST-230429 PMID: 38701131

Hussain, H. K., Tariq, A., Gill, A. Y., & Ahmad, A. (2022). Transforming healthcare: The rapid rise of artificial intelligence revolutionizing healthcare applications. *BULLET: Jurnal Multidisiplin Ilmu, 1*(02), 592216.

Hwang, E. J., Jeong, W. G., David, P. M., Arentz, M., Ruhwald, M., & Yoon, S. H. (2024). AI for detection of tuberculosis: implications for global health. Radiology: Artificial Intelligence, 6(2), e230327.

Ibrahim, A., Lashen, A., Toss, M., Mihai, R., & Rakha, E. (2022). Assessment of mitotic activity in breast cancer: Revisited in the digital pathology era. *Journal of Clinical Pathology, 75*(6), 365–372. DOI: 10.1136/jclinpath-2021-207742 PMID: 34556501

Integrative Physiology of Pneumonia | Physiological Reviews | American Physiological Society. (n.d.). Retrieved May 28, 2026, from https://journals.physiology.org/doi/full/10.1152/physrev.00032.2017

Islam, M. T., Al Mamun, M. A., Khan, O. U., Akeem, A. B., Mohammad, H., Hamdache, A., & Elmouki, I. (2024). Emerging Trends In Artificial Intelligence Learning Methods: Deep Learning And Machine Learning Innovation In Computer Science. *Nanotechnology Perceptions, 20*(13), 1150–1173. DOI: 10.62441/nano-ntp.vi.2598

Jahrami, H., Husain, W., Trabelsi, K., Penzel, T., Hirshkowitz, M., Razjouyan, J., BaHammam, A. S., & Sharafkhaneh, A. (2025). Artificial intelligence and sleep medicine II: A scoping review of applications, advancements, and future directions. *Sleep Medicine Reviews, 85*, 102212. DOI: 10.1016/j.smrv.2025.102212 PMID: 41330180

Jaime, F. J., Muñoz, A., Rodríguez-Gómez, F., & Jerez-Calero, A. (2023). Strengthening privacy and data security in biomedical microelectromechanical systems by IoT communication security and protection in smart healthcare. *Sensors (Basel), 23*(21), 8944. DOI: 10.3390/s23218944 PMID: 37960646

Jaroensri, R., Wulczyn, E., Hegde, N., Brown, T., Flament-Auvigne, I., Tan, F., Cai, Y., Nagpal, K., Rakha, E. A., Dabbs, D. J., Olson, N., Wren, J. H., Thompson, E. E., Seetao, E., Robinson, C., Miao, M., Beckers, F., Corrado, G. S., Peng, L. H., & Chen, P. H. C. (2022). Deep learning models for histologic grading of breast cancer and association with disease prognosis. *NPJ Breast Cancer, 8*(1), 113. DOI: 10.1038/s41523-022-00478-y PMID: 36192400

Jayaratne, M., Nallaperuma, D., De Silva, D., Alahakoon, D., Devitt, B., Webster, K. E., & Chilamkurti, N. (2019). A data integration platform for patient-centered e-healthcare and clinical decision support. *Future Generation Computer Systems, 92*, 996–1008. DOI: 10.1016/j.future.2018.07.061

Jayatunga, M. K., Xie, W., Ruder, L., Schulze, U., & Meier, C. (2022). AI in small-molecule drug discovery: A coming wave. *Nature Reviews. Drug Discovery*, *21*(3), 175–176. DOI: 10.1038/d41573-022-00025-1 PMID: 35132242

Jiang, J., Lu, A., Ma, X., Ouyang, D., & Williams, R. O.III. (2023). The applications of machine learning to predict the forming of chemically stable amorphous solid dispersions prepared by hot-melt extrusion. *International Journal of Pharmaceutics: X*, *5*, 100164. DOI: 10.1016/j.ijpx.2023.100164 PMID: 36798832

Jiang, J., Ma, X., Ouyang, D., & Williams, R. O.III. (2022). Emerging artificial intelligence (AI) technologies used in the development of solid dosage forms. *Pharmaceutics*, *14*(11), 2257. DOI: 10.3390/pharmaceutics14112257 PMID: 36365076

Jiang, W., Zhang, H., Li, Z., Jiang, X., Shao, J., Yang, X., Xiong, J., Zhou, P., Zhang, H., Wang, H., Yu, J., Su, X., Wang, Y., Liu, J., & Li, Z. (2025). AI-Powered Chest X-Ray for Diagnosing Pulmonary Tuberculosis in County and Township Health Care Facilities in Yichang: Retrospective, Real-World Study. *Journal of Medical Internet Research*, *27*, e83041. DOI: 10.2196/83041 PMID: 41328508

JMIR Bioinformatics and Biotechnology—Use of Artificial Intelligence in the Search for New Information Through Routine Laboratory Tests: Systematic Review. (n.d.). Retrieved May 28, 2026, from https://bioinform.jmir.org/2022/1/e40473

Joeris, A., Zhu, T. Y., Lambert, S., Wood, A., & Jayakumar, P. (2023). Real-world patient data: Can they support decision making and patient engagement? *Injury*, *54*, S51–S56. DOI: 10.1016/j.injury.2021.12.012 PMID: 34949460

Jones, B. E., Jones, J., Bewick, T., Lim, W. S., Aronsky, D., Brown, S. M., Boersma, W. G., van der Eerden, M. M., & Dean, N. C. (2011). CURB-65 Pneumonia Severity Assessment Adapted for Electronic Decision Support. *Chest*, *140*(1), 156–163. DOI: 10.1378/chest.10-1296 PMID: 21163875

Jyothi, P., & Singh, A. R. (2023). Deep learning models and traditional automated techniques for brain tumor segmentation in MRI: A review. *Artificial Intelligence Review*, *56*(4), 2923–2969. DOI: 10.1007/s10462-022-10245-x

Kamrul, S. M., Jobair, H. F. M., Bofan, H., Cheng, J. Q., & Huanying, G. (2025). Multimodal Models in Healthcare: Methods, Challenges, and Future Directions for Enhanced Clinical Decision Support. *Information (Basel)*, *16*(11), 971. DOI: 10.3390/info16110971

Kanchepu, N. (2025). Unveiling the Black Box: The Crucial Role of Interpretability in Machine Learning Models. In *Cutting-Edge Solutions for Advancing Sustainable Development: Exploring Technological Horizons for Sustainability-Part 1* (pp. 22-44). Bentham Science Publishers.

Kaplan, A., Cao, H., FitzGerald, J. M., Iannotti, N., Yang, E., Kocks, J. W., Kostikas, K., Price, D., Reddel, H. K., Tsiligianni, I., Vogelmeier, C. F., Pfister, P., & Mastoridis, P. (2021). Artificial intelligence/machine learning in respiratory medicine and potential role in asthma and COPD diagnosis. *The Journal of Allergy and Clinical Immunology. In Practice*, *9*(6), 2255–2261. DOI: 10.1016/j.jaip.2021.02.014 PMID: 33618053

Kasoju, N., Remya, N., Sasi, R., Sujesh, S., Soman, B., Kesavadas, C., Muraleedharan, C., Varma, P. H., & Behari, S. (2023). Digital health: Trends, opportunities and challenges in medical devices, pharma and bio-technology. *CSI Transactions on ICT*, *11*(1), 11–30. DOI: 10.1007/s40012-023-00380-3

Kerasidou, A. (2021). Ethics of artificial intelligence in global health: Explainability, algorithmic bias and trust. *Journal of Oral Biology and Craniofacial Research*, *11*(4), 612–614. DOI: 10.1016/j.jobcr.2021.09.004 PMID: 34567966

Khalifa, M., & Albadawy, M. (2024). Artificial Intelligence for Clinical Prediction: Exploring Key Domains and Essential Functions. *Computer Methods and Programs in Biomedicine Update*, *5*, 100148. DOI: 10.1016/j.cmpbup.2024.100148

Khan, A., Rauf, Z., Sohail, A., Khan, A. R., Asif, H., Asif, A., & Farooq, U. (2023). A survey of the vision transformers and their CNN-transformer based variants. *Artificial Intelligence Review*, *56*(3), 2917–2970. DOI: 10.1007/s10462-023-10595-0

Khemasuwan, D., Sorensen, J. S., & Colt, H. G. (2020). Artificial intelligence in pulmonary medicine: Computer vision, predictive model and COVID-19. *European Respiratory Review : an Official Journal of the European Respiratory Society*, *29*(157), 200181. DOI: 10.1183/16000617.0181-2020 PMID: 33004526

Khosravi, P., Kazemi, E., Imielinski, M., Elemento, O., & Hajirasouliha, I. (2018). Deep convolutional neural networks enable discrimination of heterogeneous digital pathology images. *EBioMedicine*, *27*, 317–328. DOI: 10.1016/j.ebiom.2017.12.026 PMID: 29292031

Kim, J.-C., & Chung, K. (2019). Prediction model of user physical activity using data characteristics-based long short-term memory recurrent neural networks. [TIIS]. *KSII Transactions on Internet and Information Systems*, *13*(4), 2060–2077.

Kim, Y., Kim, H., Choi, J., Cho, K., Yoo, D., Lee, Y., Park, S. J., Jeong, M. H., Jeong, S. H., Park, K. H., Byun, S.-Y., Kim, T., Ahn, S.-H., Cho, W. H., & Lee, N. (2023). Early prediction of need for invasive mechanical ventilation in the neonatal intensive care unit using artificial intelligence and electronic health records: A clinical study. *BMC Pediatrics, 23*(1), 525. Advance online publication. DOI: 10.1186/s12887-023-04350-1 PMID: 37872515

KNVC, L. (2024). FORMULATION AND EVALUATION OF PROPRANOLOL HYDROCHLORIDE FLOATING TABLETS BY 32 FACTORIAL DESIGN. *INTERNATIONAL JOURNAL, 14*(4), 1716-1721.

Kole, E., Jadhav, K., Shirsath, N., Dudhe, P., Verma, R. K., Chatterjee, A., & Naik, J. (2023). Nanotherapeutics for pulmonary drug delivery: An emerging approach to overcome respiratory diseases. *Journal of Drug Delivery Science and Technology, 81*, 104261. DOI: 10.1016/j.jddst.2023.104261

Korostin, O. (2025). Optimising machine learning integration in real-time text analytics platforms: Technical approaches and performance criteria. *COMPUTER-INTEGRATED TECHNOLOGIES: EDUCATION, SCIENCE. Production*, (58), 38–45.

Kothinti, R. R.Rishi Reddy Kothinti. (2024). Deep learning in healthcare: Transforming disease diagnosis, personalized treatment, and clinical decision-making through AI-driven innovations. *World J Adv Res Rev, 24*(2), 2841–2856. DOI: 10.30574/wjarr.2024.24.2.3435

Krauss, C., Do, X. A., & Huck, N. (2017). Deep neural networks, gradient-boosted trees, random forests: Statistical arbitrage on the S&P 500. *European Journal of Operational Research, 259*(2), 689–702. DOI: 10.1016/j.ejor.2016.10.031

Labaki, W. W., Martinez, C. H., Martinez, F. J., Galbán, C. J., Ross, B. D., Washko, G. R., Barr, R. G., Regan, E. A., Coxson, H. O., Hoffman, E. A., Newell, J. D.Jr, Curran-Everett, D., Hogg, J. C., Crapo, J. D., Lynch, D. A., Kazerooni, E. A., & Han, M. K. (2017). The role of chest computed tomography in the evaluation and management of the patient with chronic obstructive pulmonary disease. *American Journal of Respiratory and Critical Care Medicine, 196*(11), 1372–1379. DOI: 10.1164/rccm.201703-0451PP PMID: 28661698

Labarere, J., Bertrand, R., & Fine, M. J. (2014). How to derive and validate clinical prediction models for use in intensive care medicine. *Intensive Care Medicine, 40*(4), 513–527. DOI: 10.1007/s00134-014-3227-6 PMID: 24570265

Lai, G., Chang, W.-C., Yang, Y., & Liu, H. (2018). Modeling long-and short-term temporal patterns with deep neural networks. The 41st international ACM SIGIR conference on research & development in information retrieval, Levy, J. I., Quirós-Alcalá, L., Fabian, M. P., Basra, K., & Hansel, N. N. (2018). Established and emerging environmental contributors to disparities in asthma and chronic obstructive pulmonary disease. *Current Epidemiology Reports*, *5*(2), 114–124. PMID: 30319934

Lambin, P., Rios-Velazquez, E., Leijenaar, R., Carvalho, S., van Stiphout, R. G., Granton, P., Zegers, C. M., Gillies, R., Boellard, R., Dekker, A., & Aerts, H. J. (2012). Radiomics: Extracting more information from medical images using advanced feature analysis. *European Journal of Cancer*, *48*(4), 441–446. DOI: 10.1016/j.ejca.2011.11.036 PMID: 22257792

Lavorini, F., Pistolesi, M., & Usmani, O. S. (2017). Recent advances in capsule-based dry powder inhaler technology. *Multidisciplinary Respiratory Medicine*, *12*, 1–7. DOI: 10.4081/mrm.2017.236

Lee, G., Park, H., Bak, S. H., & Lee, H. Y. (2020). Radiomics in Lung Cancer from Basic to Advanced: Current Status and Future Directions. *Korean Journal of Radiology*, *21*(2), 159–171. DOI: 10.3348/kjr.2019.0630 PMID: 31997591

Lee, J. H., Sun, H. Y., Park, S., Kim, H., Hwang, E. J., Goo, J. M., & Park, C. M. (2020). Performance of a deep learning algorithm compared with radiologic interpretation for lung cancer detection on chest radiographs in a health screening population. *Radiology*, *297*(3), 687–696. DOI: 10.1148/radiol.2020201240 PMID: 32960729

Leelavati, T. S.. (2023). Revolutionizing healthcare delivery: Telemedicine's influence on access and patient satisfaction. *International Journal of Chemical and Biochemical Science*, *24*(5), 106–115.

Leelavati, T. S., Madhavi, S., & Aminabee, S. (2025). Fostering ethical decision-making skills in pharmaceutical education: Vital for future pharmacists. *Indian Journal of Pharmaceutical Education and Research*, *59*(2), 433–440. DOI: 10.5530/ijper.20254872

Leelavati, T. S., Madhavi, S., Susmitha, K., Kumar, K. S. V., Goud, P. V. P., & Raju, K. G. (2023). Exploring university student attitudes, beliefs, and alcohol usage patterns: An investigation into alcohol and drug use within the student lifestyle. *Journal of Drug and Alcohol Research*, *12*(6).

Lee, M. (2023). Recent advancements in deep learning using whole slide imaging for cancer prognosis. *Bioengineering (Basel, Switzerland)*, *10*(8), 897. DOI: 10.3390/bioengineering10080897 PMID: 37627783

Lennerz, J. K., Salgado, R., Kim, G. E., Sirintrapun, S. J., Thierauf, J. C., Singh, A., Indave, I., Bard, A., Weissinger, S. E., Heher, Y. K., de Baca, M. E., Cree, I. A., Bennett, S., Carobene, A., Ozben, T., & Ritterhouse, L. L. (2023). Diagnostic quality model (DQM): An integrated framework for the assessment of diagnostic quality when using AI/ML. [CCLM]. *Clinical Chemistry and Laboratory Medicine*, *61*(4), 544–557. DOI: 10.1515/cclm-2022-1151 PMID: 36696602

Levenson, A. R., Morales Nebreda, L., Alexander, M. J., & Schroedl, C. J. (2020). Harnessing machine learning to improve patient outcomes in pulmonary and critical care medicine. *American Journal of Respiratory and Critical Care Medicine*, *202*(1), 30–39. DOI: 10.1164/rccm.201912-2486RR PMID: 32752881

Liang, Z., Ni, R., Zhou, J., & Mao, S. (2015). Recent advances in controlled pulmonary drug delivery. *Drug Discovery Today*, *20*(3), 380–389. DOI: 10.1016/j.drudis.2014.09.020 PMID: 25281854

Li, S., Yue, R., Lu, S., Luo, J., Wu, X., Zhang, Z., Liu, M., Fan, Y., Zhang, Y., Pan, C., Huang, X., & He, H. (2025). Artificial intelligence and machine learning in acute respiratory distress syndrome management: Recent advances. *Frontiers in Medicine*, *12*, 1597556. DOI: 10.3389/fmed.2025.1597556 PMID: 40740956

Litjens, G., Kooi, T., Bejnordi, B. E., Setio, A. A. A., Ciompi, F., Ghafoorian, M., van der Laak, J. A. W. M., van Ginneken, B., & Sánchez, C. I. (2017). A survey on deep learning in medical image analysis. *Medical Image Analysis*, *42*, 60–88. DOI: 10.1016/j.media.2017.07.005 PMID: 28778026

Liu, Z., Lin, Y., Cao, Y., Hu, H., Wei, Y., Zhang, Z., . . . Guo, B. (2021). Swin transformer: Hierarchical vision transformer using shifted windows. In Proceedings of the IEEE/CVF international conference on computer vision (pp. 10012-10022).

Liu, D., Pang, Z., & Lloyd, S. (2008). A neural network method for detection of obstructive sleep apnea and narcolepsy based on pupil size and EEG. *IEEE Transactions on Neural Networks*, *19*(2), 308–318. DOI: 10.1109/TNN.2007.908634 PMID: 18269961

Liu, S., Xu, Q., Xu, Z., Liu, Z., Sun, X., Xie, G., Feng, M., & See, K. C. (2024). Reinforcement learning to optimize ventilator settings for patients on invasive mechanical ventilation: Retrospective study. *Journal of Medical Internet Research*, *26*, e44494. DOI: 10.2196/44494 PMID: 39219230

Liu, Y., Stojadinovic, S., Hrycushko, B., Wardak, Z., Lau, S., Lu, W., Yan, Y., Jiang, S. B., Jia, X., Wang, X., & Gu, X. (2017). A deep convolutional neural network-based automatic delineation strategy for multiple brain metastases stereotactic radiosurgery. *PLoS One*, *12*(10), e0185844. DOI: 10.1371/journal.pone.0185844 PMID: 28985229

Liu, Z. Y., Zhang, X. Y., Shi, Y. J., Wang, L., Zhu, H. T., Tang, Z. C., Wang, S., Li, X. T., Tian, J., & Sun, Y. S. (2017). Radiomics analysis for evaluation of pathological complete response to neoadjuvant chemoradiotherapy in locally advanced rectal cancer. *Clinical Cancer Research, 23*(23), 7253–7262. DOI: 10.1158/1078-0432.CCR-17-1038 PMID: 28939744

Li, W., Milletari, F., Xu, D., Rieke, N., Hancox, J., Zhu, W., Baust, M., Cheng, Y., Ourselin, S., Cardoso, M. J., & Feng, A. (2019). *Privacy-Preserving Federated Brain Tumour Segmentation.*, DOI: 10.1007/978-3-030-32692-0_16

Li, X. M., Nguyen, T., Sparks, H. D., Sung, K., & Chiang, J. (2025). Quantitative Dynamic Contrast-Enhanced Magnetic Resonance Imaging (DCE-MRI) in Hepatocellular Carcinoma: A Review of Emerging Applications for Locoregional Therapy. *Bioengineering (Basel, Switzerland), 12*(8), 870. DOI: 10.3390/bioengineering12080870 PMID: 40868383

Lococo, F., Ghaly, G., Flamini, S., Campanella, A., Chiappetta, M., Bria, E., Vita, E., Tortora, G., Evangelista, J., Sassorossi, C., Congedo, M. T., Valentini, V., Sala, E., Cesario, A., Margaritora, S., Boldrini, L., & Mohammed, A. (2024). Artificial intelligence applications in personalizing lung cancer management: State of the art and future perspectives. *Journal of Thoracic Disease, 16*(10), 7096–7110. DOI: 10.21037/jtd-24-244 PMID: 39552872

Lopez, R., Doukkali, A., Barateau, L., Evangelista, E., Chenini, S., Jaussent, I., & Dauvilliers, Y. (2017). Test-retest reliability of the multiple sleep latency test in central disorders of hypersomnolence. *Sleep (Basel), 40*(12), zsx164. Advance online publication. DOI: 10.1093/sleep/zsx164 PMID: 29099966

Low, C. A. (2020). Harnessing consumer smartphone and wearable sensors for clinical cancer research. npj. *Digital Medicine, 3*(1), 140. DOI: 10.1038/s41746-020-00351-x PMID: 33134557

Lucia, F., Visvikis, D., Desseroit, M. C., Miranda, O., Malhaire, J. P., Robin, P., Pradier, O., Hatt, M., & Schick, U. (2018). Prediction of outcome using pretreatment 18F-FDG PET/CT and MRI radiomics in locally advanced cervical cancer treated with chemoradiotherapy. *European Journal of Nuclear Medicine and Molecular Imaging, 45*(5), 768–786. DOI: 10.1007/s00259-017-3898-7 PMID: 29222685

Lundberg, S. M., & Lee, S.-I. (2017). A unified approach to interpreting model predictions. *Advances in Neural Information Processing Systems, 30*, 4765–4774.

Luo, X., Zeng, W., Tang, J., Liu, W., Yang, J., Chen, H., Jiang, L., Zhou, X., Huang, J., Zhang, S., Du, L., Shen, X., Chi, H., & Wang, H. (2024). Multi-modal transcriptomic analysis reveals metabolic dysregulation and immune responses in chronic obstructive pulmonary disease. *Scientific Reports*, *14*(1), 22699. DOI: 10.1038/s41598-024-71773-w PMID: 39349929

Machine Learning for Antimicrobial Resistance Prediction: Current Practice, Limitations, and Clinical Perspective | Clinical Microbiology Reviews. (n.d.). Retrieved May 28, 2026, from https://journals.asm.org/doi/full/10.1128/cmr.00179-21

MacLeod, M., Papi, A., Contoli, M., Beghé, B., Celli, B. R., Wedzicha, J. A., & Fabbri, L. M. (2021). Chronic obstructive pulmonary disease exacerbation fundamentals: Diagnosis, treatment, prevention and disease impact. *Respirology (Carlton, Vic.)*, *26*(6), 532–551. DOI: 10.1111/resp.14041 PMID: 33893708

Madhavi, S.. (2024). Unravelling the impact of alcohol use on college students' educational success: A systematic analysis. *Journal of Drug and Alcohol Research*, *13*(2), 1–5.

Magrabi, F., Ammenwerth, E., McNair, J. B., De Keizer, N. F., Hyppönen, H., Nykänen, P., Rigby, M., Scott, P. J., Vehko, T., Wong, Z. S.-Y., & Georgiou, A. (2019). Artificial intelligence in clinical decision support: Challenges for evaluating AI and practical implications. *Yearbook of Medical Informatics*, *28*(01), 128–134. DOI: 10.1055/s-0039-1677903 PMID: 31022752

Mahmood, S., Hasan, R., Hussain, S., & Adhikari, R. (2025). An Interpretable and Generalizable Machine Learning Model for Predicting Asthma Outcomes: Integrating AutoML and Explainable AI Techniques. *WORLD (Oakland, Calif.)*, *6*(1), 15. DOI: 10.3390/world6010015

Maleki, F., Muthukrishnan, N., Ovens, K., Reinhold, C., & Forghani, R. (2020). Machine learning algorithm validation: From essentials to advanced applications and implications for regulatory certification and deployment. *Neuroimaging Clinics of North America*, *30*(4), 433–445. DOI: 10.1016/j.nic.2020.08.004 PMID: 33038994

Mamalakis, M., Dwivedi, K., Sharkey, M., Alabed, S., Kiely, D., & Swift, A. J. (2023). A transparent artificial intelligence framework to assess lung disease in pulmonary hypertension. Scientific Reports, 13, 3812. PMID: N/A. https://doi.org/ DOI: 10.1038/s41598-023-30503-4

Mamdouh, D., Attia, M., Osama, M., Mohamed, N., Lotfy, A., Arafa, T., Rashed, E. A., & Khoriba, G. (2025). Advancements in Radiology Report Generation: A Comprehensive Analysis. *Bioengineering (Basel, Switzerland)*, *12*(7), 693. DOI: 10.3390/bioengineering12070693 PMID: 40722385

Mangal, S., Gao, W., Li, T. L., & Zhou, Q. (2017). Pulmonary delivery of nanoparticle chemotherapy for the treatment of lung cancers: Challenges and opportunities. *Acta Pharmacologica Sinica*, *38*(6), 782–797. DOI: 10.1038/aps.2017.34 PMID: 28504252

Manik, M. M. T. G., Hossain, S., Ahmed, M. K., Rozario, E., Miah, M. A., Moniruzzaman, M., & Saimon, A. S. M.Mia Md Tofayel Gonee Manik. (2022). Integrating genomic data and machine learning to advance precision oncology and targeted cancer therapies. *Nanotechnology Perceptions*, *18*(2), 219–243. DOI: 10.62441/nano-ntp.v18i2.5443

Mannumadam Venugopal, S. (2024). Can Vision Transformers Be the Next State-of-the-Art Model for Oncology Medical Image Analysis? *AI in Precision Oncology*, *1*(6), 286–305. DOI: 10.1089/aipo.2024.0023

Marinakis, I., Karampidis, K., & Papadourakis, G. (2024). Pulmonary nodule detection, segmentation and classification using deep learning: A comprehensive literature review. *BioMedInformatics*, *4*(3), 2043–2106. DOI: 10.3390/biomedinformatics4030111

Marouf, A. A., Rokne, J. G., & Alhajj, R. (2025). Integrating Multi-Omics and Medical Imaging in Artificial Intelligence-Based Cancer Research: An Umbrella Review of Fusion Strategies and Applications. *Cancers (Basel)*, *17*(22), 3638. DOI: 10.3390/cancers17223638 PMID: 41301005

Martell, M. B., Linton-Reid, K., Chen, M., & Aboagye, E. O. (2025). Radiomics for lung cancer diagnosis, management, and future prospects. *Clinical Radiology*, *86*, 106926. DOI: 10.1016/j.crad.2025.106926 PMID: 40344812

Martínez-García, M., & Hernández-Lemus, E. (2022). Data integration challenges for machine learning in precision medicine. *Frontiers in Medicine*, *8*, 784455. DOI: 10.3389/fmed.2021.784455 PMID: 35145977

Maslove, D. M., Elbers, P. W. G., & Clermont, G. (2021). Artificial intelligence in telemetry: What clinicians should know. *Intensive Care Medicine*, *47*(2), 150–153. DOI: 10.1007/s00134-020-06295-w PMID: 33386857

Masood, A., Naseem, U., & Razzak, I. (2023, April). Multi-scale swin transformer enabled automatic detection and segmentation of lung metastases using CT images. In 2023 IEEE 20th international symposium on biomedical imaging (ISBI) (pp. 1-5). IEEE. DOI: 10.1109/ISBI53787.2023.10230663

Mathias, N. R., & Hussain, M. A. (2010). Non-invasive systemic drug delivery: Developability considerations for alternate routes of administration. *Journal of Pharmaceutical Sciences*, *99*(1), 1–20. DOI: 10.1002/jps.21793 PMID: 19499570

Mathrani, A., Susnjak, T., Ramaswami, G., & Barczak, A. (2021). Perspectives on the challenges of generalizability, transparency and ethics in predictive learning analytics. *Computers and Education Open*, *2*, 100060. DOI: 10.1016/j.caeo.2021.100060

Matthew, B. (2025). Smart Inhalers and Respiratory IoTs for Asthma Management Gene.

May, C., Myall, M., Lund, S., Campling, N., Bogle, S., Dace, S., & Richardson, A. (2020). Managing patient preferences and clinical responses in acute pathophysiological deterioration: What do clinicians think treatment escalation plans do? *Social Science & Medicine*, *258*, 113143. DOI: 10.1016/j.socscimed.2020.113143 PMID: 32599414

May, S. M., & Li, J. T. (2015). Burden of chronic obstructive pulmonary disease: healthcare costs and beyond. Allergy and asthma proceedings, Mitta, N. R. (2021). AI-Based Personalized Therapeutic Monitoring Systems in Chronic Disease Management: Leveraging Machine Learning for Patient Adherence Prediction, Medication Optimization, and Real-Time Intervention. *Los Angeles Journal of Intelligent Systems and Pattern Recognition*, *1*, 190–228.

McCormack, M. C., Bascom, R., Brandt, M., Burgos, F., Butler, S., Caggiano, C., Dimmock, A. E. F., Fineberg, A., Goldstein, J., Guzman, F. C., Halldin, C. N., Johnson, J. D., Kerby, G. S., Krishnan, J. A., Kurth, L., Morgan, G., Mularski, R. A., Pasquale, C. B., Ryu, J., & Drummond, M. B. (2021). Electronic health records and pulmonary function data: Developing an interoperability roadmap. An official American Thoracic Society workshop report. *Annals of the American Thoracic Society*, *18*(1), 1–11. DOI: 10.1513/AnnalsATS.202010-1318ST PMID: 33385224

Meeradevi, T., Sasikala, S., Murali, L., Manikandan, N., & Ramaswamy, K. (2025). Lung cancer detection with machine learning classifiers with multi-attribute decision-making system and deep learning model. *Scientific Reports*, *15*(1), 8565. DOI: 10.1038/s41598-025-88188-w PMID: 40075131

Megat Ramli, P. N., Aizuddin, A. N., Ahmad, N., Abdul Hamid, Z., & Ismail, K. I. (2025). A Systematic Review: The Role of Artificial Intelligence in Lung Cancer Screening in Detecting Lung Nodules on Chest X-Rays. *Diagnostics (Basel)*, *15*(3), 246. DOI: 10.3390/diagnostics15030246 PMID: 39941176

Meissner, A. K., Gutsche, R., Galldiks, N., Kocher, M., Junger, S. T., Eich, M. L., Kessing, M., Ruge, M. I., Goldbrunner, R., & Lohmann, P. (2023). Radiomics for the non-invasive prediction of PD-L1 expression in patients with brain metastases secondary to non-small cell lung cancer. *Journal of Neuro-Oncology*, *163*(3), 597–605. DOI: 10.1007/s11060-023-04367-7 PMID: 37382806

Mei, X., Liu, Z., Singh, A., Lange, M., Boddu, P., Gong, J. Q. X., Lee, J., DeMarco, C., Cao, C., Platt, S., Sivakumar, G., Gross, B., Huang, M., Masseaux, J., Dua, S., Bernheim, A., Chung, M., Deyer, T., Jacobi, A., & Yang, Y. (2023). Interstitial lung disease diagnosis and prognosis using an AI system integrating longitudinal data. *Nature Communications*, *14*(1), 2272. DOI: 10.1038/s41467-023-37720-5 PMID: 37080956

Mekov, E., Miravitlles, M., & Petkov, R. (2020). Artificial intelligence and machine learning in respiratory medicine. *Expert Review of Respiratory Medicine*, *14*(6), 559–564. DOI: 10.1080/17476348.2020.1743181 PMID: 32166988

Michaud, C. M. (2009). Global Burden of Infectious Diseases. *Encyclopedia of Microbiology*, 444–454. DOI: 10.1016/B978-012373944-5.00185-1

Misseri, G., Piattoli, M., Cuttone, G., Gregoretti, C., & Bignami, E. G. (2024). Artificial intelligence for mechanical ventilation: A transformative shift in critical care. *Therapeutic Advances in Pulmonary and Critical Care Medicine*, *19*, 29768675241298918. Advance online publication. DOI: 10.1177/29768675241298918 PMID: 39534716

Mlodzinski, E., Stone, D. J., & Celi, L. A. (2020). Machine learning for pulmonary and critical care medicine: A narrative review. *Pulmonary Therapy*, *6*(1), 67–77. DOI: 10.1007/s41030-020-00110-z PMID: 32048244

Mo, Q., Cui, J., Jia, S., Zhang, Y., Xiao, Y., Liu, C., . . . Zhao, M. (2025). Stacking Ensemble Learning-based Models Enabling Accurate Diagnosis of Cardiac Amyloidosis using SPECT/CT: an International and Multicentre Study. medRxiv, 2025-06.

Mok, T. S. K., Wu, Y. L., Kudaba, I., Kowalski, D. M., Cho, B. C., Turna, H. Z., Castro, G.Jr, Srimuninnimit, V., Laktionov, K. K., Bondarenko, I., Kubota, K., Lubiniecki, G. M., Zhang, J., Kush, D., Lopes, G., Adamchuk, G., Ahn, M.-J., Alexandru, A., Altundag, O., & Zippelius, A.KEYNOTE-042 Investigators. (2019). Pembrolizumab versus chemotherapy for previously untreated, PD-L1-expressing, locally advanced or metastatic non-small-cell lung cancer (KEYNOTE-042): A randomised, open-label, controlled, phase 3 trial. *Lancet*, *393*(10183), 1819–1830. DOI: 10.1016/S0140-6736(18)32409-7 PMID: 30955977

Molfino, N. A., Turcatel, G., & Riskin, D. (2024). Machine learning approaches to predict asthma exacerbations: A narrative review. *Advances in Therapy*, *41*(2), 534–552. DOI: 10.1007/s12325-023-02743-3 PMID: 38110652

Mondal, R. S., Akter, L., & Bhuiyan, M. N. A. (2024). Artificial intelligence in drug development and delivery: Opportunities, challenges, and future directions. *Journal of Angiotherapy*, *8*(1), 1–10. DOI: 10.25163/angiotherapy.8810326

Mondal, R. S., Bhuiyan, M. N. A., & Akter, L. (2025). AI-driven innovations in cancer research and personalized healthcare. [Journal of Angiotherapy]. *Integrative Biomedical Research*, *9*(1), 1–10. DOI: 10.25163/angiotherapy.9110321

Moon, C., Smyth, H. D. C., Watts, A. B., & Williams, R. O.III. (2019). Delivery technologies for orally inhaled products: An update. *AAPS PharmSciTech*, *20*(3), 117. DOI: 10.1208/s12249-019-1314-2 PMID: 30783904

Moor, M., Banerjee, O., Abad, Z. S. H., Krumholz, H. M., Leskovec, J., Topol, E. J., & Rajpurkar, P. (2023). Foundation models for generalist medical artificial intelligence. *Nature*, *616*(7956), 259–265. DOI: 10.1038/s41586-023-05881-4 PMID: 37045921

Morin, C. M., & Jarrin, D. C. (2022). Epidemiology of insomnia: Prevalence, course, risk factors, and public health burden. *Sleep Medicine Clinics*, *17*(2), 173–191. DOI: 10.1016/j.jsmc.2022.03.003 PMID: 35659072

Moscalu, M., Moscalu, R., Dascălu, C. G., arcă, V., Cojocaru, E., Costin, I. M., arcă, E., & erban, I. L. (2023). Histopathological images analysis and predictive modeling implemented in digital pathology—Current affairs and perspectives. *Diagnostics (Basel)*, *13*(14), 2379. DOI: 10.3390/diagnostics13142379 PMID: 37510122

Muzny, M., Henriksen, A., Giordanengo, A., Muzik, J., Grøttland, A., Blixgård, H., Hartvigsen, G., & Årsand, E. (2020). Wearable sensors with possibilities for data exchange: Analyzing status and needs of different actors in mobile health monitoring systems. *International Journal of Medical Informatics*, *133*, 104017. DOI: 10.1016/j.ijmedinf.2019.104017 PMID: 31778885

Nagy, B., Galata, D. L., Farkas, A., & Nagy, Z. K. (2022). Application of artificial neural networks in the process analytical technology of pharmaceutical manufacturing—A review. *The AAPS Journal*, *24*(4), 74. DOI: 10.1208/s12248-022-00706-0 PMID: 35697951

Nahar, K., Hossain, M. Z., Islam, R., Khan, M. M., & Hossain, M. S. (2024). Operationalizing Predictive Modeling in Clinical Workflows: Design, Integration, and Validation of Decision Support Mechanisms within US Healthcare Infrastructure. *Frontiers in Computer Science and Artificial Intelligence*, *3*(2), 37–45. DOI: 10.32996/fcsai.2022.1.2.8

Nakajo, M., Hirahara, D., Hirahara, M., Eizuru, Y., Tani, A., Kanzaki, F., & Yoshiura, T. (2025). Artificial intelligence in oncological positron emission tomography: Advancing image analysis and interpretation. *Clinical Radiology*, •••, 107187. PMID: 41401681

National Academies of Sciences, Engineering, and Medicine. (2023). Advances in the diagnosis and evaluation of disabling physical health conditions. National Academies Press.

Navarro-Garcia, D., Marcos, A., Beets-Tan, R., Blomqvist, L., Bodalal, Z., Deandreis, D., Crispin-Ortuzar, M., Gallagher, F., Giandini, T., Graves, M. J., Lassau, N., Maier-Hein, K., Prelaj, A., Schader, P., Schlemmer, H.-P., Sedlaczek, O., Vaiani, M., & Perez-Lopez, R. (2025). Real-world radiology data for artificial intelligence-driven cancer support systems and biomarker development. *ESMO Real World Data and Digital Oncology*, *8*, 100120. DOI: 10.1016/j.esmorw.2025.100120 PMID: 41647703

Nayak, K., Kadavigere, R., Pendem, S., Mane, P. R., Sampathila, N., Pattath Sankaran, P., & Siddeshappa, N. (2026). Diagnostic Accuracy of Artificial Intelligence Models for Differentiation of Squamous Cell Carcinoma and Adenocarcinoma of Lung—A Systematic Review. *Diagnostics (Basel)*, *16*(3), 500. DOI: 10.3390/diagnostics16030500 PMID: 41681818

Newman, S. P. (2005). Principles of metered-dose inhaler design. *Respiratory Care*, *50*(9), 1177–1190. DOI: 10.4187/respcare.05501177 PMID: 16122401

Nguyen, H. T. T., Le-Quy, V., Dinh-Xuan, A. T., & Nguyen, L. N. (2026). Artificial Intelligence for Tuberculosis Screening and Detection: From Evidence to Policy and Implementation. *Diagnostics (Basel)*, *16*(8), 1127. DOI: 10.3390/diagnostics16081127 PMID: 42072753

Nguyen, P. L., Uddin, M. M., Mir, T., Khalil, A., Regmi, N., Pervaiz, A., Hussain, T., Babu, M. A., Ullah, I., Patel, P., Lohia, P., Saydain, G., Koul, P. A., & Soubani, A. O. (2021). Trends in incidence, and mortality of acute exacerbation of chronic obstructive pulmonary disease in the United States Emergency Department (2010–2018). *COPD*, *18*(5), 567–575. DOI: 10.1080/15412555.2021.1979500 PMID: 34530662

Nhat-Duc, H., & Van-Duc, T. (2023). Comparison of histogram-based gradient boosting classification machine, random Forest, and deep convolutional neural network for pavement raveling severity classification. *Automation in Construction, 148*, 104767. DOI: 10.1016/j.autcon.2023.104767

Nici, L., Mammen, M. J., Charbek, E., Alexander, P. E., Au, D. H., Boyd, C. M., Criner, G. J., Donaldson, G. C., Dreher, M., Fan, V. S., Gershon, A. S., Han, M. L. K., Krishnan, J. A., Martinez, F. J., Meek, P. M., Morgan, M., Polkey, M. I., Puhan, M. A., Sadatsafavi, M., & Aaron, S. D. (2020). Pharmacologic management of chronic obstructive pulmonary disease. An official American Thoracic Society clinical practice guideline. *American Journal of Respiratory and Critical Care Medicine, 201*(9), e56–e69. DOI: 10.1164/rccm.202003-0625ST PMID: 32283960

Nicolò, A., Massaroni, C., Schena, E., & Sacchetti, M. (2020). The importance of respiratory rate monitoring: From healthcare to sport and exercise. *Sensors (Basel), 20*(21), 6396. DOI: 10.3390/s20216396 PMID: 33182463

Nikkonen, S., Korkalainen, H., Leino, A., Myllymaa, S., Duce, B., Leppänen, T., & Toyras, J. (2021). Automatic respiratory event scoring in obstructive sleep apnea using a long short-term memory neural network. *IEEE Journal of Biomedical and Health Informatics, 25*(8), 2917–2927. DOI: 10.1109/JBHI.2021.3064694 PMID: 33687851

Obermeyer, Z., Powers, B., Vogeli, C., & Mullainathan, S. (2019). Dissecting racial bias in an algorithm used to manage the health of populations. *Science, 366*(6464), 447–453. DOI: 10.1126/science.aax2342 PMID: 31649194

Ogut, E. (2025). Artificial intelligence in clinical medicine: Challenges across diagnostic imaging, clinical decision support, surgery, pathology, and drug discovery. *Clinics and Practice, 15*(9), 169. DOI: 10.3390/clinpract15090169 PMID: 41002784

Oks, M., Sachdeva, R., Davenport, M., Husain, A. M., Kalra, M., Krishnan, V., Le, T., Parekh, A. A., Park, H., Prasad, B., Ryals, S. M., Zia, S., Anastasi, M., Shelgikar, A. V., Abbasi-Feinberg, F., Abreu, A. R., Bandyopadhyay, A., Gurubhagavatula, I., Kapur, V. K., & Wickwire, E. M. (2025). Artificial intelligence in sleep medicine: An updated American Academy of Sleep Medicine position statement. *Journal of Clinical Sleep Medicine : JCSM : Official Publication of the American Academy of Sleep Medicine, 21*(11), 1953–1962. DOI: 10.5664/jcsm.11832 PMID: 40742116

Olyanasab, A., & Annabestani, M. (2024). Leveraging machine learning for personalized wearable biomedical devices: A review. *Journal of Personalized Medicine, 14*(2), 203. DOI: 10.3390/jpm14020203 PMID: 38392636

Organization, W. H. (2024). *Ethics and governance of artificial intelligence for health: Large multi-modal models. WHO guidance*. World Health Organization.

Ortuño-Miquel, S., Roca, R., Alenda, C., Aranda, F., Martínez-Banaclocha, N., Amador, S., & Gil, D. (2025). Deep Learning Model-Based Architectures for Lung Tumor Mutation Profiling: A Systematic Review. *Cancers (Basel), 17*(22), 3619. DOI: 10.3390/cancers17223619 PMID: 41300986

Oudkerk, M., Liu, S., Heuvelmans, M. A., Walter, J. E., & Field, J. K. (2021). Lung cancer LDCT screening and mortality reduction—Evidence, pitfalls and future perspectives. *Nature Reviews. Clinical Oncology, 18*(3), 135–151. DOI: 10.1038/s41571-020-00432-6 PMID: 33046839

Owens, C. A. R. A., Hindocha, S. U. M. E. E. T., Lee, R. I. C. H. A. R. D., Millard, T. H. O. M. A. S., & Sharma, B. H. U. P. I. N. D. E. R. (2023). The lung cancers: staging and response, CT, 18F-FDG PET/CT, MRI, DWI: review and new perspectives. *The British Journal of Radiology, 96*(1148), 20220339. DOI: 10.1259/bjr.20220339 PMID: 37097296

Palani, M., Rajagopal, S., & Chintanpalli, A. K. (2024). A systematic review on feature extraction methods and deep learning models for detection of cancerous lung nodules at an early stage–the recent trends and challenges. *Biomedical Physics & Engineering Express, 11*(1), 012001. DOI: 10.1088/2057-1976/ad9154 PMID: 39530659

Pan, F., Feng, L., Liu, B., Hu, Y., & Wang, Q. (2023). Application of radiomics in diagnosis and treatment of lung cancer. *Frontiers in Pharmacology, 14*, 1295511. Advance online publication. DOI: 10.3389/fphar.2023.1295511 PMID: 38027000

Parra-Medina, R., Guerron-Gomez, G., Mendivelso-González, D., Gil-Gómez, J. H., Alzate, J. P., Gomez-Suarez, M., Polo, J. F., Sprockel, J. J., & Mosquera-Zamudio, A. (2025). Deep learning in histopathology images for prediction of oncogenic driver molecular alterations in lung cancer: A systematic review and meta-analysis. *Translational Lung Cancer Research, 14*(5), 1756–1769. DOI: 10.21037/tlcr-2024-1196 PMID: 40535093

Parreco, J., Hidalgo, A., Parks, J. J., Kozol, R., & Rattan, R. (2018). Using artificial intelligence to predict prolonged mechanical ventilation and tracheostomy placement. *The Journal of Surgical Research, 228*, 179–187. DOI: 10.1016/j.jss.2018.03.028 PMID: 29907209

Parsonage, M., Nathwani, D., Davey, P., & Barlow, G. (2009). Evaluation of the performance of CURB-65 with increasing age. *Clinical Microbiology and Infection, 15*(9), 858–864. DOI: 10.1111/j.1469-0691.2009.02908.x PMID: 19702590

Pastorino, U., Silva, M., Sestini, S., Sabia, F., Boeri, M., Cantarutti, A., Sverzellati, N., Sozzi, G., Corrao, G., & Marchiano, A. (2019). Prolonged lung cancer screening reduced 10-year mortality in the MILD trial: New confirmation of lung cancer screening efficacy. *Annals of Oncology : Official Journal of the European Society for Medical Oncology*, *30*(7), 1162–1169. DOI: 10.1093/annonc/mdz117 PMID: 30937431

Patanaik, A., Ong, J. L., Gooley, J. J., Ancoli-Israel, S., & Chee, M. W. L. (2018). An end-to-end framework for real-time automatic sleep stage classification. *Sleep (Basel)*, *41*(5). Advance online publication. DOI: 10.1093/sleep/zsy041 PMID: 29590492

Patton, J. S., Fishburn, C. S., & Weers, J. G. (2004). The lungs as a portal of entry for systemic drug delivery. *Proceedings of the American Thoracic Society*, *1*(4), 338–344. DOI: 10.1513/pats.200409-049TA PMID: 16113455

Paudyal, R., Grkovski, M., Oh, J. H., Schöder, H., Nunez, D. A., Hatzoglou, V., Deasy, J. O., Humm, J. L., Lee, N. Y., & Shukla-Dave, A. (2021). Application of community detection algorithm to investigate the correlation between imaging biomarkers of tumor metabolism, hypoxia, cellularity, and perfusion for precision radiotherapy in head and neck squamous cell carcinomas. *Cancers (Basel)*, *13*(15), 3908. DOI: 10.3390/cancers13153908 PMID: 34359810

Peberdy, M. A., Cretikos, M., Abella, B. S., DeVita, M., Goldhill, D., Kloeck, W., Kronick, S. L., Morrison, L. J., Nadkarni, V. M., Nichol, G., Nolan, J. P., Parr, M., Tibballs, J., van der Jagt, E. W., & Young, L. (2007). Recommended guidelines for monitoring, reporting, and conducting research on medical emergency team, outreach, and rapid response systems: an Utstein-style scientific statement: a scientific statement from the International Liaison Committee on Resuscitation (American Heart Association, Australian Resuscitation Council, European Resuscitation Council, Heart and Stroke Foundation of Canada, InterAmerican Heart Foundation, Resuscitation Council of Southern Africa, and the New Zealand Resuscitation Council); the American Heart Association Emergency Cardiovascular Care Committee; the Council on Cardiopulmonary, Perioperative, and Critical Care; and the Interdisciplinary Working Group on Quality of Care and Outcomes Research. *Circulation*, *116*(21), 2481–2500. DOI: 10.1161/CIRCULATIONAHA.107.186227 PMID: 17993478

Peeken, J. C., Nüsslin, F., & Combs, S. E. (2017). "Radio-oncomics": The potential of radiomics in radiation oncology. *Strahlentherapie und Onkologie*, *193*(10), 767–779. DOI: 10.1007/s00066-017-1175-0 PMID: 28687979

Peine, A., Hallawa, A., Bickenbach, J., Dartmann, G., Fazlic, L. B., Schmeink, A., Ascheid, G., Thiemermann, C., Schuppert, A., Kindle, R., Celi, L., Marx, G., & Martin, L. (2021). Development and validation of a reinforcement learning algorithm to dynamically optimize mechanical ventilation in critical care. *NPJ Digital Medicine*, *4*(1), 32. DOI: 10.1038/s41746-021-00388-6 PMID: 33608661

Peng, C., Goswami, P., & Bai, G. (2020). A literature review of current technologies on health data integration for patient centered health management. *Health Informatics Journal*, *26*(3), 1926–1951. DOI: 10.1177/1460458219892387 PMID: 31884843

Peng, J., Chen, C., Zhou, M., Xie, X., Zhou, Y., & Luo, C.-H. (2020). A machine-learning approach to forecast aggravation risk in patients with acute exacerbation of chronic obstructive pulmonary disease with clinical indicators. *Scientific Reports*, *10*(1), 3118. DOI: 10.1038/s41598-020-60042-1 PMID: 32080330

Penha, D., Pinto, E. G., Matos, F., Hochhegger, B., Monaghan, C., Taborda-Barata, L., Irion, K., & Marchiori, E. (2021). CO-RADS: Coronavirus Classification Review. *Journal of Clinical Imaging Science*, *11*, 9. DOI: 10.25259/JCIS_192_2020 PMID: 33767901

Perlis, M. L., Posner, D., Riemann, D., Bastien, C. H., Teel, J., & Thase, M. (2022). Insomnia. *Lancet*, *400*(10357), 1047–1060. DOI: 10.1016/S0140-6736(22)00879-0 PMID: 36115372

Pesapane, F., Codari, M., & Sardanelli, F. (2018). Artificial intelligence in medical imaging: Threat or opportunity? Radiologists again at the forefront of innovation in medicine. *European Radiology Experimental*, *2*(1), 35. DOI: 10.1186/s41747-018-0061-6 PMID: 30353365

Pesapane, F., Codari, M., & Sardanelli, F. (2021). Artificial intelligence and machine learning for medical imaging: A technology review. *Physica Medica*, *83*, 242–256. DOI: 10.1016/j.ejmp.2021.04.016 PMID: 33979715

Piccialli, F., di Cola, V. S., Giampaolo, F., & Cuomo, S. (2021). The Role of Artificial Intelligence in Fighting the COVID-19 Pandemic. *Information Systems Frontiers*, *23*(6), 1467–1497. DOI: 10.1007/s10796-021-10131-x PMID: 33935585

Pierce, J. D., Rosipko, B., Youngblood, L., Gilkeson, R. C., Gupta, A., & Bittencourt, L. K. (2021). Seamless integration of artificial intelligence into the clinical environment: Our experience with a novel pneumothorax detection artificial intelligence algorithm. *Journal of the American College of Radiology*, *18*(11), 1497–1505. DOI: 10.1016/j.jacr.2021.08.023 PMID: 34597622

Pilard, C., Ancion, M., Delvenne, P., Jerusalem, G., Hubert, P., & Herfs, M. (2021). Cancer immunotherapy: It's time to better predict patients' response. *British Journal of Cancer, 125*(7), 927–938. DOI: 10.1038/s41416-021-01413-x PMID: 34112949

Pilcer, G., & Amighi, K. (2010). Formulation strategy and use of excipients in pulmonary drug delivery. *International Journal of Pharmaceutics, 392*(1-2), 1–19. DOI: 10.1016/j.ijpharm.2010.03.017 PMID: 20223286

Pinsky, M. R., Bedoya, A., Bihorac, A., Celi, L., Churpek, M., Economou-Zavlanos, N. J., Elbers, P., Saria, S., Liu, V., Lyons, P. G., Shickel, B., Toral, P., Tscholl, D., & Clermont, G. (2024). Use of artificial intelligence in critical care: Opportunities and obstacles. *Critical Care, 28*(1), 113. DOI: 10.1186/s13054-024-04860-z PMID: 38589940

Pinto-de-Sá, R., Sousa-Pinto, B., & Costa-de-Oliveira, S. (2024). Brave New World of Artificial Intelligence: Its Use in Antimicrobial Stewardship—A Systematic Review. *Antibiotics (Basel, Switzerland), 13*(4), 307. DOI: 10.3390/antibiotics13040307 PMID: 38666983

Pleasants, R. A., Riley, I. L., & Mannino, D. M. (2016). Defining and targeting health disparities in chronic obstructive pulmonary disease. *International Journal of Chronic Obstructive Pulmonary Disease*, 2475-2496. Martínez-García, M., & Hernández-Lemus, E. (2022). Data integration challenges for machine learning in precision medicine. *Frontiers in medicine, 8*, 784455.

Prasanth, D. S. N. B. K., Aminabee, S. K., Rao, A. L., Guntupalli, C., Reddy, A. R., Kulandaivelu, U., Koteswara, S. N., & Rajeshwari, P. (2021). Inhibitory effects of Manosa alliacea in Freund's adjuvant arthritis on inflammatory markers and its confirmation by In-silico strategy. *Thaiphesatchasan, 45*(6), 532–544. DOI: 10.56808/3027-7922.2535

Prasanth, D. S. N. B. K., Aminabee, S. K., Rao, A. L., Teja, N., Bhargavi, K., Monika, C., Pujitha, B., Sandhya, T., Lalitha, A., & Panda, S. P. (2020). Anthelmintic activity of Mansoa alliacea against Pheretima posthuma: In vitro and in silico approach. *Thaiphesatchasan, 44*(3), 186–196. DOI: 10.56808/3027-7922.2451

Price, D., Brusselle, G., Roche, N., Freeman, D., & Chisholm, A. (2015). Real-world research and its importance in respiratory medicine. *Breathe (Sheffield, England), 11*(1), 26–38. DOI: 10.1183/20734735.015414 PMID: 26306101

Qin, Z. Z., Ahmed, S., Sarker, M. S., Paul, K., Adel, A. S. S., Naheyan, T., Barrett, R., Banu, S., & Creswell, J. (2021). Tuberculosis detection from chest x-rays for triaging in a high tuberculosis-burden setting: An evaluation of five artificial intelligence algorithms. *The Lancet. Digital Health*, *3*(9), e543–e554. DOI: 10.1016/S2589-7500(21)00116-3 PMID: 34446265

Qureshi, R., Irfan, M., Gondal, T. M., Khan, S., Wu, J., Hadi, M. U., Heymach, J., Le, X., Yan, H., & Alam, T. (2023). AI in drug discovery and its clinical relevance. *Heliyon*, *9*(7), e17575. DOI: 10.1016/j.heliyon.2023.e17575 PMID: 37396052

Rajendran, A., Angelin Rajan, R., Balasubramaniyam, S., & Elumalai, K. (2025). AI-Enhanced Predictive Imaging in Precision Medicine: Advancing Diagnostic Accuracy and Personalized Treatment. *iRadiology*, *3*(4), 261–278. DOI: 10.1002/ird3.70027

Raju, K. G., Goud, P. V., Parween, S., Ramarao, M., Leelavati, T. S., Madhavi, S., & Aminabee, S. (2024). Economic Analysis of Pharmacological Interventions for Substance Use Disorders Cost-effectiveness and Market Dynamics. *Ashdin Publishing Journal of Drug and Alcohol Research, 13*(29), 01-04.

Rangel, G., Cuevas-Tello, J. C., Nunez-Varela, J., Puente, C., & Silva-Trujillo, A. G. (2024). A survey on convolutional neural networks and their performance limitations in image recognition tasks. *Journal of Sensors*, *2024*(1), 2797320. DOI: 10.1155/2024/2797320

Raptis, S., Ilioudis, C., & Theodorou, K. (2024). Uncovering the diagnostic power of radiomic feature significance in automated lung cancer detection: An integrative analysis of texture, shape, and intensity contributions. *BioMedInformatics*, *4*(4), 2400–2425. DOI: 10.3390/biomedinformatics4040129

Restrepo, J. C., Dueñas, D., Corredor, Z., & Liscano, Y. (2023). Advances in genomic data and biomarkers: Revolutionizing NSCLC diagnosis and treatment. *Cancers (Basel)*, *15*(13), 3474. DOI: 10.3390/cancers15133474 PMID: 37444584

Revolutionizing healthcare: The role of artificial intelligence in clinical practice | BMC Medical Education | Springer Nature Link. (n.d.). Retrieved May 28, 2026, from https://link.springer.com/article/10.1186/s12909-023-04698-z

Ribeiro, M. T., Singh, S., & Guestrin, C. (2016). "Why Should I Trust You?": Explaining the Predictions of Any Classifier. *Proceedings of the 22nd ACM SIGKDD International Conference on Knowledge Discovery and Data Mining. KDD : Proceedings / International Conference on Knowledge Discovery & Data Mining. International Conference on Knowledge Discovery & Data Mining*, *16*, 1135–1144. DOI: 10.1145/2939672.2939778

Rieke, N., Hancox, J., Li, W. *et al.* (2020). The future of digital health with federated learning. *npj Digit. Med. 3*, 119. https://doi.org/10.1038/s41746-020-00323-1

Rieke, N., Hancox, J., Li, W., Milletarì, F., Roth, H. R., Albarqouni, S., Bakas, S., Galtier, M. N., Landman, B. A., Maier-Hein, K., Ourselin, S., Sheller, M., Summers, R. M., Trask, A., Xu, D., Baust, M., & Cardoso, M. J. (2020). The future of digital health with federated learning. *NPJ Digital Medicine*, *3*(1), 119. DOI: 10.1038/s41746-020-00323-1 PMID: 33015372

Rodak, O., Peris-Diaz, M. D., Olbromski, M., Podhorska-Okołów, M., & Dzięgiel, P. (2021). Current landscape of non-small cell lung cancer: Epidemiology, histological classification, targeted therapies, and immunotherapy. *Cancers (Basel)*, *13*(18), 4705. DOI: 10.3390/cancers13184705 PMID: 34572931

Rosenfeld, L. S., Goldmann, F., & Kaprio, L. A. (1957). Reasons for prolonged hospital stay: A study of need for hospital care. *Journal of Chronic Diseases*, *6*(2), 141–152. DOI: 10.1016/0021-9681(57)90048-6 PMID: 13449139

Rouvinov, K., Naamneh, R., Yakobson, A., Najjar, W., Abu Amna, M., Soklakova, A., Abu Zeid, E. E. D., Brenner, R., Asla, M., Ghalion, F. A., Abu Juma'a, A., Meirovitz, A., & Shalata, W. (2026). The Transformative Potential of Liquid Biopsies and Circulating Tumor DNA (ctDNA) in Modern Oncology. *Diagnostics (Basel)*, *16*(4), 523. DOI: 10.3390/diagnostics16040523 PMID: 41750672

Rutsch, N., Amrein, P., Exadaktylos, A. K., Benneker, L. M., Schmaranzer, F., Müller, M., Albers, C. E., & Bigdon, S. F. (2023). Cervical spine trauma – Evaluating the diagnostic power of CT, MRI, X-Ray and LODOX. *Injury*, *54*(7), 110771. DOI: 10.1016/j.injury.2023.05.003 PMID: 37164902

Saba, L., Biswas, M., Kuppili, V., Cuadrado Godia, E., Suri, H. S., Edla, D. R., & Suri, J. S. (2019). The present and future of deep learning in radiology. *European Journal of Radiology*, *114*, 14–24. DOI: 10.1016/j.ejrad.2019.02.038 PMID: 31005165

Safarian, A., Mirshahvalad, S. A., Nasrollahi, H., Jung, T., Pirich, C., Arabi, H., & Beheshti, M. (2025). Impact of [18F]FDG PET/CT radiomics and artificial intelligence in clinical decision making in lung cancer: Its current role. *Seminars in Nuclear Medicine*, *55*(2), 156–166. DOI: 10.1053/j.semnuclmed.2025.02.006 PMID: 40050131

Saha, P. K., Nadeem, S. A., & Comellas, A. P. (2023). A survey on artificial intelligence in pulmonary imaging. *Wiley Interdisciplinary Reviews. Data Mining and Knowledge Discovery*, *13*(6), e1510. DOI: 10.1002/widm.1510 PMID: 38249785

Saha, S., Kumar, A., & Nandi, D. (2024). ViT-ILD: A vision transformer-based neural network for detection of interstitial lung disease from CT images. *Procedia Computer Science*, *235*, 779–788. DOI: 10.1016/j.procs.2024.04.074

Sait, A. R. W., & Shaikh, M. A. (2025). Artificial Intelligence-Powered Chronic Obstructive Pulmonary Disease Detection Techniques—A Review. *Diagnostics (Basel)*, *15*(20), 2562. DOI: 10.3390/diagnostics15202562 PMID: 41153235

Sakagianni, A., Koufopoulou, C., Feretzakis, G., Kalles, D., Verykios, V. S., Myrianthefs, P., & Fildisis, G. (2023). Using Machine Learning to Predict Antimicrobial Resistance—A Literature Review. *Antibiotics (Basel, Switzerland)*, *12*(3), 452. DOI: 10.3390/antibiotics12030452 PMID: 36978319

Salmanpour, M. R., Mehrnia, S. S., Jabarzadeh Ghandilu, S., Safahi, Z., Falahati, S., Taeb, S., Mousavi, G., Maghsudi, M., Shariftabrizi, A., Hacihaliloglu, I., & Rahmim, A. (2026). Handcrafted vs. Deep Radiomics vs. Fusion vs. Deep Learning: A Comprehensive Review of Machine Learning-Based Cancer Outcome Prediction in PET and SPECT Imaging. *Journal of Imaging Informatics in Medicine*, •••, 1–50. DOI: 10.1007/s10278-025-01804-z PMID: 41612111

Salvi, S. (2014). Tobacco smoking and environmental risk factors for chronic obstructive pulmonary disease. *Clinics in Chest Medicine*, *35*(1), 17–27. DOI: 10.1016/j.ccm.2013.09.011 PMID: 24507834

Salwei, M. E., Carayon, P., & Hoonakker, P. L. T. (2021a). Workflow integration analysis of a human factors-based clinical decision support in the emergency department. Applied Ergonomics, 97, 103498. PMID: N/A. https://doi.org/DOI: 10.1016/j.apergo.2021.103498

Salwei, M. E., Carayon, P., & Hoonakker, P. L. T. (2021b). Usability barriers and facilitators of a human factors engineering-based clinical decision support technology for diagnosing pulmonary embolism. International Journal of Medical Informatics, 158, 104657. PMID: N/A. https://doi.org/DOI: 10.1016/j.ijmedinf.2021.104657

San José Estépar, R. (2022). Artificial intelligence in functional imaging of the lung. *The British Journal of Radiology*, *95*(1132), 20210527. DOI: 10.1259/bjr.20210527 PMID: 34890215

Sanchez-Morillo, D., Fernandez-Granero, M. A., & Leon-Jimenez, A. (2016). Use of predictive algorithms in-home monitoring of chronic obstructive pulmonary disease and asthma: A systematic review. *Chronic Respiratory Disease*, *13*(3), 264–283. DOI: 10.1177/1479972316642365 PMID: 27097638

Sartor, O., de Bono, J., Chi, K. N., Fizazi, K., Herrmann, K., Rahbar, K., Tagawa, S. T., Nordquist, L. T., Vaishampayan, N., El-Haddad, G., Park, C. H., Beer, T. M., Armour, A., Pérez-Contreras, W. J., DeSilvio, M., Kpamegan, E., Gericke, G., Messmann, R. A., Morris, M. J., & Krause, B. J. (2021). Lutetium-177–PSMA-617 for metastatic castration-resistant prostate cancer. *The New England Journal of Medicine*, *385*(12), 1091–1103. DOI: 10.1056/NEJMoa2107322 PMID: 34161051

Satapathy, P., Padhi, B. K., & Al Khathlan, N. (2023). Artificial intelligence in respiratory therapy: Opportunities and ethical challenges. *Respiratory Medicine*, *217*, 107342. DOI: 10.1016/j.rmed.2023.107342 PMID: 37380092

Saul, E. E., Guerra, R. B., Saul, M. E., da Silva, L. L., Aleixo, G. F. P., Matuda, R. M. K., & Lopes, G. (2020). The challenges of implementing low-dose computed tomography for lung cancer screening in low- and middle-income countries. *Nature Cancer*, *1*(12), 1140–1152. DOI: 10.1038/s43018-020-00142-z PMID: 35121933

Selvaraju, R. R., Cogswell, M., Das, A., Vedantam, R., Parikh, D., & Batra, D. (2017). Grad-cam: Visual explanations from deep networks via gradient-based localization. In *Proceedings of the IEEE international conference on computer vision* (pp. 618-626). DOI: 10.1109/ICCV.2017.74

Sendak, M., Balu, S., & Hernandez, A. F. (2023). Proactive algorithm monitoring to ensure health equity. JAMA Network Open, 6(12), e2345022. PMID: N/A. https://doi.org/DOI: 10.1001/jamanetworkopen.2023.45022

Seyam, E. A. (2025). Predicting High-Cost Healthcare Utilization Using Machine Learning: A Multi-Service Risk Stratification Analysis in EU-Based Private Group Health Insurance. *Risks*, *13*(7), 133. DOI: 10.3390/risks13070133

Seyyed-Kalantari, L., Zhang, H., McDermott, M. B. A., Chen, I. Y., & Ghassemi, M. (2021). Underdiagnosis bias of artificial intelligence algorithms applied to chest radiographs in under served patient populations. *Nature Medicine*, *27*(12), 2176–2182. DOI: 10.1038/s41591-021-01595-0 PMID: 34893776

Shafiq-Ul-Hassan, M., Latifi, K., Zhang, G., Ullah, G., Gillies, R., & Moros, E. (2018). Voxel size and gray level normalization of CT radiomic features in lung cancer. *Scientific Reports*, *8*(1), 10545. DOI: 10.1038/s41598-018-28895-9 PMID: 30002441

Shamji, M. H., Ollert, M., Adcock, I. M., Bennett, O., Favaro, A., Sarama, R., Riggioni, C., Annesi-Maesano, I., Custovic, A., Fontanella, S., Traidl-Hoffmann, C., Nadeau, K., Cecchi, L., Zemelka-Wiacek, M., Akdis, C. A., Jutel, M., & Agache, I. (2023). EAACI guidelines on environmental science in allergic diseases and asthma–leveraging artificial intelligence and machine learning to develop a causality model in exposomics. *Allergy*, *78*(7), 1742–1757. DOI: 10.1111/all.15667 PMID: 36740916

Shao, W., Rowe, S. P., & Du, Y. (2021). SPECTnet: A deep learning neural network for SPECT image reconstruction. *Annals of Translational Medicine*, *9*(9), 819. DOI: 10.21037/atm-20-3345 PMID: 34268432

Sharma, M., Taweesedt, P. T., & Surani, S. (2021). Utilizing artificial intelligence in critical care: Adding a handy tool to our armamentarium. *Cureus*, *13*(6), e15531. DOI: 10.7759/cureus.15531 PMID: 34268051

Sharma, P., Mehta, M., Dhanjal, D. S., Kaur, S., Gupta, G., Singh, H., Thangavelu, L., Rajeshkumar, S., Tambuwala, M., Bakshi, H. A., Chellappan, D. K., Dua, K., & Satija, S. (2019). Emerging trends in the novel drug delivery approaches for the treatment of lung cancer. *Chemico-Biological Interactions*, *309*, 108720. DOI: 10.1016/j.cbi.2019.06.033 PMID: 31226287

Sheetal, A., Jiang, Z., & Di Milia, L. (2023). Using machine learning to analyze longitudinal data: A tutorial guide and best-practice recommendations for social science researchers. *Applied Psychology*, *72*(3), 1339–1364. DOI: 10.1111/apps.12435

Sheller, M. J., Reina, G. A., Edwards, B., Martin, J., & Bakas, S. (2019). Multi-Institutional Deep Learning Modeling Without Sharing Patient Data: A Feasibility Study on Brain Tumor Segmentation. *Brainlesion: Glioma, Multiple Sclerosis, Stroke and Traumatic Brain Injuries. Lecture Notes in Computer Science*, *11383*, 92–104. DOI: 10.1007/978-3-030-11723-8_9 PMID: 31231720

Shung, D. L., Au, B., Taylor, R. A., Tay, J. K., Laursen, S. B., Stanley, A. J., Dalton, H. R., Ngu, J., Schultz, M., & Laine, L. (2020). Validation of a machine learning model that outperforms clinical risk scoring systems for upper gastrointestinal bleeding. *Gastroenterology*, *158*(1), 160–167. DOI: 10.1053/j.gastro.2019.09.009 PMID: 31562847

Siegel, R. L., Miller, K. D., & Jemal, A. (2019). Cancer statistics, 2019. *CA: a Cancer Journal for Clinicians*, *69*(1), 7–34. DOI: 10.3322/caac.21551 PMID: 30620402

Silva, M., Schaefer-Prokop, C. M., Jacobs, C., & Prokop, M. (2018). Detection of subsolid pulmonary nodules in lung cancer screening: Complementary sensitivity of visual reading and computer-aided diagnosis. *Investigative Radiology*, *53*(8), 441–449. DOI: 10.1097/RLI.0000000000000464 PMID: 29543693

Singh, A., Sengupta, S., & Lakshminarayanan, V. (2020). Explainable deep learning models in medical image analysis. *Journal of Imaging*, *6*(6), 52. DOI: 10.3390/jimaging6060052 PMID: 34460598

Sinha, P., Calfee, C. S., & Delucchi, K. L. (2020). Practitioner's guide to latent class analysis: Methodological considerations and common pitfalls. *Critical Care Medicine*, *49*(1), e63–e79. DOI: 10.1097/CCM.0000000000004710 PMID: 33165028

Sjoding, M. W., Dickson, R. P., Iwashyna, T. J., Gay, S. E., & Valley, T. S. (2020). Racial bias in pulse oximetry measurement. *The New England Journal of Medicine*, *383*(25), 2477–2478. DOI: 10.1056/NEJMc2029240 PMID: 33326721

Slavakis, K., Giannakis, G. B., & Mateos, G. (2014). Modeling and optimization for big data analytics:(statistical) learning tools for our era of data deluge. *IEEE Signal Processing Magazine*, *31*(5), 18–31. DOI: 10.1109/MSP.2014.2327238

Sluimer, I., Schilham, A., Prokop, M., & van Ginneken, B. (2006). Computer analysis of computed tomography scans of the lung: A survey. *IEEE Transactions on Medical Imaging*, *25*(4), 385–405. DOI: 10.1109/TMI.2005.862753 PMID: 16608056

Smeltzer, M. P., Wynes, M. W., Lantuejoul, S., & Govindan, R. (2020). The International Association for the Study of Lung Cancer global survey on molecular testing in lung cancer. *Journal of Thoracic Oncology*, *15*(9), 1434–1448. DOI: 10.1016/j.jtho.2020.05.002 PMID: 32445813

Smyth, H. D. C. (2003). The influence of formulation variables on the performance of alternative propellant-driven metered dose inhalers. *Advanced Drug Delivery Reviews*, *55*(7), 807–828. DOI: 10.1016/S0169-409X(03)00079-6 PMID: 12842602

Soenksen, L. R., Ma, Y., Zeng, C., Boussioux, L., Villalobos Carballo, K., Na, L., Wiberg, H. M., Li, M. L., Fuentes, I., & Bertsimas, D. (2022). Integrated multimodal artificial intelligence framework for healthcare applications. npj. *Digital Medicine*, *5*(1), 149. Advance online publication. DOI: 10.1038/s41746-022-00689-4 PMID: 36127417

Sollini, M., Cozzi, L., Chiti, A., & Kirienko, M. (2017). Texture analysis and machine learning to characterize suspected lung nodules and lung cancer: A narrative review. *European Journal of Radiology*, *90*, 1–9. PMID: 29362138

Soriano, J. B., Kendrick, P. J., Paulson, K. R., Gupta, V., Abrams, E. M., Adedoyin, R. A., & Moradi, M. (2020). Prevalence and attributable health burden of chronic respiratory diseases, 1990–2017: A systematic analysis for the Global Burden of Disease Study 2017. *The Lancet. Respiratory Medicine*, *8*(6), 585–596. DOI: 10.1016/S2213-2600(20)30105-3 PMID: 32526187

Sparrow, D., Aloia, M., Demolles, D. A., & Gottlieb, D. J. (2010). A telemedicine intervention to improve adherence to continuous positive airway pressure: A randomised controlled trial. *Thorax*, *65*(12), 1061–1066. DOI: 10.1136/thx.2009.133215 PMID: 20880872

Stephansen, J. B., Olesen, A. N., Olsen, M., Ambati, A., Leary, E. B., Moore, H. E., Carrillo, O., Lin, L., Han, F., Yan, H., Sun, Y. L., Dauvilliers, Y., Scholz, S., Barateau, L., Hogl, B., Stefani, A., Hong, S. C., Kim, T. W., Pizza, F., & Mignot, E. (2018). Neural network analysis of sleep stages enables efficient diagnosis of narcolepsy. *Nature Communications*, *9*(1), 5229. DOI: 10.1038/s41467-018-07229-3 PMID: 30523329

Steyerberg, E. W., van der Ploeg, T., & Van Calster, B. (2014). Risk prediction with machine learning and regression methods. *Biometrical Journal. Biometrische Zeitschrift*, *56*(4), 601–606. DOI: 10.1002/bimj.201300297 PMID: 24615859

Strassberger, C., Hedner, J., Sands, S. A., Tolbert, T. M., Taranto-Montemurro, L., Marciniak, A., Zou, D., & Grote, L. (2023). Night-to-night variability of PSG-derived physiological endotypic traits in patients with moderate to severe Obstructive Sleep Apnea. *Chest*. Advance online publication. DOI: 10.1016/j.chest.2022.12.029 PMID: 36610664

Strielkowski, W., Vlasov, A., Selivanov, K., Muraviev, K., & Shakhnov, V. (2023). Prospects and challenges of the machine learning and data-driven methods for the predictive analysis of power systems: A review. *Energies*, *16*(10), 4025. DOI: 10.3390/en16104025

Subramanian, J., & Simon, R. (2010). Gene expression-based prognostic signatures in lung cancer: Ready for clinical use? *Journal of the National Cancer Institute*, *102*(7), 464–474. DOI: 10.1093/jnci/djq025 PMID: 20233996

Su, H. N., & Lee, P. C. (2010). Mapping knowledge structure by keyword co-occurrence: A first look at journal papers in technology foresight. *Scientometrics*, *85*(1), 65–79. DOI: 10.1007/s11192-010-0259-8

Sung, H., Ferlay, J., Siegel, R. L., Laversanne, M., Soerjomataram, I., Jemal, A., & Bray, F. (2021). Global cancer statistics 2020: GLOBOCAN estimates of incidence and mortality worldwide for 36 cancers in 185 countries. *CA: a Cancer Journal for Clinicians*, *71*(3), 209–249. DOI: 10.3322/caac.21660 PMID: 33538338

Sun, H., Jia, J., Goparaju, B., Huang, G. B., Sourina, O., Bianchi, M. T., & Westover, M. B. (2017). Large-scale automated sleep staging. *Sleep (Basel)*, *40*(10), zsx139. Advance online publication. DOI: 10.1093/sleep/zsx139 PMID: 29029305

Sun, W., Zheng, B., & Qian, W. (2016). Computer aided lung cancer diagnosis with deep learning algorithms. *Proceedings of SPIE Medical Imaging*, *9785*, 97850Z. DOI: 10.1117/12.2216307

Susilo, Y. K. B., & Rahman, S. A. (2025). Revolutionizing COPD and Asthma Management with Artificial Intelligence. medRxiv, 2025.2003. 2018.25324219. DOI: 10.1101/2025.03.18.25324219

Swanson, K., Wu, E., Zhang, A., Alizadeh, A. A., & Zou, J. (2023). From patterns to patients: Advances in clinical machine learning for cancer diagnosis, prognosis, and treatment. *Cell*, *186*(8), 1772–1791. DOI: 10.1016/j.cell.2023.01.035 PMID: 36905928

Sweatt, A. J., Hedlin, H. K., Balasubramanian, V., Hsi, A., Blum, L. K., Robinson, W. H., Haddad, F., Hickey, P. M., Condliffe, R., Lawrie, A., Nicolls, M. R., Rabinovitch, M., Khatri, P., & Zamanian, R. T. (2019). Discovery of distinct immune phenotypes using machine learning in pulmonary arterial hypertension. *Circulation Research*, *124*(6), 904–919. DOI: 10.1161/CIRCRESAHA.118.313911 PMID: 30661465

Swinckels, L., Bennis, F. C., Ziesemer, K. A., Scheerman, J. F., Bijwaard, H., de Keijzer, A., & Bruers, J. J. (2024). The use of deep learning and machine learning on longitudinal electronic health records for the early detection and prevention of diseases: Scoping review. *Journal of Medical Internet Research*, *26*, e48320. DOI: 10.2196/48320 PMID: 39163096

Takamatsu, M. (2025). Transforming histologic assessment: artificial intelligence in cancer diagnosis and personalized treatment: Molecular Diagnostics. *British Journal of Cancer*, *133*(12), 1765–1775. DOI: 10.1038/s41416-025-03206-y PMID: 40993310

Tang, J., Ouyang, Q., Li, Y., Zhang, P., Jin, W., Qu, S., Yang, F., He, Z., & Qin, M. (2022). Nanomaterials for delivering antibiotics in the therapy of pneumonia. *International Journal of Molecular Sciences*, *23*(24), 15738. DOI: 10.3390/ijms232415738 PMID: 36555379

Tanoli, Z., Vähä-Koskela, M., & Aittokallio, T. (2021). Artificial intelligence, machine learning, and drug repurposing in cancer. *Expert Opinion on Drug Discovery*, *16*(9), 977–989. DOI: 10.1080/17460441.2021.1883585 PMID: 33543671

Tao, G., Zhu, L., Chen, Q., Yin, L., Li, Y., Yang, J., Ni, B., Zhang, Z., Koo, C. W., Patil, P. D., Chen, Y., Yu, H., Xu, Y., & Ye, X. (2022). Prediction of future imagery of lung nodule as growth modeling with follow-up computed tomography scans using deep learning: A retrospective cohort study. *Translational Lung Cancer Research*, *11*(2), 250–262. DOI: 10.21037/tlcr-22-59 PMID: 35280310

Tejani, A. S., Cook, T. S., Hussain, M., Sippel Schmidt, T., O'Donnell, K. P., & Arzen, S. (2024). Integrating and Adopting AI in the Radiology Workflow: A Primer for Standards and Integrating the Healthcare Enterprise (IHE) Profiles. *Radiology*, *311*(3), e232653. DOI: 10.1148/radiol.232653 PMID: 38888474

Thandra, K. C., Barsouk, A., Saginala, K., Aluru, J. S., & Barsouk, A. (2021). Epidemiology of lung cancer. *Contemporary Oncology = Współczesna Onkologia*, *25*(1), 45–52. DOI: 10.5114/wo.2021.103829 PMID: 33911981

Tiwari, A., Ghose, A., Hasanova, M., Faria, S. S., Mohapatra, S., Adeleke, S., & Boussios, S. (2025). The current landscape of artificial intelligence in computational histopathology for cancer diagnosis. *Discover. Oncology*, *16*(1), 438. DOI: 10.1007/s12672-025-02212-z PMID: 40167870

Tizhoosh, H. R., & Pantanowitz, L. (2018). Artificial intelligence and digital pathology: Challenges and opportunities. *Journal of Pathology Informatics*, *9*(1), 38. DOI: 10.4103/jpi.jpi_53_18 PMID: 30607305

Togunwa, T. O., Babatunde, A. O., Fatade, O. E., Olatunji, R., Ogbole, G., & Falade, A. (2025). Detection of pneumonia in children through chest radiographs using artificial intelligence in a low-resource setting: A pilot study. *PLOS Digital Health*, *4*(9), e0000713. DOI: 10.1371/journal.pdig.0000713 PMID: 40991626

Topol, E.J. (2019) Deep Medicine How Artificial Intelligence Can Make Healthcare Human Again. Basic Books. - References—Scientific Research Publishing. (n.d.-a). Retrieved March 2, 2026, from https://www.scirp.org/reference/referencespapers?referenceid=3758241

Topol, E. J. (2019). High-performance medicine: The convergence of human and artificial intelligence. *Nature Medicine*, *25*(1), 44–56. DOI: 10.1038/s41591-018-0300-7 PMID: 30617339

Touvron, H., Cord, M., Douze, M., Massa, F., Sablayrolles, A., & Jégou, H. (2021, July). Training data-efficient image transformers & distillation through attention. In *International conference on machine learning* (pp. 10347-10357). PMLR.

Tran, T. K., Tran, M. C., Joseph, A., Phan, P. A., Grau, V., & Farmery, A. D. (2024). A systematic review of machine learning models for management, prediction and classification of ARDS. *Respiratory Research*, *25*(1), 232. Advance online publication. DOI: 10.1186/s12931-024-02834-x PMID: 38834976

Trenkwalder, C., Allen, R., Béné Harbé, E., Bhatt, D., Bhattacharyya, A., & Bhattacharyya, B.. (2016). Restless legs syndrome associated with major diseases. *Neurology*, *86*(14), 1336–1343. DOI: 10.1212/WNL.0000000000002542 PMID: 26944272

Triantafyllidis, A. K., Koutkias, V. G., Chouvarda, I., & Maglaveras, N. (2012). A pervasive health system integrating patient monitoring, status logging, and social sharing. *IEEE Journal of Biomedical and Health Informatics*, *17*(1), 30–37. DOI: 10.1109/TITB.2012.2227269 PMID: 23193318

Trivedi, A., Hall, C., Hoffman, E. A., Woods, J. C., Gierada, D. S., & Castro, M. (2017). Using imaging as a biomarker for asthma. *The Journal of Allergy and Clinical Immunology*, *139*(1), 1–10. DOI: 10.1016/j.jaci.2016.11.009 PMID: 28065276

Tsang, K. C., Pinnock, H., Wilson, A. M., & Shah, S. A. (2022). Application of machine learning algorithms for asthma management with mHealth: A clinical review. *Journal of Asthma and Allergy*, *15*, 855–873. DOI: 10.2147/JAA.S285742 PMID: 35791395

Tsao, M., Laikijrung, C., Tran, A., Pon, T., Roach, D., Liu, B., & Le, K. (2022). Optimizing quality of care in patients admitted with chronic obstructive pulmonary disease exacerbation. *Chronic Respiratory Disease*, *19*, 14799731211073348. DOI: 10.1177/14799731211073348 PMID: 35041553

Tufael, A. R. S., & Sunny, A. R. (2022). Transforming healthcare with artificial intelligence: Innovations, applications, and future challenges. *Journal of Primeasia*, *3*(1), 1–6.

Tunali, I., Gillies, R. J., & Schabath, M. B. (2019). Application of radiomics and artificial intelligence for lung cancer precision medicine. *Cold Spring Harbor Molecular Case Studies*, *5*(6), a003111.

Tunali, I., Gray, J. E., Qi, J. D., Abdalah, M., Jeong, D. K., Guvenis, A., Gillies, R. J., & Schabath, M. B. (2019). Novel clinical and radiomic predictors of rapid disease progression phenotypes among lung cancer patients treated with immunotherapy: An early report. *Lung Cancer (Amsterdam, Netherlands)*, *129*, 75–79. DOI: 10.1016/j.lungcan.2019.01.010 PMID: 30797495

Turcatel, G., Xiao, Y., Caveney, S., Gnacadja, G., Kim, J., & Molfino, N. A. (2025). Predicting asthma exacerbations using machine learning models. *Advances in Therapy*, *42*(1), 362–374. DOI: 10.1007/s12325-024-03053-y PMID: 39556295

Upadhyay, P., & Ahlawat, P. (2022). Improvement in Quality of Life of Survivors of Chronic Obstructive Pulmonary Disease with Minimal Interventions. *Journal of Palliative Care & Medicine*, *12*(440), 2.

Vaid, A., Somani, S., Russak, A. J., Freitas, J. K., Chaudhry, F., Paranjpe, I., Johnson, K. W., Lee, S. J., & Miotto, R. (2021). Machine learning to predict mortality and critical events in COVID-19 positive New York City patients. *NPJ Digital Medicine*, *3*, 40.

Vaishya, R., Javaid, M., Khan, I. H., & Haleem, A. (2020). Artificial Intelligence (AI) applications for COVID-19 pandemic. *Diabetes & Metabolic Syndrome*, *14*(4), 337–339. DOI: 10.1016/j.dsx.2020.04.012 PMID: 32305024

van Boven, J. F., Lavorini, F., Agh, T., Sadatsafavi, M., Patino, O., & Muresan, B. (2024). Cost-effectiveness and impact on health care utilization of interventions to improve medication adherence and outcomes in asthma and chronic obstructive pulmonary disease: A systematic literature review. *The Journal of Allergy and Clinical Immunology. In Practice*, *12*(5), 1228–1243. DOI: 10.1016/j.jaip.2023.12.049 PMID: 38182099

van de Sande, D., van Genderen, M. E., Huiskens, J., Gommers, D., & van Bommel, J. (2021). Moving from bytes to bedside: A systematic review on the use of artificial intelligence in the intensive care unit. *Intensive Care Medicine*, *47*(7), 750–760. DOI: 10.1007/s00134-021-06446-7 PMID: 34089064

van Eck, N. J., & Waltman, L. (2014). Visualizing bibliometric networks. In Ding, Y., Rousseau, R., & Wolfram, D. (Eds.), *Measuring scholarly impact: Methods and practice* (pp. 285–320). Springer. DOI: 10.1007/978-3-319-10377-8_13

Vasey, B., Nagendran, M., Campbell, B., Clifton, D. A., Collins, G. S., Denaxas, S., ... & McCulloch, P. (2022). Reporting guideline for the early stage clinical evaluation of decision support systems driven by artificial intelligence: DECIDE-AI. *bmj, 377*.

Vaswani, A., Shazeer, N., Parmar, N., Uszkoreit, J., Jones, L., Gomez, A. N., & Polosukhin, I. (2017). Attention is all you need. *Advances in Neural Information Processing Systems*, •••, 30.

Villaruz, L. C., & Socinski, M. A. (2013). The role of anti-angiogenesis in non-small-cell lung cancer: An update. *Current Oncology Reports*, *15*, 346–355. PMID: 25947099

Vliegenthart, R., Fouras, A., Jacobs, C., & Papanikolaou, N. (2022). Innovations in thoracic imaging: CT, radiomics, AI and x-ray velocimetry. *Respirology (Carlton, Vic.)*, *27*(10), 818–833. DOI: 10.1111/resp.14344 PMID: 35965430

Von Platen, P., Pomprapa, A., Lachmann, B., & Leonhardt, S. (2020). The dawn of physiological closed-loop ventilation—A review. *Critical Care*, *24*(1), 121. DOI: 10.1186/s13054-020-2810-1 PMID: 32223754

Vora, L. K., Gholap, A. D., Jetha, K., Thakur, R. R. S., Solanki, H. K., & Chavda, V. P. (2023). Artificial intelligence in pharmaceutical technology and drug delivery design. *Pharmaceutics*, *15*(7), 1916. DOI: 10.3390/pharmaceutics15071916 PMID: 37514102

Wahidi, M. M., Haywood, H. B., Bass, G. D., Nathanson, I., Chowdhury, A., & Sangvai, D. (2023). Value-based care for chest physicians. *Chest*, *163*(5), 1193–1200. DOI: 10.1016/j.chest.2022.12.041 PMID: 36627080

Wang, J., Shen, L., Zhong, H., Zhou, Z., Hu, P., Gan, J., Luo, R., Hu, W., & Zhang, Z. (2019). Radiomics features on radiotherapy treatment planning CT can predict patient survival in locally advanced rectal cancer patients. *Scientific Reports*, *9*(1), 15346. DOI: 10.1038/s41598-019-51629-4 PMID: 31653909

Wang, L., Alexander, C. A., Wu, H., & Wang, J. (2021). Integrating artificial intelligence in lung cancer care: Current applications and future directions. *Seminars in Cancer Biology*, *72*, 216–230.

Wang, M., Greenberg, M., Forkert, N. D., Chekouo, T., Afriyie, G., Ismail, Z., Smith, E. E., & Sajobi, T. T. (2022). Dementia risk prediction in individuals with mild cognitive impairment: A comparison of Cox regression and machine learning models. *BMC Medical Research Methodology*, *22*(1), 284. DOI: 10.1186/s12874-022-01754-y PMID: 36324086

Wang, S., & Summers, R. M. (2012). Machine learning and radiology. *Medical Image Analysis*, *16*(5), 933–951. DOI: 10.1016/j.media.2012.02.005 PMID: 22465077

Wang, S., Yu, H., Gan, Y., Wu, Z., Li, E., Li, X., Chen, J., Liu, S., Zhang, L., Lang, J., Tian, J., Liang, C., & Liu, Z. (2022). Mining whole-lung information by artificial intelligence for predicting EGFR genotype and targeted therapy response in lung cancer: A multicohort study. *The Lancet. Digital Health*, *4*(5), e309–e319. DOI: 10.1016/S2589-7500(22)00024-3 PMID: 35341713

Wang, W., Feng, S., Ye, Z. Y. F., Gao, H. L., Lin, J. Z., & Ouyang, D. F. (2022). Prediction of lipid nanoparticles for mRNA vaccines by the machine learning algorithm. *Acta Pharmaceutica Sinica. B*, *12*(6), 2950–2962. DOI: 10.1016/j.apsb.2021.11.021 PMID: 35755271

Wang, W., Ye, Z., Gao, H., & Ouyang, D. (2021). Computational pharmaceutics-A new paradigm of drug delivery. *Journal of Controlled Release*, *338*, 119–136. DOI: 10.1016/j.jconrel.2021.08.030 PMID: 34418520

Wan, Z., Sun, X., Li, Y., Chu, T., Hao, X., Cao, Y., & Zhang, P. (2025). Applications of artificial intelligence in drug repurposing. *Advancement of Science*, *12*(14), 2411325. DOI: 10.1002/advs.202411325 PMID: 40047357

Warnaar, R. S. P., Mulder, M. P., Fresiello, L., Cornet, A. D., & Heunks, L. M. A. (2023). Computational physiological models for individualised mechanical ventilation: A systematic literature review focussing on quality, availability, and clinical readiness. Critical Care, 27, 268. PMID: N/A. https://doi.org/DOI: 10.1186/s13054-023-04549-9

Wasinger, G., Koeller, M. C., & Compérat, E. (2025). Pathology in the artificial intelligence era: Practical insights for immunohistochemistry and molecular pathology. *Diagnostic Histopathology*, *31*(7), 416–423. DOI: 10.1016/j.mpdhp.2025.04.003

Wick, K. D., McAuley, D. F., Levitt, J. E., Beitler, J. R., Annane, D., Riviello, E. D., Calfee, C. S., & Matthay, M. A. (2021). Promises and challenges of personalized medicine to guide ARDS therapy. *Critical Care*, *25*(1), 404. DOI: 10.1186/s13054-021-03822-z PMID: 34814925

Wickwire, E. M., & Collop, N. A. (2010). Insomnia and sleep-related breathing disorders. *Chest*, *137*(6), 1449–1463. DOI: 10.1378/chest.09-1485 PMID: 20525657

Willegaignon, J., Fernandes, S. C. P., Pelissoni, R. A., Coura-Filho, G. B., Sapienza, M. T., & Buchpiguel, C. A. (2023). Radiation safety measures in diagnostic nuclear medicine, based on the potential radiation dose emitted by radioactive patients. *Radiologia Brasileira*, *56*(1), 13–20. DOI: 10.1590/0100-3984.2022.0064 PMID: 36926359

Wu, J., & Hicks, C. (2021). Breast cancer type classification using machine learning. *Journal of Personalized Medicine*, *11*(2), 61. DOI: 10.3390/jpm11020061 PMID: 33498339

Wu, W., Parmar, C., Grossmann, P., Quackenbush, J., Lambin, P., Bussink, J., & Aerts, H. J. W. L. (2016). Exploratory study to identify radiomics classifiers for lung cancer histology. *Frontiers in Oncology*, *6*, 71. DOI: 10.3389/fonc.2016.00071 PMID: 27064691

Wu, X.-W., Yang, H.-B., Yuan, R., Long, E.-W., & Tong, R.-S. (2020). Predictive models of medication non-adherence risks of patients with T2D based on multiple machine learning algorithms. *BMJ Open Diabetes Research & Care*, *8*(1), e001055. DOI: 10.1136/bmjdrc-2019-001055 PMID: 32156739

Xie, T., Huang, A., Yan, H., Ju, X., Xiang, L., & Yuan, J. (2024). Artificial intelligence: Illuminating the depths of the tumor microenvironment. *Journal of Translational Medicine*, *22*(1), 799. DOI: 10.1186/s12967-024-05609-6 PMID: 39210368

Xiong, L., Li, X., Lu, X., Zhang, Z., Zhang, Y., Wu, W., & Wang, C. (2024). Inhaled multilevel size-tunable, charge-reversible and mucus-traversing composite microspheres as trojan horse: Enhancing lung deposition and tumor penetration. *Chinese Chemical Letters*, *35*(9), 109384. DOI: 10.1016/j.cclet.2023.109384

Xu, J., Glicksberg, B. S., Su, C., Walker, P., Bian, J., & Wang, F. (2021). Federated learning for healthcare informatics. *Journal of Healthcare Informatics Research*, *5*(1), 1–19. DOI: 10.1007/s41666-020-00082-4 PMID: 33204939

Xu, S., Deo, R. C., Soar, J., Barua, P. D., Faust, O., Homaira, N., Jaffe, A., Kabir, A. L., & Acharya, U. R. (2023). Automated detection of airflow obstructive diseases: A systematic review of the last decade (2013–2022). *Computer Methods and Programs in Biomedicine*, *241*, 107746. DOI: 10.1016/j.cmpb.2023.107746 PMID: 37660550

Xu, Y., Hosny, A., Zeleznik, R., Parmar, C., Coroller, T., Franco, I., Mak, R. H., & Aerts, H. J. W. L. (2019). Deep learning predicts lung cancer treatment response from serial medical imaging. *Clinical Cancer Research*, *25*(11), 3266–3275. DOI: 10.1158/1078-0432.CCR-18-2495 PMID: 31010833

Xu, Y., Quan, R., Xu, W., Huang, Y., Chen, X., & Liu, F. (2024). Advances in medical image segmentation: A comprehensive review of traditional, deep learning and hybrid approaches. *Bioengineering (Basel, Switzerland)*, *11*(10), 1034. DOI: 10.3390/bioengineering11101034 PMID: 39451409

Yang, H., Yang, M., Chen, J., Yao, G., Zou, Q., & Jia, L. (2025). Multimodal deep learning approaches for precision oncology: A comprehensive review. *Briefings in Bioinformatics*, *26*(1), bbae699. DOI: 10.1093/bib/bbae699 PMID: 39757116

Yang, J., Zeng, S., Cui, S., Zheng, J., & Wang, H. (2025). Predictive modeling of acute respiratory distress syndrome using machine learning: Systematic review and meta-analysis. *Journal of Medical Internet Research*, *27*, e66615. DOI: 10.2196/66615 PMID: 40359510

Yassine, E. L., Wang, S. L., & Ali, T. A. A. (2026). Hybrid GNN-Transformer model for multi-omic cancer classification with interpretable pathway-driven feature selection. *PeerJ. Computer Science*, *12*, e3415. DOI: 10.7717/peerj-cs.3415

Yip, S. S. F., & Aerts, H. J. W. L. (2016). Applications and limitations of radiomics. *Physics in Medicine and Biology*, *61*(13), R150–R166. DOI: 10.1088/0031-9155/61/13/R150 PMID: 27269645

Yoon, J. H., Pinsky, M. R., & Clermont, G. (2022). Artificial intelligence in critical care medicine. Critical Care, 26(1), 75. PMID: N/A. https://doi.org/DOI: 10.1186/s13054-022-03915-3

Younes, M., & Hanly, P. J. (2016). Minimizing interrater variability in staging sleep by use of computer-derived features. *Journal of Clinical Sleep Medicine : JCSM : Official Publication of the American Academy of Sleep Medicine, 12*(10), 1347–1356. DOI: 10.5664/jcsm.6186 PMID: 27448418

Younes, M., Kuna, S. T., Pack, A. I., Walsh, J. K., Kushida, C. A., Staley, B., & Pien, G. W. (2018). Reliability of the American Academy of Sleep Medicine rules for assessing sleep depth in clinical practice. *Journal of Clinical Sleep Medicine : JCSM : Official Publication of the American Academy of Sleep Medicine, 14*(2), 205–213. DOI: 10.5664/jcsm.6934 PMID: 29351821

Yousefi, M., Jalilian, H., Heydari, S., Seyednejad, F., & Mir, N. (2023). Cost of lung cancer: A systematic review. *Value in Health Regional Issues, 33*, 17–26. DOI: 10.1016/j.vhri.2022.07.007 PMID: 36201970

Yu, K. H., Beam, A. L., & Kohane, I. S. (2018). Artificial intelligence in healthcare. *Nature Biomedical Engineering, 2*(10), 719–731. DOI: 10.1038/s41551-018-0305-z PMID: 31015651

Zemanick, E. T., Harris, J. K., Conway, S., Konstan, M. W., Marshall, B., Quittner, A. L., Retsch-Bogart, G., Saiman, L., & Accurso, F. J. (2010). Measuring and improving respiratory outcomes in cystic fibrosis lung disease: Opportunities and challenges to therapy. *Journal of Cystic Fibrosis, 9*(1), 1–16. DOI: 10.1016/j.jcf.2009.09.003 PMID: 19833563

Zeng, X. M., Martin, G. P., & Marriott, C. (1995). The controlled delivery of drugs to the lung. *International Journal of Pharmaceutics, 124*(2), 149–164. DOI: 10.1016/0378-5173(95)00104-Q

Zhai, B., Elder, G. J., & Godfrey, A. (2024). Challenges and opportunities of deep learning for wearable-based objective sleep assessment. npj. *Digital Medicine, 7*(1), 85. DOI: 10.1038/s41746-024-01086-9 PMID: 38575794

Zhang, J., & Zhang, Z. M. (2023). Ethics and governance of trustworthy medical artificial intelligence. BMC Medical Informatics and Decision Making, 23, 7. PMID: N/A. https://doi.org/DOI: 10.1186/s12911-023-02103-9

Zhang, B., He, X., Ouyang, F., Gu, D., Dong, Y., Zhang, L., Mo, X., Huang, W., Tian, J., & Zhang, S. (2021). Radiomic machine-learning classifiers for prognostic biomarkers of advanced nasopharyngeal carcinoma. *Cancer Letters, 403*, 21–27. DOI: 10.1016/j.canlet.2017.06.004 PMID: 28610955

Zhang, C., Yu, W., Li, Y., Sun, H., Zhang, Y., & De Vos, M. (2022). CMS2-Net: Semi-supervised sleep staging for diverse obstructive sleep apnea severity. *IEEE Journal of Biomedical and Health Informatics*, *26*(7), 3447–3457. DOI: 10.1109/JBHI.2022.3156585 PMID: 35255000

Zhang, R., Peng, W., Wang, Y., Jiang, Y., Wang, J., Zhang, S., Li, Z., Shi, Y., Chen, F., Feng, Z., & Xiao, W. (2025). MRI radiomics model for predicting tumor immune microenvironment types and efficacy of anti-PD-1/PD-L1 therapy in hepatocellular carcinoma. *BMC Medical Imaging*, *25*(1), 211. DOI: 10.1186/s12880-025-01751-9 PMID: 40597775

Zhang, X., Liu, J., Zhou, W., Lu, J., Wu, L., Li, Y., Wang, Y., Wang, Z., & Cai, J. (2025). Deep learning enhances precision diagnosis and treatment of non-small cell lung cancer: Future prospects. *Translational Lung Cancer Research*, *14*(8), 3196–3215. DOI: 10.21037/tlcr-2025-187 PMID: 40948833

Zhang, Z., Ma, P., Ahmed, R., Wang, J., Akin, D., Soto, F., Liu, B.-F., Li, P., & Demirci, U. (2022). Advanced point-of-care testing technologies for human acute respiratory virus detection. *Advanced Materials*, *34*(1), 2103646. DOI: 10.1002/adma.202103646 PMID: 34623709

Zhao, J., Li, M., Niu, L., Zhao, Y., & Song, X. (2025). Lung cancer in non-smoking women (LCINSW): From risk factors to precision therapy. *Cancer and Metastasis Reviews*, *44*(4), 74. DOI: 10.1007/s10555-025-10289-9 PMID: 41028595

Zhao, W., Yang, J., Sun, Y., Li, C., Wu, W., Jin, L., Wang, X., & Xu, Z. (2018). 3D deep learning from CT scans predicts tumor invasiveness of ground-glass nodules. *Nature Communications*, *9*, 1–8.

Zhong, Y., She, Y., Deng, J., Chen, S., Wang, T., Yang, M., Ma, M., Song, Y., Qi, H., Wang, Y., Chen, J., Ye, X., Chen, C., & Xie, D. (2022). Deep learning for prediction of N2 metastasis and survival for clinical stage I non-small cell lung cancer. *Radiology*, *302*(1), 200–211. DOI: 10.1148/radiol.2021210902 PMID: 34698568

Zhou, J., Hu, B., Feng, W., Zhang, Z., Fu, X., Shao, H., Chen, W., Li, W., & Yu, H. (2023). An ensemble deep learning model for risk stratification of invasive lung adenocarcinoma using thin-slice CT. *NPJ Digital Medicine*, *6*(1), 119. DOI: 10.1038/s41746-023-00866-z PMID: 37407729

Zhou, L., Pan, S., Wang, J., & Vasilakos, A. V. (2017). Machine learning on big data: Opportunities and challenges. *Neurocomputing*, *237*, 350–361. DOI: 10.1016/j.neucom.2017.01.026

Zhou, Q. T., Leung, S. S. Y., Tang, P., Parumasivam, T., Loh, Z. H., & Chan, H. K. (2015). Inhaled formulations and pulmonary drug delivery systems for respiratory infections. *Advanced Drug Delivery Reviews*, *85*, 83–99. DOI: 10.1016/j.addr.2014.10.022 PMID: 25451137

Zhou, Y., Wang, F., Tang, J., Nussinov, R., & Cheng, F. (2020). Artificial intelligence in COVID-19 drug repurposing. *The Lancet. Digital Health*, *2*(12), e667–e676. DOI: 10.1016/S2589-7500(20)30192-8 PMID: 32984792

Zhu, L., & Zee, P. C. (2012). Circadian rhythm sleep disorders. *Neurologic Clinics*, *30*(4), 1167–1191. DOI: 10.1016/j.ncl.2012.08.011 PMID: 23099133

Zinchuk, A. V., Gentry, M. J., Concato, J., & Yaggi, H. K. (2017). Phenotypes in obstructive sleep apnea: A definition, examples and evolution of approaches. *Sleep Medicine Reviews*, *35*, 113–123. DOI: 10.1016/j.smrv.2016.10.002 PMID: 27815038

Zou, D., Lisik, D., Bailly, S., & Verbraecken, J. (2025). Redefining telemedicine in obstructive sleep apnea management through artificial intelligence. *Frontiers in Sleep*, *4*, 1678077. DOI: 10.3389/frsle.2025.1678077 PMID: 41425184

About the Contributors

Rahul K. Patel is a seasoned cybersecurity and information systems management professional with extensive scholarly contributions highlight his thought leadership in AI, digital infrastructure, and secure system design. Dr. Patel's research spans AI-driven digital literacy where he presents a framework for higher education and workforce collaboration in response to the AI revolution as well as studies on AI-based recommendation systems, such as an analysis of the accuracy of OTC medication suggestions generated by commercial AI platforms. He is the author of AI Frameworks and Tools for Software Development (2025), which provides a comprehensive exploration of how artificial intelligence can be strategically integrated into the software development lifecycle. His work also tackles security and privacy within emerging technologies: from leveraging clustering algorithms for predictive analytics in blockchain networks to exploring privacy-preserving architectures and cloud security fortified by distributed ledger technologies. With a PhD in Management of Information Systems, Dr. Patel serves as an Adjunct Industry Associate Professor at the Illinois Institute of Technology.

***

Mohammad Aves is a Ph.D. Research Scholar in the Department of Computer Science and Engineering at Graphic Era Deemed to be University, Dehradun, India. He is UGC NET qualified and actively engaged in research in the areas of Machine Learning, Artificial Intelligence, Data Science, Remote Sensing, and Geographic Information Systems (GIS). His research focuses on data-driven intelligent systems, geospatial data analysis, and machine learning applications in remote sensing and environmental monitoring. He has experience in programming, data analysis, and academic research, and has contributed to research papers, conference publications, and book chapters in the fields of artificial intelligence, data science, and geospatial technologies.

Mukesh Kumar Dharmalingam Jothinathan, Department of Biochemistry, Saveetha Medical College and Hospital, Saveetha Institute of Medical and Technical Sciences (SIMATS), Saveetha University, Chennai, Tamil Nadu, India

Norhène Gargouri is an Associate Professor at the Digital Research Center of Sfax in Tunisia and a member of the SM@RT Laboratory within the Computers Imaging and Electronics Systems (CIELS) research team. Her work focuses on medical image processing, particularly in the development of intelligent computer-aided diagnosis systems using deep learning and machine learning techniques. She has authored numerous scientific publications in the fields of biomedical imaging, cancer detection, and artificial intelligence, contributing significantly to advances in automated medical diagnosis. Dr Gargouri holds a Professional Doctorate in Engineering from the National Engineering School of Sfax and has obtained her University Habilitation, allowing her to supervise doctoral research. In addition to her academic and research activities, she also serves as President of the Association for Scientific Research (ABORS), demonstrating her strong commitment to promoting scientific innovation and collaboration.

B. Lokeshwari, Research Scholar, PG and Research Department of Microbiology, Sacred Heart College (Autonomous), Tirupattur, Tamil Nadu, India.

P. Saranraj holds a Ph.D. in Microbiology from Annamalai University, Chidambaram, India, and is NET (ASRB–ICAR) qualified in Microbiology. He is currently serving as Assistant Professor and Head, Department of Microbiology, at Sacred Heart College (Autonomous), Tirupattur, Tamil Nadu, India. In addition, he is the Proprietor and Managing Director of JPS Scientific Publications, contributing actively to academic publishing and research dissemination. Dr. Saranraj has over 15 years of research experience and 10 years of teaching experience in the fields of Environmental Microbiology, Agricultural Microbiology, Industrial Microbiology, Bioremediation, Microbial Biotechnology, and Sustainable Ecosystem Management. His research work has focused on Microbial degradation of pollutants, Effluent treatment, Soil health improvement, Plant–microbe interactions, and Applied environmental sustainability. He has an extensive publication record, with more than 240 international research articles, over 90 books (international and national), and 70+ book chapters published with reputed academic publishers.

Kunj R. Patel, DO Candidate Osteopathic Medical Student I Aspiring Emergency Physician I Advocate for Telemedicine in Acute Care Kunj R. Patel is a dedicated osteopathic medical student pursuing his DO degree with a strong interest in Emergency Medicine and the integration of telemedicine in clinical practice. Throughout his medical education, he has focused on developing skills in acute care settings and exploring innovative ways to improve patient outcomes through technology. Passionate about advancing access to emergency care, Kunj is actively engaged in research and educational projects related to tele-emergency medicine and digital health solutions. He seeks to leverage telemedicine to enhance clinical efficiency and support underserved populations. Kunj's commitment to patient-centered care, combined with his osteopathic training emphasizing holistic and preventive approaches, positions him well for a future career in Emergency Medicine. He aims to contribute to the evolving landscape of acute care delivery by blending clinical expertise with emerging telehealth technologies.

Nikunj R. Patel is a Computer Science graduate aspiring to become a physician. His experience spans psychiatric care at UW Health, oncology shadowing at Illinois Cancer Specialists, and computational genetics research at UW–Madison. He has worked in cybersecurity operations, co-authored academic books, and built a health tech startup. Focused on human-centered, data-driven medicine.

Subhendu Rath, MD, MSHA, FACP, is an Assistant Professor in the Departments of Neurology and Internal Medicine at the University of Kentucky College of Medicine in Lexington, Kentucky. He is board-certified in neurology, epilepsy, and sleep medicine. His clinical and research interests focus on sleep-disordered breathing, central disorders of hypersomnolence, sleep–epilepsy interactions, and the application of artificial intelligence in sleep medicine. Dr. Rath is actively involved in medical education and mentorship, teaching medical students, residents, and fellows. He has authored multiple peer-reviewed publications and serves as a reviewer for several international peer-reviewed journals. Dr. Rath is engaged in national professional societies, including the American Academy of Sleep Medicine and the American Epilepsy Society, where he contributes to educational and professional initiatives aimed at advancing sleep and neurological care.

T. Elavarasi, PG and Research Department of Microbiology, Sacred Heart College (Autonomous), Tirupattur, Tamil Nadu, India

Muskan Tamboli a student researcher in respiratory sciences with a focused interest in artificial intelligence applications in pulmonary imaging

Index

www.ingramcontent.com/pod-product-compliance
Lightning Source LLC
LaVergne TN
LVHW060006031026
849161LV00025B/1501
9798337377599